Language Development
Monolingual and Bilingual Acquisition

Alejandro E. Brice

Roanne G. Brice

Allyn & Bacon
is an imprint of

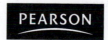

Boston   New York   San Francisco
Mexico City   Montreal   Toronto   London   Madrid   Munich   Paris
Hong Kong   Singapore   Tokyo   Cape Town   Sydney

**Vice President and
  Executive Publisher:** Jeffery W. Johnston
Executive Editor: Ann Castel Davis
Editorial Assistant: Penny Burleson
Senior Managing Editor: Pamela D. Bennett
Production Editor: Sheryl Glicker Langner
Design Coordinator: Diane C. Lorenzo

Photo Coordinator: Sandy Schaefer
Cover Designer: Aaron Dixon
Cover art: Jupiter Images
Production Manager: Laura Messerly
Director of Marketing: Quinn Perkson
Marketing Manager: Kris Ellis-Levy
Marketing Coordinator: Brian Mounts

For related titles and support materials, visit our online catalog at www.pearsonhighered.com.

Copyright © 2009 Pearson Education, Inc.

All rights reserved. No part of the material protected by this copyright notice may be reproduced or utilized in any form or by any means, electronic or mechanical, including photocopying, recording, or by any information storage and retrieval system, without written permission from the copyright owner.

To obtain permission(s) to use material from this work, please submit a written request to Pearson/Allyn & Bacon, Permissions Department, 501 Boylston Street, Suite 900, Boston, MA 02116 or fax your request to 617-671-2290.

This book was set in Garamond by S4Carlisle Publishing Services. The cover was printed by R. R. Donnelley & Sons Company

Library of Congress Cataloging in Publication Data
Brice, Alejandro E.
  Language development: monolingual and bilingual acquisition / Alejandro E. Brice, Roanne G. Brice.
    p. cm.
  Includes bibliographical references and index.
  ISBN-13: 978-0-13-170051-2 (alk. paper)
  ISBN-10: 0-13-170051-0 (alk. paper)
  1. Bilingualism. 2. Language acquisition. 3. Spanish language—Acquisition.
  4. English language—Acquisition. 5. Children with disabilities—Language. I. Brice, Roanne G. II. Title.

  P115.B75 2009
  401'.93—dc22

                                                                                  2008005957

Photo Credits: ISM/Phototake NYC, p. 1; Krista Greco/Merrill, p. 32; EyeWire Collection/Getty Images–Photodisc, p. 74; Ken Karp/PH College, p. 112; Patrick White/Merrill, p. 160; Anthony Magnacca, pp. 190, 224; David Mager/Pearson Learning Photo Studio, p. 266; Scott Cunningham/Merrill, p. 290; Hope Madden/Merrill, p. 313; Tom Watson/Merrill, p. 340; Paul Conklin/PhotoEdit Inc., p. 362

Printed in the United States of America

10 9 8 7 6 5 4 3 2 1   RRD-VA   12 11 10 09 08

Allyn & Bacon
is an imprint of

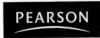

We would like to dedicate this book to all school age children and students and, in particular, to our children Jacky, Aaron, Laura, Robbie, and Brad. You have taught us innumerable lessons about life and language development.

Preface

Welcome to the first edition of *Language Development: Monolingual and Bilingual Acquisition*. Our interest in writing and editing this language development book stems from our experiences as parents of five children, and from being speech-language pathologists and educators in school and university settings. One purpose of the book is to address the topics of language acquisition among monolingual (i.e., using one language) and bilingual (i.e., using two languages) populations. The demographics of the United States are changing, and a large proportion of the culturally and linguistically diverse (CLD) growth has been in the school-age population.

Another purpose of this book is to address language-acquisition issues for infant, preschool, and school-age populations (i.e., 0 to 21 years of age). The book also incorporates various applied examples of and strategies for language development: for example, instructional strategies, case studies, and numerous illustrations of applying language development practices in classrooms.

In this era of globalization, educational professionals must know and understand language acquisition not only for the English language, but they must also have some understanding of the developmental acquisition of other languages. Classrooms across the United States are filled with a significant number of students who are from diverse cultures and who speak many languages. Speech-language pathologists, special education teachers, and general education teachers must be prepared to meet the academic needs of these students.

I (Alejandro Brice) understand the importance of this preparation because of my personal, academic, and social experiences as a young child learning to speak a second language. I spoke only Spanish until the age of 5. English is my second language. In the early 1960s, my family emigrated from Cuba to the United States when I was approximately 3 years old. We settled in a small town in Ohio where no one else spoke Spanish. We were in a foreign world where we could not comprehend what other people were saying. My parents began learning English, although they spoke only Spanish in our home. I did not begin to learn English until my entry into kindergarten. What an experience: to go from a world of total Spanish to a world of total English! I vividly recall my experiences as a young 5-year-old kindergartener in the first few months of school.

I had been in my new kindergarten classroom all morning: It was time for recess! I was excited to escape the confusing world of the classroom where I did not understand what anyone was saying. I could just play outside on the swings, the merry-go-round, the slide, and the monkey bars. Every day a boy and a girl approached me. They were getting closer and closer and saying words I did not understand. I became more and more frightened. I found myself stepping back until I was pressed up against the school building wall. These two children were speaking to me in a language that I did not understand and I was terrified! What did they want? Why were they so persistent? As I look back now, I assume that they were introducing themselves to me, asking where I was from, or inquiring if I would like to play. However, at 5 years old, I did not understand that their actions were not threatening. This scenario occurred every day for at least a month. These experiences were terrifying, and the apprehensive feelings stayed with me through my early school years.

As I progressed though elementary school, I struggled academically with both oral and written language. I was quiet and did not speak much to the teacher or my classmates. It was a constant struggle to understand and use the English language. I felt as if I was "dumb." I would observe how other children in my classes understood and knew what to do when lessons were assigned. How could these other children understand the teacher so easily? Why was it so hard for me? Why couldn't I complete assignments as quickly, without confusion? I was seldom verbally praised for good work. In first grade, I struggled with all subjects, frightened and frustrated. On my report card, the teacher indicated that in the area of language, "Alex loses trend of thought and needs individual help." In addition, she stated that I cried "over little problems." I struggled with phonemic awareness, phonological awareness, phonics, vocabulary, and comprehension in learning to read. By second grade, I was even more aware that I was not completely understanding what was said in the classroom. I felt like such a failure. I was so frustrated that I did not want to go to school. I would pretend that I was sick so that I would not have to go to school and feel that I was not as smart as the other children. In third grade, my oral language had begun to improve and I was more comfortable in the classroom and social interactions. I was beginning to more fully understand orally presented lesson directions, and my school work began to improve. In fourth grade, I earned straight A's in math! I was so excited to have received high grades, at least in one subject. However, in reading and writing I received "needs to improve" on my report card. Toward the end of the year, I did show some improvement in my reading fluency and comprehension. My writing skills were improving as well! In fifth grade, I began to excel. My teacher encouraged me and provided praise. She supported both my learning and social learning needs. My teacher must have had acute cultural understanding and language learning acquisition knowledge because she provided me with an academic environment in which I could flourish. She taught to the whole child. I believe that my success in fifth grade was due to finally grasping a working knowledge of the English language and having a teacher who cared and understood my specific language needs. None of my other teachers, from kindergarten through fourth grade, seemed to be aware of diverse cultures and second-language acquisition. Today, it would seem obvious that many of my learning difficulties could be attributed to being schooled in my second-language and not my primary language.

Near the end of sixth grade, tests were administered for class placement in junior high school (now middle school). Those tests identified me as gifted in mathematics. Language tests indicated that I was above average. Throughout junior high school, I was able to thrive and do well in my studies. By high school, I began to exceed the expectations of my teachers. My achievements were recognized by high grades, the honor roll, the National Honor Society, the Spanish Honor Society, and the French Honor Society. I was also in the French and Spanish clubs. I was recognized for my language abilities. In 12 years I had gone from a frightened little boy not knowing a word of English to a young man who was fluent in Spanish and English and learning French.

When I first entered school in 1963, bilingual education programs—indeed, any support for bilingual children—were not yet available. In addition, most teachers were not familiar with second-language learning issues coupled with academic learning as they are today. Learning a second language and succeeding in school is never an easy task for English language learners (ELLs). Academic language skills in a second language may take from four to six years or more to develop. Much has changed in the past 40 years. Educational professionals appreciate cultural diversity and the richness that other languages bring to our American culture.

Children, whether monolingual or bilingual, learn language in developmental stages, from birth to adulthood. The success of children learning language begins in the home with parents or guardians providing good models of language and a literacy-rich environment. Speech-language pathologists, general education classroom teachers, and special education teachers then facilitate language development and learning from pre-kindergarten to twelfth grade. Competent educators understand developmental language acquisition in the primary language (English); they also have a familiarity with language development and acquisition in other languages. The result is positive academic outcomes for all students. It takes time and understanding of first- and second-language development issues for school educational professionals to be able to make a positive impact on *all* students' academic success and their lives.

ORGANIZATION OF THIS BOOK

This book is divided into three parts: (1) Language Foundations and Development of Language (Chapters 1–6), (2) Content Subject Development (Chapters 7–9), and (3) Home and School Language Programs (Chapters 10–12). The different components of language, including phonology, morphology, semantics, syntax, and pragmatics, are discussed. We use the terms *language development* and *language acquisition* interchangeably. A brief overview of each chapter is next.

Chapter 1: Neurological Aspects of Language Development. Alejandro Brice and Cecyle Carson discuss brain structures and their corresponding cognitive and language attributes. Specifically, the authors discuss a neurological view of the brain, speech development and the brain, and language development and the brain.

Chapter 2: Infant and Preschool Language Development. This chapter by Jo-Anne Prendeville covers phonological development in young children, from the anatomy of the vocal tract to speech perception, stages of vowel development, sounds, phonological development, and cross-linguistic factors. Semantics is covered by examining lexical development, strategies that children use in acquiring words, and the roles of parental input. Syntax and morphology cover the traditional aspects of sentence constituents, mean length of utterances, negation, and compound/complex sentences. The chapter concludes with a discussion of pragmatics, such as the development of joint attention, communicative intents, discourse, and cross-linguistic considerations.

Chapter 3: First-Language Development. Toya A. Wyatt and Terry Irvine Saenz cover acquisition of phonology, morphology, semantics, syntax, and pragmatics during the preschool, the school-age, and the adolescent years of development. Conversational discourse and narratives relevant to adolescence and school achievement are also discussed.

Chapter 4: Second-Language Acquisition. Alejandro Brice and Roanne Brice define bilingualism as the ability to speak, listen, read, and/or write in more than one language with varying degrees of proficiency. In addition, various other concepts are defined, including (but not limited to) language proficiency, interlanguages, common and separate underlying proficiencies, and language transference. Particular attention is given to Spanish-language development in the areas of phonology, morphology, semantics, syntax, and pragmatics.

Chapter 5: School-Age Language Development. Terry Irvine Saenz covers morphological, semantic, syntactic, and narrative development of language during the primary school years. Also included is a discussion of the pragmatics of classroom discourse, which involves children's learning new interaction rules for classroom settings and deciphering the subtle clues and hints given by teachers. Narratives show development in children's use of story grammar components. Bilingual students may need additional time to adapt to classroom expectations. Students benefit greatly from a teacher's sensitivity to the child's cultural traditions in adapting to the classroom setting.

Chapter 6: Adolescent Language Development. Adolescent language development is as important to school success as earlier language development. Toya A. Wyatt discusses the growing evidence and research on adolescents that support continued language growth regarding a number of different communication aspects. Mastering the communicative expectations of adolescence is important not only for academic and school success but also for the development of social communication, personal identity, and self-esteem. The skills that develop are refined during adolescence have important implications for later life. Adolescents who experience language impairments in one or more of these areas of communication are likely to be at risk for social as well as academic difficulties. In addition, speech-language pathologists need to remain cognizant of the cultural and linguistic differences among their student populations.

Chapter 7: Reading Development in the First Language. Vicky Zygouris-Coe covers the concepts of reading development, including emergent literacy, print awareness, phonological and phonemic awareness, phonics, reading fluency skills, vocabulary, and reading comprehension skills. All of these skills need to be acquired by students for them to be successful and independent readers. Speech-language pathologists and exceptional education teachers often are primarily responsible for teaching students who have reading problems. Effective school professionals understand that developing reading skills is not automatic. They must also make instructional decisions based on their knowledge of reading and writing, scientifically based research (i.e., evidence-based practice), and their knowledge of the child's unique strengths and weaknesses. School professionals need to respect children's home language and culture and to use both to build on the child's language and literacy experiences.

Chapter 8: Reading and Writing Development for Bilingual Children (L1 and L2).
This chapter by Alejandro Brice and Roanne Brice provides information regarding reading and writing skills in students from bilingual-speaking backgrounds. Success for bilingual students occurs when they learn to read and write early and achieve academic success. This chapter addresses how the first language affects second-language literacy skills. In the United States, the vast majority of reading development with second-language learners has involved the use of Spanish and English. However, reading development in languages other than Spanish is presented in this chapter. Writing strategies for the bilingual learner are also presented, as is information regarding brain regions.

Chapter 9: Writing Development. Patricia Crawford outlines the writing process and its stages of prewriting, drafting, revising, editing, and publication. In addition, this chapter deals with spelling development as part of writing development. The author also discusses writing modifications that can be made for students with disabilities.

Chapter 10: Home and School Language Matches and Mismatches. Edward E. Heckler discusses issues of socioeconomic status, religion, and family values as cultural influences. He reviews the roles of children in communicating with family members and the roles that parents and caregivers display in communicating and also in child rearing. Matches between the home and school are presented with regard to language development.

Chapter 11: School Language Programs for Language Learning Disabled and Exceptional Needs Children. Roanne Brice and Alejandro Brice discuss the various educational reforms that have shaped school practices today, for example, inclusion, mainstreaming, collaboration, the least restrictive environment, and the No Child Left Behind Act of 2001. The different inclusion models of classroom-based team teaching or co-teaching, classroom-based complimentary teaching, and supportive teaching are also presented.

Chapter 12: School Language Programs for Bilingual Children. School language programs for bilingual students should accentuate the dynamics of bilingualism, biliteracy, and biculturalism. Elia Vazquez-Montilla discusses the common characteristics of effective programs: supportive school contexts, high expectations for success, academically challenging and engaging instruction, and school staff development programs. An effective language program for English-language learners (ELLs) is tailored to meet the linguistic, educational, and socioemotional needs of these students. Language programs should provide instruction that allows students to succeed academically and socially.

ACKNOWLEDGMENTS

We would like to acknowledge the scholarly chapter contributions from our fellow authos, colleagues, and friends: Cecyle Carson, Jo-Anne Prendeville, Toya A. Wyatt, Terry Irvine Saenz, Vicky Zygouris-Coe, Patricia Crawford, Edward E. Heckler, and

Elia Vazquez-Montilla. Their contributions have certainly enriched the contents of this book and have contributed significantly to the literature.

In addition, we gratefully thank the following reviewers for their helpful suggestions: Bonnie Abrahamsen, Old Dominion University; Ellyn Arwood, University of Portland; Linda C. Badon, University of Louisiana at Lafayette; Misha Becker, University of North Carolina, Chapel Hill; Monica C. Devers, St. Cloud State University; Ross Flom, Brigham Young University; Joseph Galasso, California State University, Northridge; Edward E. Heckler, University of Texas, Pan American; Susan Johnston, University of Utah; Diane Loeb, University of Kansas; Bonnie B. Lund, Minnesota State University, Mankato; Theresa Montano, California State University, Northridge; Carrie Mori, Boise State University; John Muma, University of Southern Mississippi; Peter V. Paul, The Ohio State University; Amanda Seidl, Purdue University; Leher Singh, Boston University; Richard A. Sprott, California State University, East Bay; and Min Wang, University of Maryland.

Alejandro E. Brice

Roanne G. Brice

Brief Contents

Contents

Chapter **3**   **First-Language Development**   74

Toya A. Wyatt and Terry Irvine Saenz

Chapter **4** **Second-Language Acquisition** **112**

Alejandro Brice and Roanne G. Brice

Chapter **5**   **School-Age Language Development**   **160**

Terry Irvine Saenz

Chapter **6**   **Adolescent Language Development**   **190**

Toya A. Wyatt

Chapter 8   Reading and Writing Development for Bilingual Children (L1 and L2)   266

Alejandro Brice and Roanne G. Brice

Chapter 9   Writing Development   290

Patricia Crawford

Chapter **12** **School Language Programs for Bilingual Children   362**

Elia Vazquez-Montilla

Part 1

Language Foundations and Development of Language

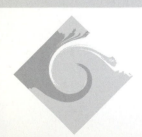

Chapter 1

Neurological Aspects of Language Development

Alejandro Brice and Cecyle Carson

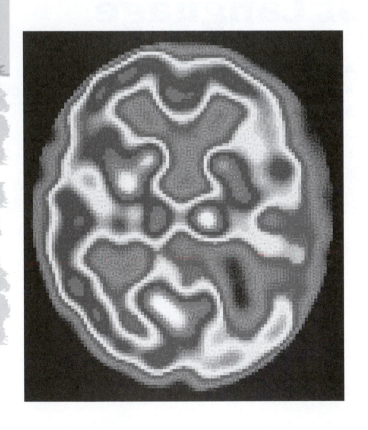

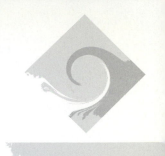

CHAPTER OUTLINE

THE BRAIN

The brain is the most complex organ in the human body. It is responsible for thought, language, emotions, memory, and perception of the world through the senses of hearing, vision, touch, movement, taste, and smell. Knowledge of the brain and neurological processes is vital to understanding cognition, communication, and language for speech-language pathologists (SLPs), special education teachers, and professionals concerned with language and learning. Four vital reasons explain why the study of the brain is important (Eliot, 2001):

1. Knowledge of the brain and its neurophysiology leads to a better understanding of child language development. Knowledge of development is critical for developmentally appropriate therapy sessions and classroom instruction. Ullman (2004) stated, "Importantly, if the systems underlying the target domains are well understood, they should yield clear predictions

about language, based solely on non-language theories and data" (p. 232). Therefore, knowledge of the brain and its structures will yield information about language;

2. The brain is sculpted by the environment and learning; hence, speech-language pathologists and teachers have a profound influence on learning and consequently on the physiology of the brain;

3. What happens in early child development has a lasting effect on the child's ability to learn and his or her success in school; and

4. When policy makers become cognizant of the fact that SLPs and teachers have a strong influence on children's learning and minds (i.e., SLPs and teachers are physically sculpting the structures of the child's brain), then more funding and quality education can be afforded to children and students.

Neurological Overview

The basis for all thought, communication, and language occurs in the brain. The nervous system is a key component to the brain. The brain, the spinal cord, the cranial nerves attached to the brain, and the spinal nerves make up the nervous system. **Afferent neurons** (also known as sensory or receptor neurons) transmit sensory information from the body to the brain. **Efferent neurons** (also known as motor or effector neurons) carry motor information from the brain to innervate muscles. The nervous system consists of a "closed loop system" where nerves receive sensory information, reactions result, and decisions regarding the information is processed. This closed loop system contains afferent neurons, **interneurons** (neurons that communicate only with other neurons), and efferent neurons.

The brain (a synonym for the brain is encephalon) and the spinal cord make up the central nervous system (CNS). The largest portion of the brain is the cerebrum (cortex). The brain is made up of the cerebrum, cerebellum, and the brain stem.

Each hemisphere is divided into four different lobes: frontal, temporal, parietal, and occipital. A **gyrus** (hill) is an elevation on the surface of the brain caused by the folding in the cortex. A **sulcus** (valley) is a groovelike depression on the brain's surface that separates the gyri. The brain and nervous system work together as an integrated unit; however, some cerebral areas are more attuned and responsible for certain cognitive and language functions. Figure 1–1 illustrates the lobes of the brain.

The frontal lobe, that is, the inferior frontal gyrus or Broca's area, has been associated with expressive oral speech. The temporal lobe has been associated with audition, memory, and innate behaviors. The temporal lobe, location of Wernicke's area (left posterior area of the superior temporal gyrus), the inferior parietal lobe, and the frontal lobe anterior to Broca's area are larger in human beings than in animals, and these areas are important for cognition, speech, and language. The temporal lobe is the seat of auditory processing (listening and comprehension). The auditory association area, the middle portion of the superior temporal gyrus, is important in the use of language. Figure 1–2 shows Broca's and Wernicke's areas.

Lobes within the brain and the two hemispheres connect via cerebral connections. Cerebral connections are made up of association fibers and commissural fibers.

FIGURE 1–1
Lobes of the Brain

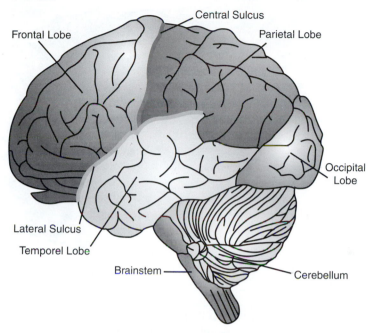

FIGURE 1–2
Broca's and Wernicke's Areas

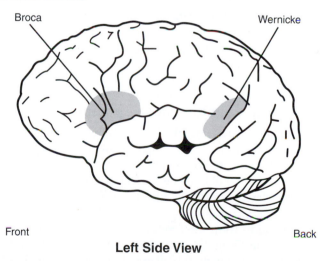

Left Side View

Association fibers connect areas within the hemispheres, while **commissural fibers** connect one area in one hemisphere with another in the other hemisphere. The **corpus callosum** is the largest commissural fiber connecting the right and left hemispheres. Figure 1–3 shows the corpus callosum.

The term *cerebellum* (see Figure 1–1) comes from Latin meaning the "little brain." It is located inferior and posterior to the cerebrum. It provides coordination to

FIGURE 1–3
Corpus Callosum

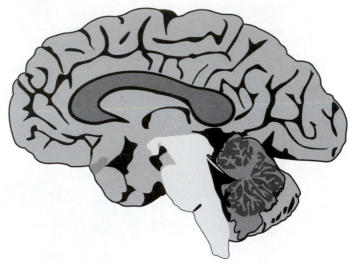

movements of the body, particularly in extremely rapid and precise movements for articulation and speech. The brainstem is the third major part of the brain. These structures are an upward extension of the spinal cord, positioned upward into the brain between the cerebral hemispheres. The caudal or lower end of the CNS is the spinal cord. The ventral or anterior portion of the spinal cord mediates motor output, while the dorsal or posterior portion mediates sensory input. Hence, the spinal nerves and extensions (called peripheral nerves) make up the peripheral nervous system (PNS).

Normal Cognitive Development

The future brain and nervous system becomes apparent at four weeks' gestation during development of a fetus. At this point a neural groove and plate develop. The neural plate groove divides into right and left halves. The plate is polarized (the head end, which will become the brain, is wider) and is bilaterally symmetrical (right and left halves mirror each other); it also regionalizes (the top becomes the brain and the bottom becomes the spinal cord). The plate forms a tube from which three swellings emerge to form the forebrain (future cortex, or prosencephalon), midbrain, (future midbrain, or mesencephalon) and hindbrain (future cerebellum, pons, medulla, and spinal cord, or rhombencephalon). See Figure 1–4 for an illustration of the embryonic forebrain, midbain, and hindbrain.

During development in utero the brain is smooth. During the last 12 weeks of development, the brain folds in on itself to create the gyri (hills) and sulci (grooves). This wrinkling of the brain accommodates more brain matter to fit within a fixed skull size. The cerebral cortex makes up approximately 70% of the

FIGURE 1–4
Embryonic Forebrain, Midbrain, and Hindbrain

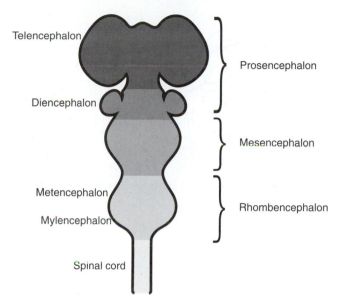

entire nervous system. A piece of cortex the size of a grain of rice contains approximately 10,000 brain cells. It is estimated that the brain contains approximately 100 billion neurons (Goswami, 2004). The brain is made up of **gray matter** (neural cortical cells on the surface of the brain) and **white matter** (the communicating filaments of neural cells containing axons, dendrites, and the **myelin sheaths,** that is, the outer covering of the axon). The myelin acts as insulation to speed the transmission of signals. Each neuron contains the axon, the cell body, and thousands of dendrites. **Axons** reach out to dendrites to send information via neural-electrical chemical reactions. The axon sends electrical signals that are converted into specific chemicals (that is, neurotransmitters), which travel across the synapse and are converted back into electrical signals to be received by the next neuron's **dendrites**. See Figure 1–5.

Mass migration is neural cell proliferation. Neural cells must connect with other neural cells in the early stages of brain development. These neural cells reach their final destination (i.e., make a connection with other neural cells) with the help of radial glia that spans the entire length of the neural tube. The neurons of the brain arrange themselves inside-out, that is, deepest neurons first. Each neuron knows its ultimate destination. Neurons are developed from **stem cells** (cells that can become any kind of human cell: brain, kidney, heart, bone, etc.). The stem cell is plastic, receiving instructions from outside itself about its transformation. Once brain cells become brain neurons, however, they remain as such forever. Defects in migration can result in neurological conditions such as epilepsy, mental handicaps, and/or physical anomalies. Children who have suffered in utero from fetal alcohol syndrome can have long-term effects because the migration pattern of the cells has been severely disrupted. Most critical aspects of brain development occur in the womb

FIGURE 1–5
Neuron

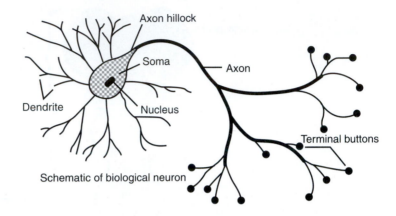

Schematic of biological neuron

and prior to the child's birth. At seven months of gestation, most brain neurons have developed (Goswami, 2004). Once the brain has developed, the neural connections are then strengthened and expanded.

Address selection refers to a period when the brain strengthens neural connections. The brain fires the neurons down a pathway, but it is not selective about which neurons are connected; that is, all the connections "light up." The brain strengthens certain connections through repetitive use and eliminates random connections. **Synaptogenesis** is the growth of connections and neuronal synapses. **Pruning** is when the brain selects strong, appropriate connections and deletes the less efficient and weak connections. Neuron density becomes 150% greater than the adult brain somewhere between four and 12 months of age. Extensive pruning then takes place between two and four years of age in the occipital lobe (i.e., the visual cortex). The density of the prefrontal cortex (planning, reasoning, language) increases more slowly and peaks after 10 to 20 years of age. Therefore, the brain continues to develop into adolescence and adulthood (Goswami, 2004).

Neurotransmitters

The brain produces specific neurotransmitters responsible for memory, cognition, and language. Neurotransmitters consist of chemicals that relay, modulate, and/or amplify electrical signals between neurons and other cells.

Neurotransmitters can generally be grouped according to two categories: (1) small molecule neurotransmitters (e.g., the biogenic amines, organic compounds containing nitrogen such as dopamine, noradrenaline, serotonin, and histamine; approximately 10 are known), and (2) larger neuropeptide neurotransmitters (neuropeptides are peptides such as endorphins found in neural tissue). Some neuropeptide neurotransmitters (approximately 50 are known) consist of corticitropin releasing hormone, corticotropin (ACTH), beta-endorphin, substance P, neurotensin, somatostatin, bradykinin, vasopressin, and angiotensin two. Neuropeptide Y and substance P have been implicated in neurological disorders such as Huntington's disease (Beal, Swartz, Finn, Bird, & Martin, 1988).

Some common small molecule neurotransmitters involved in language and cognition include dopamine, serotonin, glutamate, acetylcholine, and norepinephrine. Dopamine controls the flow of information from other areas of the brain to the frontal lobe. Dopamine disorders in the frontal lobe can cause a decline in neurocognitive functions, especially memory, attention, and problem solving (Gray's Anatomy, 2005; Zemlin, 1997). Reduced levels of dopamine in the prefrontal cortex may lead to attention deficits.

Serotonin is synthesized from the amino acid tryptophan. It is implicated in mood and anxiety disorders as selective serotonin reuptake inhibitors (SRIs). Serotonin reuptake inhibitors allow for larger doses of serotonin to remain in the brain and thus prevent serotonin from being returned to the brain's storage vesicles. SRIs are typically prescribed to individuals suffering from depression or mood disorders. Exact effects of serotonin on the hippocampus, cerebellum, and/or the cortex are unknown. Sudden infant death syndrome (SIDS) is speculated to result from serotonergic neurons being abnormal (Gray's Anatomy, 2005; Zemlin, 1997).

Glutamate is an important neurotransmitter in the brain and a profuse excitatory neurotransmitter. It is believed that glutamic acid (because of its synaptic plasticity) is involved in learning and memory (Gray's Anatomy, 2005; Zemlin, 1997). Glutamate is also a neural inhibitor responsible for reducing neurotransmissions and for aiding in the formation of new memories. When glutamate levels are high, brain neurons die. As a result, a child's brain with high levels of glutamate becomes insensitive to glutamate bursts, and her or his brain is thus unable to retain new memories. The loss of acetylcholine (a neurotransmitter linked to memory and cognition) has also been found in individuals with memory difficulties (Cowley, 1999). Acetylcholine is a neurotransmitter in both the central nervous system and the peripheral nervous system.

Norepinephrine and **dopamine** are both thought to play large roles in attention and focus (Gray's Anatomy, 2005; Zemlin, 1997). The psychostimulant ritalin (methylphenidate) is prescribed to increase levels of norepinephrine and dopamine (Zemlin, 1997). Methylphenidate is a central nervous system stimulant. It is thought to affect attention deficit hyperactivity disorder (ADHD) by acting as a dopamine reuptake inhibitor. That is, it is believed that ADHD may result from decreased dopamine levels in the frontal cortex (Gray's Anatomy, 2005; Zemlin, 1997).

Developmental Milestones Related to Neurological Development

A baby's vision is the last sense to develop. An immature brain cannot handle excess stimulation. Therefore, the brain is protected from overstimulation by damping down incoming visual stimuli. At this point the baby sees the world like a faded photograph. However, stimulation is still critical to development. Experience (from external stimulation) drives maturation and development. With experience from the environment, neuronal cells can refine their circuits or connections and influence which connections are stabilized and which connections are lost (i.e., pruned). Learning is about neuronal connections. At two days the baby can recognize his or her mother by sight alone. By four months of age, an infant recognizes an adult's face. Infants can recognize sounds and their mother's voice at birth.

Contrary to vision, hearing is more developed at birth (Eliot, 2001). A baby's hearing is fully developed at one month of age. Developmental milestones from birth to three months of age include: (1) the baby startles to loud sounds; (2) the infant becomes quiet when spoken to; (3) the baby seems to recognize the mother, father, or caregiver's voice and stops crying; and (4) the infant may increase or decrease sucking behaviors in response to sounds (American Speech-Language-Hearing Association [ASHA], 2007).

It is important to recognize that hearing is vital to the learning of speech and language. Parents should be advised to seek audiological testing if their infant does not seem responsive to sound. It is also important to mention that even newborns can be tested for hearing. The Department of Otolaryngology and Head and Neck Surgery (2007) states, "The screening of newborns and infants involves use of non-invasive, objective physiologic measures that include otoacoustic emissions (OAEs) and/or auditory brainstem response (ABR). Both procedures can be done painlessly while the infant is resting quietly" (lines 13–41).

Sensitive learning periods refer to periods of time (windows of opportunity) in the child's development that are optimal for certain types of learning. Learning can occur later; however, the brain is primed to learn or register certain information at certain times (e.g., visual stimuli in early childhood). Sensitive periods are not all-or-nothing time frames, but the ability to learn specialized skills may be best during these time periods. Neurons have opportunities of assimilating other functions than the ones they were primarily assigned if certain experiences and learning do not take place. For example, the temporal regions of brains of individuals with profound hearing losses (i.e., who are deaf) may take on visual capabilities instead of the more traditional auditory role (Goswami, 2004). Hence, some brain regions demonstrate plasticity dependent upon environmental stimulation. All modalities (e.g., vision, audition, smell, taste) are initially linked together, which may offer some explanation as to why young children tend to learn best through multimodality teaching.

Premature infants are at risk for right hemisphere and frontal lobe disturbances. In premature infants, the prefrontal lobe myelination is thinner. The right hemisphere generally governs social rule interactions (e.g., pragmatics) and the frontal lobe governs higher-order thinking and reasoning skills (e.g., deficits in attention, concentration, or focus). These deficits are observable at 23 to 24 months.

Six-month-old children are capable of differentiating sounds that are and are not in their language system. Babies are born with the capacity to learn any language. By listening, babies sort through a catalog of sounds. At seven months a baby can distinguish between sounds in his or her language and those of another language. At 11 months the baby's brain becomes specialized in her or his language and this capability is lost. By one year of age, infants lose the ability to perceive the differences across languages and instead focus on the sound perception of their own language. The brain becomes specialized in the sounds of their own language. At 12 months of age and beyond, the brain experiences a dramatic surge of luxuriant growth. Experiences determine which neural connections will be developed and strengthened.

Neural growth and pruning continues into the second year of life. Language moves from a dual-hemisphere activity (12 to 13 months) to a single-hemisphere activity (18 to 20 months). Language input sculpts the brain to create a perceptual system that highlights contrasts crucial to one particular language and deemphasizes those that are not crucial (e.g., r-l distinction for Japanese babies). Thus, babies form the sound system of their language prior to speaking at about 9 months of age.

At thirteen months, children listen and understand language with both cerebral hemispheres. Language initially begins bilaterally in both hemispheres. At 18 to 20 months, language localizes to the anterior region of the left hemisphere (Restak, 2001). This shift is driven by environmental exposure. Experience is a major player in driving differentiation of the brain (Restak, 2001).

Reading is an acquired skill. Knowledge of the alphabet, sound-letter correspondence, syllables, parsing (segmenting phonemes and syllables), and phonemic awareness are some of the bottom-up skills for reading. When listeners hear words, the information is first processed in the auditory association area (Wernicke's area and the supramarginal gyrus; see Figure 1–6) of the left temporal lobe. In order to read, a combination of visual processing, auditory processing, and making sense of the words in print (thinking skills located in Broca's area and the inferior frontal lobe) occurs.

During reading aloud, the brain processes information in the primary visual cortex (occipital lobe), then the information is transferred to the auditory association area (Wernicke's area, where speech comprehension occurs); from there it travels via a bundle of fibers called the arcuate fasciculus through the angular gyrus to Broca's area. After Broca's area processes the signal and makes sense of what was read, it travels to the motor strip area to innervate the muscles to speak. Listening to someone reading follows a similar pathway. The information is first processed in the primary auditory cortex and then goes to Wernicke's area, followed by transmission to Broca's area.

FIGURE 1–6
Supramarginal Gyrus

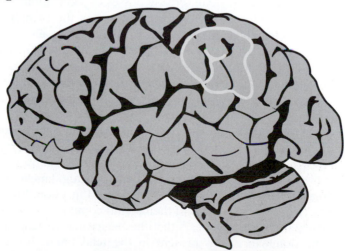

SPEECH DEVELOPMENT AND THE BRAIN

Monolingual Speech Development

The aforementioned structural and functional characteristics, with the left hemisphere as the site of language processing and production, are true for the majority of children. To fully understand the processes involved, however, a developmental perspective is required. Advances in neuroimaging technologies and recent neuropsychological or behavioral data have provided information about the brain structures and insights into how infants acquire language Positron emission tomography (PET) and functional magnetic resonance imaging (fMRI) techniques have improved our understanding of areas of brain functioning during specific activities. Both imaging techniques make use of the fact that active neurons require oxygen and glucose to fuel their energy use, and thus additional blood flow occurs to those neurons and areas that are functioning or involved in an activity (Aine, 1995). Consequently, this allows for images to be seen.

Speech Development in the Prenatal Period

The fetus begins learning the **melody** (prosody) and sounds of the language in the third trimester of pregnancy (Locke, 1997). Stress and intonation information from speech occurring in the environment are transmitted into the womb and are heard by the fetus (Lecanuet & Granier-Deferre, 1993). Newborns have been found to respond preferentially to their mother's voice over the voices of unfamiliar females and their father's voice (DeCasper & Prescott, 1984), thus implying that familiarization has occurred in the womb. Further, newborns have been found to prefer a passage read twice per day over the last 6 weeks of pregnancy by the mother over a novel passage, and to have a preference for the maternal reading over an unfamiliar female reading (DeCasper & Spence, 1986). This indicates that the fetus heard the passage and is capable of recognizing it (likely via the prosody of the passage). Thus, during the late prenatal period, the fetus already possesses some auditory perceptual capabilities.

In terms of neuroanatomy, asymmetry of the planum temporale is visible at 31 weeks of fetal life (Wada, Clarke, & Hamm, 1975), although this asymmetry favoring the left hemisphere (Foundas, Leonard, Gilmore, Fennell, & Heilman, 1994) may be related to hemispheric specialization. The planum temporale is located in the core of Wernicke's receptive language area in the temporal lobe and typically displays a greater degree of development in the left hemisphere compared to the right hemisphere (Geschwind & Levitsky, 1968; Steinmetz, 1996). Abnormal asymmetrical development (i.e., greater development in the right hemisphere or no asymmetry) of the planum temporale has been implicated in disorders such as schizophrenia and bipolar disorder (Honeycutt, Musick, Barta, & Pearlson, 2000) and in natural specialized abilities such as musical talent (Schlaug, Jancke, Huang, & Steinmetz, 1995). Further, the planum temporale is involved in phonological processing in adults or analyzing words in terms of their sound composition (Fiez, Raichle, Balota, Tallal, & Petersen, 1996). It appears that the beginnings of language lateralization (and perhaps dominance) are present in the fetal brain; however, laterality of function develops over the course of the first three years of life (Leybaert & D'Hondt, 2003).

Speech Development in the Postnatal Period

Speech in the First Year of Life

Skills appearing during the prelinguistic period, or the first 10 to 12 months of life, are vital to developing language competence (Benasich, Choudhury, Friedman, Realpe-Bonilla, Chojnowska, & Gou, 2006; Locke, 1997). At four days old, infants can distinguish differences in consonant-vowel syllables (Eimas, Siqueland, Jusczyk, & Vigorito, 1971), can identify two-syllable speech stimuli from three-syllable speech stimuli (Bertoncini, J., Floccia, C., Nazzi, T., & Mehler, 1995), and can recognize differences between two languages (Ramus, Hauser, Miller, Morris, & Mehler, 2000). The ability that newborns demonstrate in discriminating between and among subtle acoustic cues is critical for language acquisition (Kuhl, 2004). (Also refer to Chapter 2 for greater discussion of these aspects.)

Infants are sensitive to the rhythms of language; they can tell the difference between utterances produced in languages that have different rhythmic bases (Mehler et al., 1988; Nazzi, Bertoncini, & Mehler, 1998). At two months of age, infants respond differentially (orient faster) to their native language as compared to a non-native language, even when the utterance length in time is short (1.2 seconds average) (Dehaene-Lambertz & Houston, 1998). Preferences for the infant's native-language rhythmic patterns evolve between the ages of 6 and 9 months (Jusczyk, Culter, & Redanz, 1993), with the infant learning the rhythmic pattern of the native language by 9 months of age (Nazzi et al., 1998). It is hypothesized that infants use rhythmic perception as a cue in segmenting the language to which they are exposed (i.e., separating it into meaningful units such as words and syllables), and thus learn the phonological properties of the language (Ramus, Nespor, & Mehler, 1999).

The newborn comes into the world as a universal language consumer, with abilities to perceive and learn any native language. Infants can hear differences among phonetic features in foreign languages that adults cannot discriminate (e.g., Trehub, 1976). Adults cannot perceive differences in speech sounds that do not occur in their native language (i.e., differences between non-native contrasts) without extensive training (Logan, Lively, & Pisoni, 1991) because they have not needed to use those perceptual categories to understand and speak their native language. For example, whether a /t/ is produced with an alveolar placement (the tongue stops airflow by touching the alveolar ridge behind the central incisors) or produced as an interdental (the tongue is projected between the front teeth), the sound is still perceived as a /t/ in English. However, in other languages, such as Hindi or Nepali, this change in placement would represent two different sounds. The ability to detect differences in non-native contrasts begins to decline around the age of 6 months due to exposure to the ambient language (Jusczyk et al., 1993).

According to Kuhl (2000), infants use three types of learning strategies to acquire their native language. First, they detect similarities or patterns in the language. They develop a perceptual filter through which potential words are analyzed. For example, 9-month-old infants listen longer to native language words than non-native words and can discriminate between the native and non-native language through the detection of sound sequences that are allowed and not allowed in the native language (Jusczyk, Friederici, Wessels, Svenkerud, & Jusczyk, 1993). Further, 9-month-olds can detect differences between more- and less-common nonsense phoneme sequences that are allowed in their native language (e.g., "chun" [more common] versus "yush" [less common]) (Jusczyk, Luce, & Charles-Luce, 1994). This finding supports the idea that infants have some knowledge of native language phonotactics, or allowed combinations of sounds in a language (Bauman-Waengler, 2004). Further, they appear to be able to recognize which sound sequences are more likely to occur within words versus between words (Mattys, Jusczyk, Luce, & Morgan, 1999).

Second, infants use formulas in learning speech associated with their language and thus locate possible word candidates from the flow of conversational speech prior to knowing the meaning of words. The task seems burdensome given that there are around 500,000 words in English (Kuhl, 2004); however, most infants achieve this skill through what comes naturally, that is, listening. To support this second premise, 9-month-old infants have been found to have the ability to use multiple cues to parse out words, such as phonological information (consonant sequences that are more likely to occur within a word versus across a word boundary) and prosodic cues (e.g., English words begin generally with a stressed or strong first syllable followed by a weak syllable) (Mattys et al., 1999). It is apparent that the brain's growth in the early years is quite noticeable. However, the brain's growth does not stop after the child's early years.

Neurophysiological Evidence in the First Year of Life

Neuroanatomical data via fMRI images support the activation of left hemispheric cortical areas in the brains of 3-month-old infants that correspond to areas activated in adults when listening to speech (Dehanene-Lambertz et al., 2002). These areas consist of the left hemisphere superior temporal gyrus (e.g., Heschl's gyrus) and surrounding temporal areas, including the left angular gyrus. The angular gyrus is considered to be an association area because a number of neuronal axons pass through it. Damage to this area of the left, or dominant, hemisphere results in difficulty with naming, math calculations, reading, and left-right orientation. Findings from the Dehanene-Lambertz et al. study supported the dominance of the left planum temporale area over the right in infants when the infants were exposed to acoustic stimuli. The left planum temporale was significantly more active during presentation of speech stimuli than was the right, suggesting early specialization of the left over the right hemisphere for processing speech signals. Further, the right prefrontal cortex was found to be more active in infants who were awake during speech stimuli presentation compared to those who were asleep. This same activation pattern has been seen in adults when they access verbal information from memory (Fletcher & Henson, 2001), thus implying that the frontal cortex may be contributing to early language processing, even though this cortex matures later than other areas, and is not fully myelinated and connected via synapses at an early age.

Results from neurophysiological tests have provided evidence of atypical cortical activation involving both hemispheres in infants who have family histories of language learning problems or dyslexia. Benasich et al. (2006) reported differing patterns of brain activation on rapid auditory processing (RAP) stimuli between infants from families with a positive history of language-based impairments (FH+) and infants from families with no history of language-based learning problems (FH−). Infants who were in the FH+ group showed less brain activation in the fronto-central areas of the left hemisphere compared to activation in the right hemisphere; whereas those who were in the FH– group displayed no activation differences between the hemispheres. Further, Guttorm, Leppanen, Richardson, and Lyytinen (2001) found different patterns of brain activation when comparing newborn infants who had a family history of dyslexia (FH+) with control infants. Those with a negative family history for dyslexia (controls) had responses to three CV stimuli (/da/, /ga/, and /ba/) in the left hemisphere, compared to newborn infants in the FH+ group who had greater activation of the right temporal and parietal lobes. These findings are important because the left hemisphere is considered to be a more effective and efficient processor of acoustic information for speech and language than the right hemisphere (e.g., Studdert-Kennedy & Shankweiler, 1970). Thus, those children whose left hemispheres fail to establish early dominance over the right for auditory tasks may be at a distinct disadvantage in decoding and acquiring the native language. It appears that genetic predisposition plays a role in establishing neural locations that are committed to analyzing acoustic stimuli; therefore, some brains may be biased prior to birth for right hemisphere structures to assume responsibility for functions normally obligated to the left hemisphere. Regarding heritability of language abilities, genetics has been found to play a significant role in the acquisition of receptive and expressive language abilities (Benasich & Tallal, 2002).

LANGUAGE DEVELOPMENT AND THE BRAIN

Monolingual Language Development

The most sophisticated part of the brain is the frontal lobe, which is responsible for memory, thinking, and language (Eliot, 2001). The child's motor explorations in early life have a profound effect on brain development and consequent language development (Eliot, 2001). Experience actually affects brain growth by selecting certain synapses to be reinforced, making these dendrites grow and thus altering the brain's wiring. Just as "biological structures tend to evolve from already existing structure . . ." (Ullman, 2004; p. 232), language seems to have evolved from existing brain structures.

Research indicates that syntax and grammar rely more on the frontal area of the left hemisphere, while semantics and vocabulary seem to reside in the lateral regions of both hemispheres (Goswami, 2004). Phonological processing generally occurs on the temporo-partietal junction (i.e., the inferior supramarginal gyrus). Sound-to-letter correspondence (important in reading and spelling) also involves this area. Simos et al. (2002) found that reading remediation for children with reading difficulties increased activation in the temporo-partietal junction. Therefore, specific therapy programs can effect changes in the brain. Thomson, Baldeweg and Goswami (2004) stated that the brain structures of children with specific language impairments and reading disorders are immature rather than deviant from normal brains.

Language Development in the Prenatal Period

The planum temporale (located in the superior temporal gyrus; see Figure 1–7) also plays an important role in language development (Eliot, 2001) because it is larger in

FIGURE 1–7
Superior Temporal Gyrus

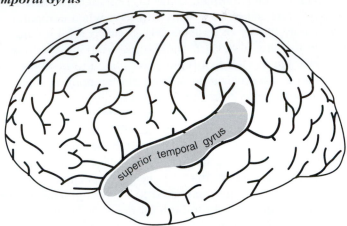

the left hemisphere than in the right hemisphere. This asymmetry in the planum temporale appears prenatally as early as 29 weeks' gestation. Broca's area is involved in syntax and phonology, while Wernicke's area is where sound is linked to words and their meaning (i.e., phonetics and semantics). Wernicke's area is appropriately situated because it lies at the juncture for the major senses of hearing, vision, and touch (Eliot, 2001), next to the auditory cortex. When the brain integrates these areas, it can unite all the mental constructs to word meaning. Since language is perceived auditorally, when a child hears a word in the temporal lobe, Wernicke's area can decode and attach meaning to the word. It is not surprising that Wernicke's area develops before Broca's area because children are able to understand words before they are able to speak (Eliot, 2001).

The right hemisphere develops earlier than the left hemisphere in utero. The right hemisphere's role in language development is its ability to focus on the tones, stress, intonation, and musical qualities of language (Soroker, Kasher, Giora, Batori, Corn, Gil, & Zaidel, 2005). This allows infants to focus on the tonality of language in their first year of life. This is not to say that the right hemisphere is not capable of developing complex language abilities. For example, children who have undergone a left **hemispherectomy** (e.g., the left hemisphere may be removed due to uncontrollable seizures) may be capable of developing language functions in the right hemisphere if the hemispherectomy was performed at an early age. For example, Vanlancker-Sidtis (2004) studied a young male who had undergone a left hemispherectomy at five years of age. As an adult he was tested, whereupon it was revealed that the participant performed normally on most aspects of language. Exceptions indicated that phonemically complex words were more effortful. In addition, comprehension of linguistics contrasts and syntax were also impaired. Children who undergo left hemispherectomy recover the ability in the right hemisphere to first comprehend (Restak, 2001). This is followed by a large lag in speaking. Kolb (1999) and Kolb and Wishaw (1990) stated that one's recovery from brain injury or trauma does not typically improve before or after the brain's period of plasticity. The type of lesion and location of the lesion also play important roles in the brain's ability to recover. However, it should also be noted that environmental influences through the principal caregiver may also have negative effects on the developing fetus.

Environmental Influences on Prenatal Development

Certain known factors have detrimental effects on the fetus's brain, affecting language, cognition, and physical development. Ulyings (2006) stated:

> The brain is susceptible to environmentally inflicted results such as irradiation, alcohol use, smoking, drug abuse (e.g., cocaine), and stress especially during the period of major neurogenesis of cerebral cortical neurons (6–18 weeks of gestation), migration, and early path-finding of growing neurons (p. 69).

A brief review of environmental influences that affect brain development during gestation or the period of susceptibility are:

1. **Alcohol.** Alcohol exposure in infants in utero affects neuronal connections and also causes extensive neuronal cell death in infants in utero. No pregnancy trimester is immune from the effects of alcohol (Uylings, 2006).

2. **Smoking.** Chronic smoking by the mother has been associated with increased risks for low birthweight and attention deficit hyperactivity disorder (Uylings, 2006).

3. **Cocaine.** Exposure to cocaine in utero can affect the child, resulting in a smaller head and impaired abilities in alertness and orientation (Uylings, 2006).

4. **Stress.** Maternal stress can lead to lower levels of intelligence and language abilities (Uylings, 2006).

5. **Exposure to irradiation.** Infants in utero during 6 to 18 weeks of gestation who were exposed to the atom bomb blasts in Hiroshima and Nagasaki in Japan showed higher incidences of mental handicaps and epileptic seizures than infant in utero exposed at later periods of gestation (i.e., 16 to 25 weeks). The former group of children developed a smaller brain, a smaller cortex, and a smaller corpus callosum (Uylings, 2006).

In sum, several environmental influences can lead to altered fetus development affecting the child's brain and consequently affecting his or her language abilities.

Language Development in the Postnatal Period

Most brain growth occurs postnatally, that is, outside the womb. At birth, the infant's brain is one fourth of the adult's brain size. The baby's brain triples its size in the first five years of life, when it will reach 90% of its target size (Eliot, 2001). The brain overproduces neuron synapses, approximately 50% more than what the adult brain maintains. The child's brain, with experience, selectively keeps the most useful connections and deletes (i.e., prunes) the least important connections. Brain development is not a single-phase process, rather it is multiphasic (Sakai, 2005; Uylings, 2006). Sakai stated, "It may be possible that different linguistics abilities are acquired in their own developmental courses and that the timing and duration of their sensitive periods differ" (p. 816). Cerebral white matter seems to increase continually in volume from 4 to 21 years of age (Giedd, 1999; Giedd, Blumenthal, Jeffries. Castellanos, Liu, Zijdnbos, Paus, Evans, & Rapport, 1999).

One measure of brain growth is dendritic growth. It can be stated that learning is based on the brain making new dendritic connections. Giedd (1999) and Giedd et al. (1999) stated that the frontal and parietal cortices keep increasing in dendritic growth into early adolescence (i.e., around 12 to 13 years of age). The exact time value for this growth has not yet been determined. Therefore, it is possible that the brain continues to develop neuronal connections into later adolescence. Dendritic variation in children becomes more individually based after 5 years of age (Giedd, 1999). Variation from one individual to the next may be due to both genetic and environmental influences. Again, the brain continues to increase in overall white matter volume from 4 to 21 years of age (Giedd, 1999). During these ages, the posterior portion of the corpus callosum (i.e., the largest commissural fiber connecting the two hemispheres) changes continuously (Giedd, 1999). In addition, it has been shown that myelin development in and below the primary motor and primary sensory areas is more advanced than the associational, frontal, and parietal lobes (Uylings, 2006). Therefore, these latter areas seem to develop myelin growth later, and it may continue into adulthood.

Synaptogenesis is the birth of new synapses. Huttenlocher and Dabholkar (cited in Uylings, 2006) reported synaptic overgrowth peaking at approximately two to four years of age and reaching maturation around 10 to 15 years of age. According to Uylings (2006), synaptic growth after 15 years of age can be expected due to environmental stimulation. Like neuron dendrite and synapses, chemical neurotransmitters are not expected to reach maturation until adolescence or later. Some examples are monoaminergic and cholinergic transmitters (which reach maturation approximately at the end of puberty); acetycholinesterase (reaches maturation around 18 years of age or later); and dopamine, noradrenaline, and serotonin (reach maturation around the end of adolescence and/or early adulthood). Consequently, cortical neuron receptors may not reach maturation until the end of adolescence and/or early adulthood. Therefore, the notion of **critical periods**—that certain language and/or cognitive abilities cannot develop after certain postnatal developmental periods—needs to be examined in light of late brain development.

Critical Periods

The critical period theory was first postulated by Penfield and Roberts (1959) when they stated that optional language learning occurred in early childhood. Lennenberg (1967) interpreted this to mean that first and second language learners encountered a critical stage around puberty where learning was severely reduced (Lennenberg, 1967). The notion of a critical period from a neurological viewpoint for language will be reviewed.

It is generally accepted that certain brain attributes develop during a critical developmental period (Eliot, 2001; Uylings, 2006). For example, vision can develop only if the occipital lobe is stimulated with a visually rich environment. With vision the brain develops elongation of new axons over a long distance. It is impossible for the brain to develop new long-distance connections after existing ones have developed

(Knudsen, 2004). However, the notion of a critical period for language has been challenged (Sakai, 2005; Uylings; 2006).

Language is experienced learning that results from the brain making local and short dendritic connections (Uylings, 2006). This type of neuron growth does not stop in adolescence. However, it appears that these types of connections decrease with age over a person's entire lifetime. If the brain were unable to make the local and short dendritic connections, then new learning would not occur.

Critical periods for socialization (i.e., involving pragmatics of language) have been shown for aspects of interaction and language. Children who have endured extensive global neglect (i.e., severely decreased social interaction during 0 to 5 years of age) have permanently smaller head sizes (i.e., head circumference), smaller brains, and difficulty learning languages and social behaviors (Uylings, 2006). In summary, it appears that certain brain connections must develop within a certain period of time (e.g., for vision), while other brain functions (such as language) may not be so developmentally tied to specific time periods. Sensitive learning periods occur when certain language and/or cognitive abilities develop best during specific postnatal developmental periods. These language and cognitive attributes can develop later, but maybe not as optimally during the sensitive period.

Neurophysiological Evidence

It should be emphasized again that language and cognition in the brain are multi-phasic operations (i.e., language and thinking develop in different phases in the brain) and that no single area of the brain is solely responsible for any language function (Uylings, 2006). Language and cognition can be double-disassociated (i.e., language can be independent from cognition and cognition can be independent from language). In some instances, language ability is impaired regardless of normal cognitive abilities (e.g., children with language learning disabilities with normal or above average IQs). In others, language abilities are intact regardless of impaired cognitive abilities (e.g., a linguistic savant in a child with mental impairments). Refer to Smith and Tsimpli's (1995) study of Christopher, a child with intact language and an IQ of 50. In conclusion, some general areas of the brain have been associated with particular language aspects:

1. **Phonology.** Auditory comprehension and phonology have been linked to the posterior superior temporal gyrus (Sakai, 2005) and the temporo-parietal junction (Goswami, 2004).

2. **Semantics.** Semantic and lexical processing has been associated with the supra-marginal gyrus, angular gyrus (see Figure 1–8), and left perisylvian (along the sylvian fissure or lateral sulcus) temporo-parietal regions (Sakai, 2005).

3. **Syntax.** Sakai reported that "the left precentral sulcus [see Figure 1–9] is significantly enhanced" for sentences (p. 816). Müller and Basho (2004), in their functional MRI study of nine participants using a semantic decision task and a tone discrimination task, reported that activation clusters were found in the superior frontal lobe, the middle and superior temporal gyri, and the inferior and middle frontal gyri for semantic decision tasks. It appears that different semantic tasks activate slightly different brain areas.

FIGURE 1–8
Angular Gyrus

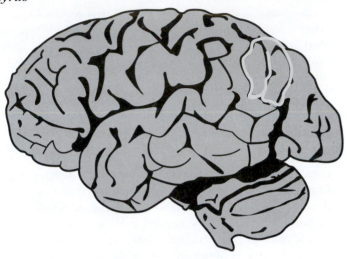

FIGURE 1–9
Precentral Sulcus

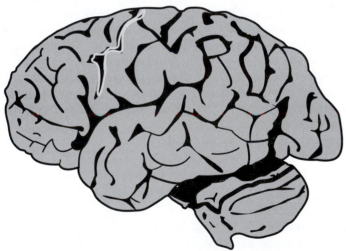

4. **Pragmatics.** Pragmatic functions seem to be implemented differently in the two hemispheres. There also appears to be localization of assertions, questions, requests, and commands with the following areas: (a) assertions in the inferior left frontal area, (b) questions in a wider left frontal region, (c) requests with a

left fronto-temporal localization, and (d) commands with a left temporo-parietal area (Soroker et al., 2004).

In sum, some pragmatic functions may be carried out by the right hemisphere, separate from phonological, semantic, or syntactic abilities.

Declarative and Procedural Memory

Language has developed in the brain according to existing biological structures. Ullman proposes a model in which language, memory, and brain neurology are integrated. The basic premise of the declarative/procedural (DP) model is that the distinction between mental lexicon and mental grammars are coupled to the distinction between declarative and procedural memory. **Lexical memory** depends on the declarative memory system, while grammar and syntax are tied to the procedural memory system.

The **declarative memory** system has been tied to the learning of facts and episodic events. It is very important for rapid learning and arbitrary information (Ullman, 2004). Declarative memory is often referred to as **explicit memory** because memory knowledge can be consciously available and retrieved. It is believed that declarative memory is accessible to various mental systems and part of declarative memory can be accessed consciously or readily (Squire & Zola, 1996). Declarative memory is essential in recalling newly learned information, for example, reciting the alphabet, or recalling one's times tables.

Declarative memory resides in the medial temporal lobe, hippocampal region, entorhinal cortex, perirhinal cortex, and parahippocampal cortex (Squire & Knowlton, 2000; Suzuki & Eichenbaum, 2000). The medial temporal region serves several memory functions, that is, encoding, consolidating, and retrieving new memories (Buckner & Wheeler, 2001; Squire & Knowlton, 2000). Declarative memory has also been linked with prefrontal regions (Buckner & Wheeler, 2001; Tulving, Kapur, Craik, Moscovitch, & Houle, 1994). Ullman (2004) states that declarative memory is interconnected to the ventral (anterior brain structures) system and to lateral temporal lobe structures. "The ventral system is thus a memory-based system, feeding representations into long-term (declarative) memory, and comparing those representations with new ones" (Ullman, 2004; p. 236).

Procedural memory assists learning of new memories and control of established sensorimotor habits and skills (e.g., tying one's shoelaces, speech articulation). Procedural memory is often referred to as implicit memory (Ullman, 2004). **Implicit memory** learning and the implicit memory knowledge are not consciously available or retrievable. Learning is generally gradual, with multiple presentations of the stimuli. Learning is also rule-like, rigid, and not generally influenced by other systems (Ullman, 2004). Information is encapsulated and also subject to stimuli to elicit a response. Procedural memory is important in learning new information and storing information. Once the alphabet has been learned and mastered, retrieving the alphabet is part of procedural memory.

Procedural memory consists of a network of certain brain regions and structures, that is, frontal/basal ganglia circuits, portions of the parietal cortex, the superior temporal cortex, and the cerebellum (Ullman, 2004). In sum, declarative and proecedural memory systems are interdependent; however, it is known that they do interact with each other in memory and language tasks (Ullman, 2004).

Bilingual Language Development

The question of whether learning a second language (L2) resides in similar or different brain structures compared to learning the first language (L1) is one of current debate and research. According to Birdsong (2006),

> The basic research issue addressed in this area of cognitive neuroscience is whether processing in the L2 is accomplished in the same way as processing in the L1. The degree of observed similarity hinges on three principal factors: the age at which L2 acquisition is begun, the level of L2 proficiency, and the type of task demanded of the subjects (p. 24).

Birdsong also reports that event related potential (ERP) studies present general support for the convergence hypothesis, which states that processing a second language (L2) becomes more nativelike as the English language learner becomes more proficient in English. An **event related potential** (ERP) is an electro-physiological brain response to a stimulus, external or internal, and the result of a sensory perception. ERPs are measured using electroencephalography (EEG). Nativelike processing has been evidenced in speech perception and other language studies measuring ultimate attainment or final attainment in L2 (Birdsong, 1992; Brice & Ryalls, 2004). Ultimate attainment in language learning is influenced by numerous internal and external factors.

Language is both an innate and a socially constructed phenomenon. Therefore, bilingual or dual language development should also contain innate and social factors (Adkison, 2001). Deacon (cited in Adkison, 2001) believes that the world's grammars are similar and easily acquired because languages have evolved from human cognitive and neurological constraints. Deacon also believes that universal grammatical features exist (Chomsky, 1965). Chomsky stated that the brain contains a restricted set of rules for organizing language. According to Chomsky, all world languages have common structural traits known as a universal grammar. Universal grammars are thought to exist because of common brain structures that have evolved, thus making language possible. According to Deacon (cited in Adkinson, 2001), the brain does not possess an overarching language acquisition device (LAD) (Chomsky, 1965), but rather each language evolves according to the brain's structures. This theory, as well as Chomsky's universal grammars and LAD, need empirical evidence. Because physiological development of the bilingual brain has not been extensively reviewed, this section reviews the neurological substrates of bilingual language development.

According to Rodriguez-Fornells, De Diego Balaguer, and Münte (2006),

> In learning (and sustaining) a second (or third) language, the brain has to build on a neural network that enables the segregation of the new language from the native one, the creation of its corresponding activation and inhibitory links at the lexical, neurological, and syntactic

level, and, finally, the development of the ability to select a word and its syntactic properties in the target language (i.e., the language currently in use) (p. 134).

It should be noted that this viewpoint espoused by Rodriguez-Fornells et al. (2006)
would seem to apply to sequential bilinguals (i.e., those who learn their native
language first, followed by their second language). It would seem that simultaneous
bilinguals (i.e., those who learn both of their languages at the same time) might be
capable of structuring both their languages in the same physical location. Lucas,
Ojemann, and Whitaker (cited in Rodriguez-Fornells et al., 2006) stated that several
perisylvian areas were found in second language learners when compared to monolinguals under conditions of picture naming. Ninety-five percent of the bilinguals in
this study had distinct and shared cortical representations in both their languages.
The areas included the inferior frontal and precentral gyrus, the posterior temporal
gyrus, and the posterior middle temporal gyrus. It seems that saying a word in one
language activates the conceptual system in the other language and consequently
activates both languages.

Simos, Billingsley-Marshall, Sakari, Pataraia, and Papanicolaou (2005) stated that
the majority of "functional neuroimaging studies have not found differences in the
brain regions which are, purportedly, parts of mechanisms of different languages . . ."
(p. 31). Simos et al. also stated that the brain regions and mechanisms in sustaining
two or more languages are related to the age at which the second language was
learned and the person's proficiency levels in his or her languages (Brice & Ryalls,
2004; Perani et al., 1998).

Kim, Relkin, Lee, and Hirsch (1997), in a functional MRI study, found that early
and late bilinguals differed in cortical areas for processing language in Broca's area,
yet not in Wernicke's area. The 12 participants spoke a variety of first languages and
had spoken English as their second language. The participants also lived in an
English-speaking country at the time of the study. The early participants initially had
been exposed to English as infants, while the late bilinguals initially had been
exposed to English in early adulthood. Kim et al. (1997) stated,

> The observation that the anatomical separation of the two languages in Broca's area varies
> with the time at which the second language was acquired, suggests that age of language
> acquisition may be a significant factor in determining the functional organization of this
> area in the human brain (p. 173).

A more exact age at which Broca's area differentiates in localization of the two languages (i.e., common versus distinct cortical areas) is yet to be determined. Simos et al.
(2005) confirm this possibility when they stated, "It may be assumed, for instance, that
acoustic, phonetic, and even semantic processes are based on common neurophysiological processes in most, if not all Indo-European languages, like English and Spanish (Illes et al., 1999)" (p. 32). This seems to support the notion that acoustics,
phonetics, and semantics (processed largely in the temporal lobe) may be more
immune to a critical period for second language learning, while syntax (processed in
the frontal lobe) may demonstrate an earlier sensitive period for language learning.
Tonal languages, such as Chinese, may involve more right hemisphere processing than
English due to the tonal and musical nature of the language (Simos et al., 2005).

CONCLUDING REMARKS

The most important part of the brain responsible for memory, thinking, and language is the frontal lobe. **Executive functioning** (i.e., higher-order thinking skills) resides in the frontal lobe. Knowledge of brain structures and their corresponding cognitive and language attributes is essential for all professionals working with young children, school-age children, adolescents, and young adults. This knowledge is applicable in preparing instructional strategies for all students, that is, students with and without disabilities, and monolingual and bilingual students.

It is important to recall that a single brain area is *not* responsible for any sole aspect of language. It is also important to recall that the brain is capable of learning new information over the course of a lifetime. However, certain periods of development may be more appropriate for acquiring language. Therefore, appropriate environmental stimulation at key points in the child's development fosters learning and, most important, actually shapes the brain's growth and neurological connections. Speech-language pathologists and educators who work with children have great opportunities to enhance a child's development, enhancements that can endure throughout a child's lifetime.

CASE STUDY PERSPECTIVES

Case Study One Background: Evelyn

Evelyn was adopted from an eastern European institution when she was 10. Evelyn was abandoned by her parents and suffered abuse, neglect, and malnutrition while she lived at the eastern European institution. She is now 13 years old and has expressive and possibly receptive language difficulties that do not appear to be primarily related to learning English as a second language, although English language issues seem to be present. Evelyn speaks only English at this time. Evelyn struggles with comprehension and expressive language. She recently had an MRI done, which showed minimal deficits in the lateral and third ventricles.

Ventricles are fluid-filled areas of the body. In the brain, these areas are filled with cerebrospinal fluid. The brain contains two lateral ventricles, the third, and fourth ventricles. The lateral ventricles are wrapped around the front, or dorsal, area of the basal ganglia. Parts of the basal ganglia receive input from the motor and prefrontal cortices. Disorders of the basal ganglia include attention deficit hyperactivity disorders (Gray's Anatomy, 2005; Zemlin, 1997). The third ventricle is a cleft between the brain's two thalami. The thalamus serves as an interpreter for the brain, for example, the processing of auditory information (Gray's Anatomy, 2005; Zemlin, 1997). Therefore, it is possible that Evelyn may have difficulties with processing auditory information and/or difficulties with attention due to proximity of the lateral and third ventricles to the basal ganglia and the thalami.

It was reported by the adoptive mother that Evelyn suffered severe physical and mental abuse and neglect while she was in the orphanage in the eastern European country. Evelyn is making gains in school, yet she struggles with classroom tasks. Her adoptive mother reports that Evelyn appears to be frustrated. In addition, the adoptive mother reports that Evelyn was not exposed to any meaningful language during her first few years and then only to very limited and poorly educated native language speakers. The adoptive mother also reported that Evelyn may have avoided communication with others in her environment because being spoken to by any adult meant that she was to be punished.

Case Study One Comments: Evelyn

Evelyn should receive a thorough speech, language, and educational diagnostic evaluation by properly trained speech-language pathologists, special educators, and school psychologists to ascertain the extent of her communication and learning difficulties. These professionals should be knowledgeable about second language development and learning issues. The evaluation should incorporate parent interviews, classroom observations, teacher input (via surveys, questionnaires, checklists, interviews, etc.), informal and formal assessment procedures, and intervention strategies documented over a period of time (e.g., response to intervention).

Evelyn appears to have suffered from abuse and neglect that could lead to decreased cognitive growth during some sensitive language learning periods (e.g., syntax and pragmatics). In addition, she may display some language and emotional issues associated with abuse (Fox, Long, & Langlois, 1988), such as being withdrawn or experiencing difficulty interacting with others.

Evelyn should receive environmentally rich stimulation because the brain can still develop in the teenage years and is never too old to benefit from stimulation (Eliot, 2001). This stimulation may take the form of enhanced reading, writing, speaking, and listening activities (refer to Chapters 3, 7, 8, and 9 for further discussion of oral and literate development). In addition, various professionals are encouraged to work with the general classroom teacher if it is found that Evelyn does display a language-based learning disability (refer to Chapters 11 and 12 for collaboration and appropriate school programs decisions for English-language-learning students). In sum, Evelyn's progress should be monitored continually because her success in middle school may be at risk at this time.

Case Study Two Background: Antonia

Antonia is a 16-year-old female who sustained a penetrating gunshot wound to the left hemisphere region of the prefrontal cortex. The bullet projectile entered through the orbital region, leaving her blind in her left eye. A craniotomy was performed immediately to clean the wound area, relieve pressure resulting from brain swelling, and remove the bullet. Antonia was in a coma for ten days immediately following the open-head traumatic brain injury (TBI). She was discharged and sent home after an extended stay of approximately one month in the hospital. As a consequence of her injury, she suffers from a severe Broca's-type aphasia, severe right-side hemiparesis (weakness), severe speech apraxia, difficulty feeding, and post-traumatic epilepsy. Her speech is complicated by a buccofacial verbal sequential apraxia (i.e., characterized by an inability to perform learned skilled movements of the face, lips, tongue, larynx, and pharynx on command [Guilmette, 1997]). This occurs in approximately 90% of individuals who have suffered from Broca's aphasia and usually results from frontal or corpus callosum lesions (Guilmette, 1997).

Antonia could not function independently upon release from the hospital. She is wheelchair-dependent, unable to speak, and incontinent. She received speech-language, occupational, and physical therapy during her hospital stay.

Case Study Two Comments: Antonia

Due to the severe nature of Antonia's disabilities, it is recommended that she receive home-based instructional services in addition to the much needed speech-language, occupational, and physical therapy. Because Antonia cannot communicate, it is recommended that she initially begin with a picture-symbol communication system. Individuals with Broca's aphasia display **agrammatism** (Kean, 1995), a distinct pattern of language characterized by short sentences typically without articles, prepositions, auxiliary verbs, and inflectional verb endings.

Initially, language therapy should focus on functional and relevant declarative and command sentences (e.g., "I want water") nonverbally through the communication board or assistive technology device. However, speech should also be emphasized. Verbal sentences may be short, that is, three to four words, increasing in length to five to six words. Antonia's sentences should include articles, prepositions, auxiliary verbs, and verb endings because she will be better understood and because her communication will be clearer and less vague.

Antonia's progress may be slow, and she may have to be retaught functional life skills, including reading, writing, and math. She should continue her occupational and physical therapy to improve her fine and gross motor coordination skills. In addition, it is recommended that she receive counseling to help her adjust to her new situation and reduce the possibility of subsequent depression. With time and appropriate therapy and instruction, Antonia's prognosis should improve.

INSTRUCTIONAL STRATEGIES

1. Learning is not a single-modality activity. Learning occurs by integrating information from the different senses (Eliot, 2001). Wernicke's area (where the temporal and parietal areas meet) lies at the juncture where hearing, vision, and touch are integrated (Eliot, 2001). In addition, the medial temporal region serves the memory functions of encoding, consolidating, and retrieving new memories (Buckner & Wheeler, 2001; Squire & Knowlton, 2000). Therefore, learning through listening, seeing, and touching activities is likely to activate the medial temporal region and the superior temporal gyrus. Repetition of the learning activities enables local and short dendritic connections to be made, in turn enabling explicit memory skills (Brice, 2004; Uylings, 2006).

2. Memories result from making brain connections, that is, short dendritic connections for learning. The more connections are made, the greater the prospect that the memories will be retained. Therefore, use of mnemonics can play a vital role in establishing

and retaining memories. Associating auditory facts with mental images incorporates the temporal, parietal, and occipital lobes. Creating mental images also increases the brain's ability to remember certain facts. For example, in remembering the difference between inductive and deductive reasoning, the first author of this chapter uses a mental image strategy that detectives use in inductive reasoning to solve mysteries, that is, finding clues to ascertain a hypothesis (i.e., who committed the crime). Memory strategies may include (1) repeating and summarizing the information, (2) segmenting and chunking the information into smaller segments, (3) use of mental rehearsal, and (4) relating new information to prior knowledge (Lash, 2000).

3. It is believed that sustained attention requires that the reticular activating system (situated between the medulla oblongata and the midbrain) produce norepinephrine in brain cells (Gray's Anatomy, 2005; Zemlin, 1997). In addition, sustained attention arises from activation of the frontal lobe, corpus callosum, and the basal ganglia (Barkley, Grodzinsky, & DuPaul, 1992; National Institute of Mental Health, 2006). Attention and concentration strategies include (1) reducing distractions in the student's classroom, (2) dividing the work into smaller segments, (3) having the student summarize recent information, and (4) establishing a nonverbal cue system to direct or redirect the student to the classroom task (Brice & Perkins, 1997; Lash, 2000).

4. The brain's ability to organize information is located in the frontal lobe (Eliot, 2001). Organizational strategies beneficial to learning include (1) allotting time for lesson review, (2) using checklists to indicate that tasks have been completed, (3) using daily routines and schedules, (4) writing down steps for organizing activities, and (5) color coding the various lessons (Brice & Perkins, 1997; Lash, 2000).

5. Following directions is crucial to classroom learning. The task of following directions includes attention, memory, and organization skills. The frontal lobe, corpus callosum, basal ganglia, reticular activating system, temporal lobe, and hippocampus most likely are involved. Strategies for following directions include (1) providing instructions orally and in written format, (2) repeating instructions to the students and having students repeat instructions back to the teacher, (3) breaking down complex instructions into smaller steps, (4) pausing and slowing the pace of instruction, and (5) circulating the room to verify that the students are on task and have understood the directions (Brice & Perkins, 1997; Lash, 2000).

REFLECTION QUESTIONS

1. Why might school professionals be confused about assessing Evelyn for possible speech and language disorders?
2. What team members should be involved in evaluating Evelyn for possible speech, language, cognitive, emotional, and learning difficulties?
3. Should Evelyn receive English as a second language (ESL) instruction if she were to be identified as having learning difficulties?

4. What functional language skills should Antonia receive as part of her overall therapeutic program?
5. What immediate language goals are appropriate for Antonia?
6. What long-term objectives are appropriate for Antonia?
7. What is Antonia's prognosis for the next year?

REFERENCES

Adkison, S. (2001). *Towards a coevolution of language theories: Linking composition with brain language studies.* Denver, CO: Annual Meeting of the Conference on College Composition and Communication. (ERIC Document Reproduction Service No. Ed. 455527).

Aine, C. J. (1995). A conceptual overview and critique of functional neuro-imaging techniques in humans: I. MRI/fMRI and PET. *Critical Reviews in Neurobiology, 9*(2–3), 229–309.

American Speech-Language-Hearing Association. (2007). Year 2007 position statement: Principles and guidelines for hearing detection and intervention programs. Retrieved December 18, 2007, from http://www.asha.org/docs/html/PS2007-00281.html.

Barkley, R. A., Grodzinsky, G., & DuPaul, G. J. (1992). Frontal lobe functions in attention deficit disorder with and without hyperactivity: A review and research report. *Journal of Abnormal Child Psychology, 20*(2), 163–188.

Bauman-Waengler, J. (2004). *Articulatory and phonological impairments* (2nd ed.). Boston: Allyn & Bacon.

Beal, M. F., Swartz, K. J., Finn, S. F., Bird, E. D., & Martin, J. B. (1988). Amino acid and neuropeptide neurontransmitters in Huntington's disease cerebellum. *Brain Research, 454,* 393–396.

Benasich, A., Choudhury, N., Friedman, J., Realpe-Bonilla, T., Chojnowska, C., & Gou, Z. (2006). The infant as a prelinguistic model for language learning impairments: Predicting from event-related potentials to behavior. *Neuropsychologia, 44*(3), 396–411.

Benasich, A., & Tallal, D. (2002). Infant discrimination of rapid auditory cues predicts later language impairment. *Behavioral Brain Research, 136,* 31–49.

Bertoncini, J., Floccia, C., Nazzi, T., & Mehler, J. (1995). Morae and syllables: Rhythmical basis of speech representations in neonates. *Language and Speech, 38,* 311–329.

Birdsong, D. (1992). Ultimate attainment in second language acquisition. *Language, 68*(4), 706–755.

Birdsong, D. (2006). Age and second language acquisition and processing: A selective overview. *Language Learning, 56*(1), 9–49.

Brice, A., & Perkins, C. (1997). What is required for transition from the ESL classroom to the general education classroom? A case study of two classrooms. *Journal of Children's Communication Development, 19*(1), 13–22.

Brice, A., & Ryalls, J. (2004). Recognition of code-mixed words by Spanish/English bilinguals: A focus on proficiency levels. *Conference Proceedings of the 26th World Congress of the International Association of Logopedics and Phoniatrics, 6,* 53–56.

Brice, R. (2004). Connecting oral and written language through applied writing strategies. *Intervention in School and Clinic, 40*(1), 38–47.

Buckner, R. L., & Wheeler, M. E. (2001). The cognitive neuroscience of remembering. *Nature Review Neuroscience, 2*(9), 624–634.

Chomsky, N. (1965). *Aspects of the theory of syntax.* Cambridge, MA: MIT Press.

Cowley, G. (1999, November). An Alzheimer's advance. *Newsweek, 134*(18), 76.

DeCasper, A. J., & Prescott, P. (1984). Human newborns' perception of male voices: Preference, discrimination, and reinforcing value. *Developmental Psychobiology, 17,* 481–491.

DeCasper, A. J., & Spence, M. J. (1986). Prenatal maternal speech influences newborns' perception of speech sounds. *Infant Behavior and Development, 9,* 133–150.

Dehaene-Lambertz, G., Dehaene, S., & Hertz-Pannier, L. (2002). Functional neuroimaging of speech perception in infants. *Science, 298,* 2013–2015.

Dehaene-Lambertz, G., & Houston, D. (1998). Language discrimination response latencies in two-month-old infants. *Language and Speech, 41,* 21–43.

Department of Otolaryngology Head and Neck Surgery. (2007). Hearing screening for newborns and infants. Retrieved December 18, 2007, from http://www.entcolumbia.org/babyscrn.html.

Eimas, P. D., Siqueland, E. R., Jusczyk, P., & Vigorito, J. (1971). Speech perception in infants. *Science, 171,* 303–306.

Eliot, L. (2001). Language and the developing brain. *The NAMTA Journal, 26* (2), 8–60.

Fiez, J. A., Raichle, M. E., Balota, D. A., Tallal, D., & Petersen, S. E. (1996). PET activation of posterior temporal regions during auditory word presentation and verb generation. *Cerebral Cortex, 6,* 1–10.

Fletcher, P. C., & Henson, R. N. (2001). Frontal lobes and human memory: Insights from functional neuroimaging. *Brain, 124,* 849–881.

Foundas, A., Leonard, C., Gilmore, R., Fennell, E., & Heilman, K. (1994). Planum temporale asymmetry and language dominance. *Neuropsychologia, 32,* 1225–1231.

Fox, L., Long, S. H., & Langlois, A. (1988). Patterns of language comprehension deficit in abused and neglected children. *Journal of Speech and Hearing Disorders, 53* (3), 239–244.

Geschwind, N., & Levitsky, W. (1968). Human brain: Left-right asymmetries in temporal speech region. *Science, 161,* 186–187.

Giedd, J. N. (1999). Development of the human corpus callosum during childhood and adolescence: A longitudinal MRI study. *Progress in Neuropsychopharmacology & Biological Psychiatry, 23,* 571–588.

Giedd, J. N., Blumenthal, J., Jeffries, N. O., Castellanos, F. X., Liu, H., Zijdenbos, A., Paus, T., Evans, E., & Rapoport, J. L. (1999). Brain development during childhood and adolescence: A longitudinal MRI study. *Nature Neuroscience, 2,* 861–863.

Goswami, U. (2004). Neuroscience, education, and special education. *British Journal of Special Education, 31* (4), 175–183.

Gray's Anatomy. (2005). *The classic collector's edition. Gray's anatomy.* New York: Crown Publishers.

Grosjean, F. (1994). Individual bilingualism. In R. E. Asher (Ed.), *The encyclopedia of language and linguistics* (pp. 1656–1660). Oxford, UK: Pergamon Press.

Guilmette, H. (1997). *Pocketguide to brain injury, cognitive, and neurobehavioral rehabilitation.* San Diego, CA: Singular.

Guttorm, T., Leppanen, P. H. T., Richardson, U., & Lyytinen, H. (2001). Event-related potentials and consonant differences in newborns with familial risk for dyslexia. *Journal of Learning Disabilities, 34,* 534–544.

Halsband, U. (2006). Bilingual and multilingual language processing. *Journal of Physiology—Paris, 99* (4–6), 355–369.

Honeycutt, N. A., Musick, A., Barta, P. E., & Pearlson, G. D. (2000). Measurement of the planum temporale (PT) on magnetic resonance imaging scans: Temporal PT alone and with parietal extension. *Psychiatric Research, 98* (2), 103–116.

Illes, J., Francis, W. S., Desmond, J. E., Gabrieli, J. D. E., Glover, G. H., Poldrack, R., et al. (1999). Convergent cortical representation of semantic processing in bilinguals. *Brain and Language, 70,* 347–363.

Jusczyk, P., Culter, A., & Redanz, N. (1993). Infants' preference for the predominant stress patterns of English words. *Child Development, 64,* 675–687.

Jusczyk, P. W., Friederici, A. D., Wessels, J. M., Svenkerud, V. Y., & Jusczyk, A. M. (1993). Infants' sensitivity to the sound patterns of native language words. *Journal of Memory and Language, 32,* 402–420.

Jusczyk, P. W., Luce, P. A., & Charles-Luce, J. (1994). Infants' sensitivity to phonotactic patterns in the native language. *Journal of Memory and Language, 33,* 630–645.

Kean, M. L. (1995). The elusive character of agrammatism. *Brain and Language, 50* (3), 369–384.

Kim, K. H. S., Relkin, N. R., Lee, K., & Hirsch, J. (1997). Distinct cortical areas associated with native and second languages. *Nature, 388,* 171–174.

Knudsen, E. I. (2004). Sensitive periods in the development of the brain and behavior. *Journal of Cognitive Neuroscience, 16,* 1412–1425.

Kolb, B. (1999). Brain development, plasticity and behavior. *American Psychologist, 44,* 1203–1212.

Kolb, B., & Whishaw, I. Q. (1990). *Fundamentals of human neuropsychology.* San Francisco: W. H. Freeman.

Kuhl, P. K. (2000). A new view of language acquisition. *Proceedings of the National Academy of Sciences of the United States of America, 97,* 11850–11857.

Kuhl, P. K. (2004). Early language acquisition: Cracking the speech code. *Nature Reviews, 5,* 831–843.

Lash, M. (2000). Teaching strategies for students with brain injuries. *TBI Challenge, 4* (2), 1–4.

Lecanuet, J. P., & Granier-Deferre, C. (1993). *Developmental neurocognition: Speech and face processing in the first year of life.* Dordrecht, The Netherlands: Kluwer.

Lennenberg, E. (1967). *Biologic foundations of language.* New York: Wiley.

Leybaert, J., & D'Hondt, M. (2003). Neurolinguistic development in deaf children: The effect of early language experience. *International Journal of Audiology, 42,* S34–S40.

Locke, J. L. (1997). A theory of neurolinguistic development. *Brain and Language, 58*(2) 265–326.

Logan, J. S., Lively, S. E., & Pisoni, D. B. (1991). Training Japanese listeners to identify English /r/ and /l/: A first report. *Journal of the Acoustic Society of America, 89,* 874–886.

Mattys, S. L., Jusczyk, P. W., Luce, P. A., & Morgan, J. L. (1999). Phonotactic and prosodic effects on word segmentation in infants. *Cognitive Psychology, 38,* 465–494.

Mehler, J., Jusczyk, P. W., Lambertz, G., Halsted, N., Bertoncini, J., & Amiel-Tison, C. (1988). A precursor of language acquisition in young infants. *Cognition, 29,* 143–178.

Müller, R., & Basho, S. (2004). Are nonlinguistic functions in "Broca's area" prerequisites for language acquisition? FMRI findings from an ontogenetic viewpoint. *Brain and Language, 89,* 329–336.

National Institute of Mental Health. (2006). *Attention deficit hyperactivity disorder.* Bethesda, MD: Department of Health and Human Services.

Nazzi, T., Bertoncini, J., & Mehler, J. (1998). Language discrimination by newborns: Toward an understanding of the role of rhythm. *Journal of Educational Psychology, 24*(3), 756–766.

Penfield, W., & Roberts, L. 1959. *Speech and brain mechanisms.* Princeton, NJ: Princeton University Press.

Perani, D., Paulesu, E., Galles, N. S., Dupoux, E., Dehaene, S., Bettinardi, V., Cappa, S. F., Fazio, F., & Mehler, J. (1998). The bilingual brain. Proficiency and age of acquisition of the second language. *Brain, 121,* 1841–1852.

Ramus, F., Hauser, M. D., Miller, C., Morris, D., & Mehler, J. (2000). Language discrimination by human newborns and by cotton-top tamarin monkeys. *Science, 288,* 349–351.

Ramus, F., Nespor, M., & Mehler, J. (1999). Correlates of linguistic rhythm in the speech signal. *Cognition, 73,* 265–292.

Restak, R. (2001). *The secret life of the brain.* New York: Joseph Henry Press.

Rodriguez-Fornells, A., De Diego Balaguer, R., & Münte, T. F. (2006). Executive control in bilingual language processing. *Language Learning, 56*(1), 133–190.

Sakai, K. L. (2005). Language acquisition and brain development. *Science, 310*(4), 815–819.

Simos, P. G., Billingsley-Marshall, R. L., Sakari, S., Pataraia, E., & Papanicolaou, A. C. (2005). Brain mechanisms supporting distinct languages. *Learning Disabilities Research and Practice, 20*(1), 31–38.

Simos, P. G., Fletcher, J. M., Bergman, E., Breier, J. L., Foorman, B. R., Castillo, E. M., Davis, R. N., Fitzgerald, M., & Papanicolaou, A. C. (2002). Dyslexia specific brain activation profile becomes normal following successful remedial training. *Neurology, 58,* 1203–1213.

Smith, N. V., & Tsimpli, I. M. (1995). *The mind of a savant: Language learning and modularity.* Oxford, UK: Blackwell.

Soroker, N., Kasher, A., Giora, R., Batori, G., Corn, C., Gil, M., & Zaidel, E. (2005). Processing of basic speech acts following localized brain damage: A new light on neuroanatomy of language. *Brain and Cognition 57,* 215–217.

Squire, L. R., & Knowlton, B. J. (2000). The medial temporal lobe, the hippocampus, and the memory systems of the brain. In M. S. Gazzaniga (Ed.), *The new cognitive neurosciences* (pp. 765–780). Cambridge, MA: MIT Press.

Squire, L. R., & Zola, S. M. (1996). Structure and function of declarative and nondeclarative memory systems. *Proceedings of the National Academy of Sciences of the United States of America, 93,* 13515–13522.

Steinmetz, H. (1996). Structure, function and cerebral asymmetry: In vivo morphometry of the planum temporale. *Neuroscience and Biobehavioral Reviews, 20,* 587–591.

Studdert-Kennedy, M., & Shankweiler, D. P. (1970). Hemispheric specialization for speech perception. *Journal of the Acoustical Society of America, 48,* 579–595.

Suzuki, W. A., & Eichenbaum, H. (2000). The neurophysiology of memory. *Annals of the New York Academy of Sciences, 911,* 175–191.

Thomson, J., Baldeweg, T., & Goswami, U. (2004, June). *Amplitude envelope onsets and dyslexia: A behavioural and electrophysiological study.* Paper presented at the Annual Meeting of the Society for the Scientific Study of Reading, Amsterdam, The Netherlands.

Trehub, S. E. (1976). The discrimination of foreign speech contrasts by infants and adults. *Child Development, 47,* 466–472.

Tulving, E., Kapur, S., Craik, F. I. M., Moscovitch, M., & Houle, S. (1994). Hemispheric encoding/retrieval asymmetry in episodic memory: Positron emission tomography findings. *Proceedings of the National*

Academy of Sciences of the United States of America, 91, 2016–2020.

Ullman, M. T. (2004). Contributions of memory circuits to language: The declarative/procedural model. *Cognition, 92*, 231–270.

Uylings, H. B. M. (2006). Development of the human cortex and the concept of "critical" or "sensitive" periods. *Language Learning, 56* (1), 59–90.

Vanlancker-Sidtis, D. (2004). When only the right hemisphere is left: Studies in language and communication. *Brain and Language, 91*, 199–211.

Wada, J. A., Clarke, R., & Hamm, A. (1975). Cerebral hemispheric asymmetry in humans: Cortical speech zones in 100 adult and 100 infant brains. *Archives of Neurology, 32*, 239–246.

Zemlin, W. R. (1997). *Speech and hearing science: Anatomy and physiology* (4th ed.). Boston, MA: Allyn & Bacon.

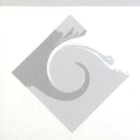

Chapter 2

Infant and Preschool Language Development

Jo-Anne Prendeville

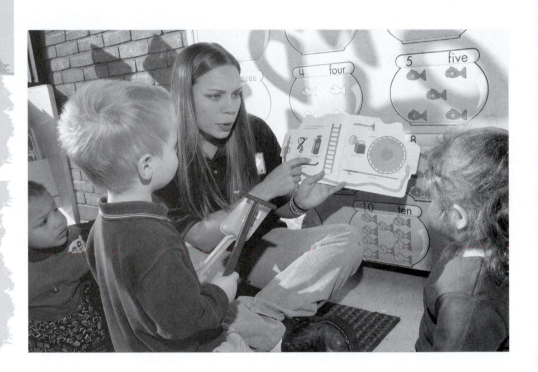

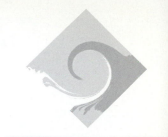

CHAPTER OUTLINE

Introduction

Phonology
    Anatomy of the Infant Vocal Tract
    Speech Perception
    Stages of Vocal Development
    Sounds, Words, and Meaningful Speech
    Phonological Development
    Cross-Linguistic Considerations

Semantics
    Principles of Early Lexical Development
    Nature of the Early Lexicon
    Referential Versus Expressive Styles
    Overextension, Underextension, Overlap, and Mismatch
    Relational Terms
    Parental Input and Lexical Development
    Cross-Linguistic Considerations

Case Study Perspectives
    Case Study One Background: Chad
    Case Study One Comments: Chad
    Case Study Two Background: Tess
    Case Study Two Comments: Tess

Syntax and Morphology
    Sentence Constituents
    Mean Length of Utterance
    Interrogative Forms
    Negation
    Compound and Complex Sentences
    Cross-Linguistic Considerations

Pragmatics
    Joint Attention and Joint Action Routines
    Nonverbal Communication and Gestures
    Conversation and Discourse: Protoconversations
    Cross-Linguistic Considerations

Concluding Remarks

INTRODUCTION

Language is a dynamic system that, when embedded in context, provides children access into the social world of interpersonal communication. Children, from birth, begin to develop the components of language: phonology, semantics, syntax, morphology, and pragmatics. They continue to refine and expand skills in these areas throughout the preschool years, school years, and beyond.

Children learn that language is intricate and that it is more than the sum of its components. Two processes are at work in language acquisition: (1) children do not merely learn each of the components separately, and (2) they learn how these components are intertwined and how the interaction of these components leads to proficient and successful communication (Refer to Chapter 1 for additional discussion of the multiphasic properties of language development and brain neurophysiology).

Phonological Abilities

Developing phonological abilities involves learning the sounds and phoneme system of a language. **Phonemes** are the smallest unit of language that provides contrastive meaning and allows an individual to make distinctions between words. Thus, when children produce the words *cat* (/kæt/) and *sat* (/sæt/) the listener differentiates one word from another based on the contrast between the two phonemes of /k/ and /s/. Children learn how to combine phonemes of their language to create words.

Minimal pairs are pairs of words that differ by only one phoneme that changes the meaning of each word. For example, minimal pairs can be classified according to distinctive features of the word. Distinctive features of words can be classified according to (1) major class features (consonants, vowels, or syllables), (2) laryngeal features (voicing, spread glottis, and restricted glottis), (3) manner features (manner of articulation to include the features of continuants, nasals, stridents, laterals, and stops/fricatives), and (4) place features (place of articulation to include labials, coronals, dorsal, and sounds produced with the root of the tongue). The distinctive feature of voicing or not voicing differentiates an initial voiced consonant in the word *bat* [+ voicing CVC] versus the initial voiceless consonant in the word *pat* [−voicing CVC]. Thus, the distinctive feature of voicing differentiates these two words (*bat* versus *pat*).

As part of combining sounds to produce words, children learn the syllable structure of language. **Syllables** are comprised of sequences of consonants (C) and vowels (V) and can include strings such as CV (to: /tu/), CVC (mitt /mit/), and CCVC (stack: /stæk/), to name a few. Phonemes and syllable structures are all language-specific, and children must learn which forms are appropriate for the language or languages they are learning to speak.

Semantic Abilities

One aspect of developing semantic abilities entails children's discovery of word meanings and their referents as they increase and broaden their lexicons. Word learning is more than just attaching a label to objects or events. It involves a deeper understanding that incorporates the perceptual, nonperceptual, and functional qualities of the words, and that leads to stronger concept knowledge (Anglin, 1977). This aspect of semantic development is termed **referential knowledge**.

Semantic development extends beyond referential knowledge to relational knowledge. **Relational meaning** encompasses the associations between words in utterances and the interplay of roles with respect to each other. Thus, the meaning of an utterance is more than the sum of the individual words that comprise it (Wells, 1985). For example, the word *dog* changes roles within the following utterances: The dog is running; I gave food to my dog; or That dog is big. In the first sentence, *dog* is an agent that is doing an action. In the second, *dog* is a recipient that is receiving an object due to the action of an agent. In the third, *dog* is an entity that is being described with respect to an attribute. Thus, even though the referential meaning of the word *dog* has not changed, its relationship with the other words in the utterance is different from one sentence to the next.

Syntactic and Morphological Abilities

Development of syntactic abilities provides children with the knowledge needed to combine words in the order that is accepted by the languages used in their environment. By combining words, children produce sentences to convey their thoughts and ideas. Although simple sentences predominate in children's early utterances, as they develop and mature, they learn to produce compound and complex sentences as well. **Independent clauses** are those that can stand alone, whereas dependent clauses are those that need to be combined with an independent clause. A **simple sentence** is made up of one independent clause, a **compound sentence** is a combination of two independent clauses, and a **complex sentence** is comprised of an independent and a minimum of one dependent clause (Justice & Ezell, 2002). As children's syntactic abilities progress, so do the types of sentences they can produce. They learn to juxtapose information in sentences through a range of syntactic markers and clauses used to convey various relationships.

The morphological component of language relates to word structure. Content words and function words are types of morphemes. **Content words** consist of nouns, verbs, adjectives, and adverbs, whereas **function words** are the small words that connect the content words together, for example, articles, prepositions, conjunctions, and relative pronouns (Lahey, 1988). Morphemes can be attached to nouns and verbs. **Morphemes** can change the syntactic class of the word or modify aspects such as the word's number or tense.

Pragmatic Abilities

Children may develop phonological, semantic, morphological, and syntactic skills, but without pragmatic skills, they would not know how to use language in conversation. The knowledge of how to carry on a conversation and how to accomplish one's wants and needs through language is the domain of **pragmatics.** Children need to request, comment, and access information. They must know the rules of discourse or how to engage in conversation, how to link their turns with their partners' turns, how to initiate and maintain topics, and how to take conversational turns. In addition, children must be able to adjust their talk to contextual variations, such as different environments (e.g., home, school) or different partners (e.g., parents, peers). They also need to be able to presuppose their partner's knowledge (i.e., make assumptions about what their conversational partner knows about the topic) and information and adjust the way they talk and the information they share accordingly.

In summary, all aspects of language are critical to enable children to communicate. Language gives children a way to share life experiences, past and present. Language skills provide children with a means to interact in play with peers. Oral language also provides children access to literacy and written language.

PHONOLOGY

Anatomy of the Infant Vocal Tract

As infants enter into the realm of producing sounds, they begin with a vocal tract that is structurally different from the vocal tract of an adult. Infants have a short pharyngeal area and an oral cavity that is broad. The mass of an infant's tongue sits further forward and fills a large portion of the mouth, making the tongue better suited to move back and forth. The larynx is high, causing the velum and epiglottis to almost touch. These differences diminish at four to six months of age as the infant's vocal tract develops (Kent & Miolo, 1995; Vihman, 2004). The structure of the infant's vocal tract affects sound production. Initially vocalizations are nasal (Vihman, 2004), and vowels are produced at a higher frequency than those of adults (Kent, 1992). In addition to structural changes in the vocal tract that facilitate vocalizations, infant's cortical development contributes to increased motor control, so as infants get older, they can prolong sequences of cooing and babbling (Kent & Miolo, 1995). (Refer to Chapter 1 for further discussion of cortical development and speech development.)

Speech Perception

Speech perception is the ability to identify various parameters of speech, including sounds and prosodic features. Speech perception skills are present from the very beginning of life and increase as infants get older. As young as birth to one month of age, infants can differentiate the phonetic contrasts in speech (Kent & Miolo, 1995; Vihman, 2004). Their sensitivity extends to individual speech patterns as well as overall speech patterns (Kent & Miolo, 1995). Place and manner of articulation can be discriminated by infants as young as two months old. With respect to place, in English they can differentiate among /b/, /d/, and /g/ in the initial position of syllables. In terms of manner, infants can distinguish stops from nasals, from glides (Vihman, 2004). From one to four months, infants can discriminate vowel contrasts (Kent & Miolo, 1995) such as /a/ versus /i/, versus /u/ (Vihman, 2004). During this period, they can even make the distinction among different intonation patterns (Kent & Miolo, 1995). From four to six months, infants demonstrate a sensitivity to the prosodic characteristics of language. They can perceive prosodic indicators of clauses, and they can discriminate prosodic features in their parents' language from those features in another language (Kent & Miolo, 1995). The ability to distinguish between native and non-native speech perception begins to appear from seven to ten months of age, when infants are beginning to differentiate words in other languages from words spoken in their environment and are less likely to distinguish sound contrasts in other languages (Kent & Miolo, 1995). By 10 to 12 months, they are no longer able to discriminate sound contrasts in words that are not in their native language, but their speech perception abilities in their native language become increasingly well developed (Kent & Miolo, 1995). Oller and Eilers (1983) determined that 2-year-old Spanish-speaking children could identify natural contrasts in Spanish better than in English, while English-speaking 2-year-olds could identify natural contrasts better in English than in Spanish. It is apparent from this developmental progression of speech perception that there is a movement from perceiving global language features to perceiving language features that are specific to the language in the child's environment. This has an effect on the acquisition of the speech system.

Stages of Vocal Development

A developmental stage model approach (or theory) has been applied to describe infant speech development (Stark, 1979; Oller, 1980; Stoel-Gammon, 1998; Oller, 2000). Stage models trace the course of infant speech acquisition through a developmental progression that begins at birth and proceeds through to the production of first words. Although the stages may be subdivided differently across these models, there is a general consensus about the vocal and speech behaviors produced by infants across the first year of life. The earliest types of vocalizations are sounds that are reflexive and vegetative in nature, followed by cooing and gooing sounds. Subsequently, infants engage in vocal play and marginal babbling. The production of babbled syllables follow in the form of reduplicated (e.g., baba) and variegated babbling (e.g., badaga). A discussion of Oller's stage model follows (Oller, 1980; Oller, Eilers, Neal & Schwartz, 1999; Oller, 2000).

Oller's stages of speech development are grounded in the concept of **infraphonology** and the distinction between fixed signals and vegetative sounds and **protophones**. Infant speech infraphonology incorporates three properties of speech: phonation, articulation, and consonant-vowel combinations (Oller et al., 1999). There is an additive progression for infants incorporating these properties into their vocalizations. The properties of infraphonology are not noted in fixed signals or vegetative sounds but are apparent in protophones. Fixed signals include sounds behaviors such as crying, laughing, or moaning; vegetative sounds include bodily functions such as coughing, sneezing, burping, grunting, and the like (Oller, 2000). Fixed signals and vegetative sounds are distinguished from protophones, which are precursors to speech and lead to the development of the lexicon. Infants who are typically developing engage in producing protophones for an extended period of time prior to the onset of word production (Oller et al., 1999; Oller, 2000).

Oller's four stages of infant speech development consist of (1) the phonation stage (0 to 2 months), (2) the primitive articulation stage (1 to 4 months), (3) the expansion stage (3 to 8 months), and (4) the canonical stage (5 to 10 months). During the phonation stage, infants' productions include not only vegetative and fixed sounds, but also early vocalizations, including the protophone labeled a quasivowel. This protophone incorporates the infraphonological property of phonation (Oller, 2000). The vocalization is termed a **quasivowel** because it shares some but not all the characteristics of fully formed vowels. Quasivowels and fully-formed vowels are comparable because they are produced with normal phonation. The difference resides in the positioning of the tongue, lips, and jaws. With fully-formed vowels, there is a change in the position of the tongue, lips, and jaw that translates to the production of a range of vowel types. With quasivowels, infants do not move their tongue, lips, and jaw; rather, their vocal tract is at rest and thus does not vary the quality of the vowel (Oller et al., 1999; Oller, 2000).

Oller's second stage of development is the primitive articulation stage. During this stage, between 1 and 4 months of age, infants begin to produce limited articulation (Oller, 2000) in conjunction with normal phonation (Oller et al., 1999). Most of the sounds that infants produce in English at this time use the back of the tongue placed against the back part of the mouth or velum (Oller, 2000). Thus, these sounds are called velar sounds and at this stage, infants demonstrate a preference for this type of sound (Oller, 1980). Although velar sounds dominate, other sound productions do occur (Oller, 2000). The protophone produced by this limited articulation is called gooing or cooing (Oller, 1980; Oller et al., 1999; Oller, 2000). Infants produce gooing and cooing when they are alone and when they engage in protoconversations with adults (Oller, 2000). The infraphonological property that infants master during this stage is limited articulation produced with normal phonation already mastered during the phonation stage (Oller et al., 1999; Oller, 2000).

The third stage of speech development is the expansion stage (Oller et al., 1999; Oller, 2000), which occurs between 3 and 8 months of age (Oller, 2000). This stage is characterized by infants practicing with different positions of the vocal tract, such as using complete openness or different positions of the lips and tongue as they use normal phonation. These movements create full vowel-like protophones (Oller et al., 1999; Oller, 2000). The term **full vowel** is used because during this stage, vowels are formed with full resonance (Oller, 2000). These sounds are also termed vocants, which are precursors to adultlike vowels (Kent & Bauer, 1985). Infants also begin to use **closants**, which are precursors to adultlike consonants (Kent & Bauer, 1985). Closants are produced by interrupting the vocal tract and interrupting the airstream, creating consonantlike protophones. Infants also use sequences of full vowels and closed sounds to produce the protophone of marginal babbling. These sequences are labeled marginal babbling because the timing of the sequence of full vowels and closed sounds is slow (Oller, 2000), whereas well-formed syllables have a rapid transition between sounds (Oller et al., 1999).

At this time, infants experiment with other types of sounds, such as raspberries, squealing and growling, and yelling and whispering (Oller, 1980; Oller, 2000). Raspberries are friction sounds that are produced with air blown through lips that are tightly closed. Raspberries can be produced with or without voicing (Oller, 2000). Squeals are produced using a high-pitched, falsetto voice that is initiated or terminated using a full voice (Oller, 1980; Oller, 2000). In contrast, growls are low-pitched with vocal tension that creates a noisy sound (Oller, 2000). Yelling and whispering are contrastive sounds that range from maximum loudness to minimum loudness. Infants engage in using this range of protophones during the expansion stage. Infants' productions now incorporate three of the infraphonological properties: normal phonation, limited articulation, and full resonance.

The final speech developmental stage is called the canonical stage and occurs from 5 to 10 months of age. Infants produce well-timed, consonantlike, and vowel-like sequences with normal phonation (Oller et al., 1999). The most prominent feature of these vocalizations is that they are reduplicated syllables (i.e., baba, dada). The transitions between consonants and vowels are rapid, in contrast with those in the previous stage that are slow-yielding vocalizations identified by adults as speech-like (Oller et al., 1999). Indeed, these syllables seem wordlike (Stoel-Gammon, 1998), and adults often mistake these syllables as efforts by infants to produce meaningful words (Oller, 2000). Even though these syllable sounds appear wordlike, there is no indication that there is an association between sound and meaning at this time (Stoel-Gammon, 1998). From an infraphonological perspective, this stage is the culmination of previous stages, with infants using normal phonation, full resonance, well-timed articulation, and rapid transitions between sounds (Oller, 2000).

Babbling is a vocal behavior milestone produced by infants. Babbling is a multi-syllabic production (Mitchell & Kent, 1990) that can be reduplicated or variegated in structure (Stark, 1979; Mitchell & Kent, 1990). In **reduplicated babbling** infants produce a series of alternating consonant and vowel syllables (Stoel-Gammon, 1998), repeating the same consonants and vowels across the vocalization (e.g., bababa) (Stark, 1979). In contrast, **nonreduplicated or variegated babbling** is characterized by the use of variation in the syllable structure. In these syllables, the consonants and vowels differ across syllables (e.g., badaga) (Stark, 1979; Oller, 1980; Stoel-Gammon, 1998). These two types of babbling have been described as sequential stages, with reduplicated babbling occurring first, followed by variegated babbling (Stark, 1979; Stoel-Gammon, 1998). This stagelike sequence of development has been questioned, and it has been demonstrated that indeed phonetic variation is apparent in the early babbling of infants (Mitchell & Kent, 1990). Furthermore, the amount of variation in babbling is similar for infants at 7, 9, and 11 months of age.

As infants move through the stages of babbling to the production of first words, the sound inventory and their syllable shapes that they use change and evolve. For infants at 13 months, the greatest number of syllables are in the form of a single vocant, the precursor to vowels (V) or two vocants produced in sequence (VV). These syllables are not produced with any closant, the precursor to consonants. The next most frequent syllable for 13-month-olds is combinations of closants, vocants, and CVs. Two other syllable types are observed but with much lesser frequency: VCV and CVCV. It is notable that the CV syllable is used by itself or embedded in other syllable sequences: CVC, VCV, CVCV, or VCVCV. No syllables with consonant clusters are observed (Kent & Bauer, 1985). Of the vowel syllables (V or VV) used in these sequences, there is a tendency to use central and front vowels rather than back vowels. Also more low vowels are produced than high vowels (Kent & Bauer, 1985). Vowels are used in the following order of frequency: /ʌ/ or /ə/, /ɛ/, /æ/, /u/, /e/, /a/, and /o/.

Consonant vowel syllables are the second most frequently used syllables, and they are common syllable types observed across languages. In these syllables, stops are the most frequently used closant, produced 74% of the time; followed by fricatives and nasals, produced only 11% and 10% of the time, respectively; and the least frequent closants are glides. Of the sounds described, most that are produced are bilabials (those produced with both lips) and those produced with the tip of the tongue. Although not as frequent, sounds produced in the back of the mouth (velars) occur as well. Of these closants, the greatest number produced by the infant are voiced to the extent that 85% of the sounds produced are voiced. The most frequently used closants are /b/ or /d/, sounds that are voiced and produced with both lips and the tongue tip. The vocants used in conjunction with the closants in these CV syllables are usually midcentral, mid or low front, or low back (Kent & Bauer, 1985). The third most frequently used syllable type is CVCV. It is possible that these syllable types are just a chain of CV syllables linked together. By and large, the closants and vocants that are used in CV syllables are also those noted in CVCV syllables (Kent & Bauer, 1985).

Across languages, six syllables occur most frequently in children's vocal productions: /da/, /ba/, /wa/, /də/, /ha/, and /hə/. Of these syllables, /da/ is the most frequently used. When focusing exclusively on vowels, /a/æ/ and /ʌ/ are the most common vowels produced (Vihman, 1992). As children progress from babbling to the use of words, the influence of the adult language system is brought to bear on the syllable shapes that they use. Two factors have an effect on the syllables that children begin to use in their first words: the saliency of syllables that they hear and the ease with which the syllables can be produced motorically (Vihman, 1992). Thus, the linguistic environment has an impact on the sounds used in babbling and in first words. This can be seen as early as 10 months of age (Stoel-Gammon, 1992). By the time children's vocabularies are comprised of fifteen different words, the sounds in the language they hear have a definite impact on their own sound repertoires and sound production (Vihman et al., 1986).

Sounds, Words, and Meaningful Speech

Even before children begin to use adultlike words, they produce wordlike utterances. These forms have been called **phonetically consistent forms** (PCFs) (Dore, Franklin, Miller, & Ramer, 1976), protowords (Menyuk & Menn, 1979; Vihman, 1988; Vihman, 2004), or vocables (Elbers & Wijnen, 1992). These are prelinguistic vocal patterns that bridge babbling and true word production (Dore et al., 1976). These vocalizations are different from babbling because they (1) are comprised of consistent vocal patterns (Vihman, 2004), (2) can be isolated by the pause boundaries that surround them, (3) recur in children's inventory of sound productions, and (4) may be associated with specific situations. And they contain what is termed protophonemic structure, which is a more stable phonetic structure than babbling (Dore et al., 1976). **Protowords** may not have any relationship to adult words. Often they are in the form of CV syllables that incorporate glottals /ʔ/ or /h/ or stops in the consonant position (Vihman, 2004). From a sentence structure perspective, children may use protowords as a placeholder in an utterance. They may also be used in conjunction with other words and chained together with protowords. Elbers and Wijnen (1992) use the term *positional vocable* to describe this particular function. Children may also use a protoword to fill their conversational turn (Vihman, 1988). At first they are used in narrow, context-specific situations and then are generalized and used more broadly (Menyuk & Menn, 1979). Children may even continue to use these forms once they begin to use true words (Vihman, 2004). Of great importance is the communicative function of these vocalizations. Children use them to signal a range of intentional (i.e., purposeful) communication even before they are using true words. Children may use these forms to gain attention, focus attention on an object or an action, express feelings, or cause others to do something for them (Dore et al., 1976; Vihaman, 2004). Therefore, it can be said that pragmatic intents or functions develop before the appearance of words.

Phonological Development

As children begin to use words and continue to expand their vocabularies and sentence length, they apply certain modifications to the adult word structure. These modifications are termed **phonological processes** and reflect a set of phonological rules that children apply as they produce their version of an adult word. Phonological process productions should not be viewed as errors. Rather they should be seen as part of the developmental sequence of word production. Rules that are applied fall into three categories: syllable structure rules, consonant harmony rules, and substitution rules (Prater & Swift, 1982). **Syllable structure rules** modify the syllable in the direction of a CV (Kahn, 1982; Prater & Swift, 1982) or CVCV (Prater & Swift, 1982) configuration. Syllable structure processes include deletion of final consonants, cluster reduction, weak syllable deletion, and glottal replacement. **Consonant harmony rules** include processes that create a similarity in phonetic features of sounds (Grunwell, 1982). Harmony processes include final consonant devoicing, velar assimilation, and prevocalic voicing. **Substitution processes** are those where one sound is replaced by another sound. The sound can be in the initial, medial, or final position (Ingram, 1974). Substitution processes include stopping, fronting, vocalization, gliding, affrication, and denasalization (Prater & Swift, 1982). Phonological processes can be applied individually or in combination with other processes. For example, a child says /bæt/ for *black* by reducing the consonant cluster to /b/ and fronting the /k/ to /t/. When the child says /bɛt/ for *peg*, she or he is voicing the /p/ and devoicing the /g/ (Grunwell, 1982).

As children get older, their use of these processes diminishes along a developmental sequence. The six processes of deletion of final consonants, cluster reduction, weak syllable deletion, gliding, vocalization, and final consonant devoicing occur 35 to 55% of the time and have the greatest impact on children's word productions in English (Prater & Swift, 1982). The greatest decline in the use of phonological processes occurs between the ages of 2;6 and 4. The processes used the most during this time frame are deletion of final consonants, cluster reduction, fronting, stopping, and liquid gliding. By the time children have reached 4;0 cluster reduction and liquid gliding do not occur frequently, and deletion of final consonants, fronting, and stopping are seldom used (Roberts, Burchinal, & Footo, 1990; Haelsig & Madison, 1986).

The consistent use of processes has been documented for specific ages. The following is a list of common phonological processes and the ages through which they are consistently used in English: (1) weak syllable deletion through age 3;6; (2) final consonant deletion through approximately 2;8; (3) reduplication through age 2;0; (4) harmony through approximately 2;4; (5) cluster reduction through approximately 3;4; (6) fronting through 2;6; (7) gliding through 3;0; and (8) context sensitive voicing through approximately 2;4. The continued use of stopping varies by consonant. For example, stopping that affects /f/ only occurs through 2;0, while it affects /ð/ consistently until 4;6. Although these ages represent consistent use of these processes, they do continue to be noted in words beyond these ages; they do so, however, at a substantially lower frequency (Grunwell, 1982).

Cross-Linguistic Considerations

Phonological processes are a sensitive measure for describing the structural patterns of young children's early words. This is true for children speaking various English dialects (e.g., African American English [AAE], Spanish-influenced English) and languages other than English (e.g., Spanish, Taiwanese). Phonological processes have been used to capture the developmental speech patterns of African American English–(AAE) (Bland-Stewart, 2003) and Spanish-speaking children (Brice & de la Paz, 1997; Goldstein & Iglesias, 1998). The syllables reflected in words produced by two-year-old African American children are CV, CVC, and CVCV. Many of the phonological processes used by toddler speakers of AAE are similar to those used by adults speaking AAE. These phonological processes are cluster reduction, final consonant deletion, stopping of fricatives and affricates, velarization and vowelization of /r/.

Two-year-old children also produce phonological processes that are similar to children of the same age learning Standard American English (SAE). These processes include cluster reduction and deletion of final consonants (Bland-Stewart, 2003).

Spanish phoneme acquisition has been systematically researched, along with the use of phonological processes (Brice, 1996). The general acquisition process is the same across the Spanish language, but dialectical trends and variations differentiate the phonological development and processes used within the Spanish language. All dialects of a particular language are rule-governed and mutually intelligible. Therefore, any dialect should be considered changes from a standard (i.e., a standard Spanish) from which one can measure specific variations (Goldstein & Iglesias, 2001).

Because Spanish dialects differ greatly from each other, and these differences are characterized by consonant distinctions (the basis for typically diagnosing a phonological disorder), the consequences of not considering dialect may be more serious for Spanish-speaking children. Although Spanish dialects show differences on vowels, dialects in Spanish are characterized mainly through consonant differences that affect large consonant sound classes—particularly fricatives, liquids, glides, and nasals (Cotton & Sharp, 1988).

Research on Spanish phonological acquisition has been limited to a few isolated dialects. It is reported that there are seven major dialects of American Spanish: Mexican and southwestern United States; Central American; American; Caribbean; Highlandian; Chilean; and southern Paraguayan, Uruguayan, and Argentinean (Stockwell & Bowen, 1965). Fricatives and liquids show greater variation by these dialectical features (Goldstein & Iglesias, 1998). The dialectical feature may inflate a phonological process of occurrence score and thus make the child look disordered when, in fact, she or he may have a language difference (Brice, 1996).

By 3 years of age, the most prevalent phonological processes in Spanish are cluster reduction, gliding of the liquid, and deletion of the stop with retention of the liquid. By 4, most speakers of Spanish master consonants and vowels (Goldstein & Iglesias, 1996). Jimenez (1987) studied the articulation of Spanish-speaking children from the Sacramento Valley in California and found a larger number of phonemes mastered after age 4 than did Acevedo (cited in Mann & Hodson, 1994).

According to Martinez (1986), tap-trill /r/ deficiencies, consonant sequence reductions, de-affrication, stopping, affrication, fronting, assimilations, palatalization, metathesis, migration, vowel deviations, and sibilant distortions are the only processes evident after the age of 4 in children of Mexican descent. Consonant sequence reduction, de-affrication, and a number of nonphonemic deviations and tap-trill deficiencies are evident after age 4 in monolingual children of Mexican descent (Becker, 1982).

Goldstein and Iglesias (1998) noted that the processes used in words more than 10% of the time are cluster reduction and liquid simplification. Those used to a lesser extent—less than 10%—are palatal fronting, assimilation, and final consonant deletion, while de-affrication, backing, spirantization, denasalization, addition, and palatalization are extremely rare. Generally, by the time that Spanish-speaking children reach age 3, they have suppressed most of the phonological processes (Goldstein & Iglesias, 1998). An inventory of the use of phonological processes in children of Spanish-speaking Puerto Rican descent indicates that at age 3 the only phonological process used more than 10% of the time is cluster reduction. Other processes are used less than 10% of the time by 3-year-olds. These include liquid simplification, stopping, weak syllable deletion, velar fronting, and assimilation. By 4 years old, all of the children use all processes less than 10% of the time (Goldstein & Iglesias, 1996).

Dialect also affects the production of phonological processes and must be taken into account when determining the developmental appropriateness of children's word productions. Differences have been documented in the use of phonological processes by 3- and 4-year-old children speaking standard Spanish and Puerto Rican Spanish speakers (from Philadelphia, Pennsylvania). Final consonant deletion and liquid simplification reflected the greatest difference in percentage of use, with general Spanish-speaking children using the processes to a greater extent than Puerto Rican Spanish-speaking children. A difference was present for weak syllable deletion but not to a great extent (Goldstein & Iglesias, 2001). As described previously, as children's phonological systems develop, use of phonological processes is suppressed or discontinued. The percentage of children speaking standard Spanish using final consonant deletion, liquid simplification, and weak syllable deletion more than 20% of the time was 98%, 43%, and 7%, respectively, while the percentage of children speaking Puerto Rican Spanish using the same processes was 17%, 6%, and 0%, respectively. The differences in suppression of processes noted between children speaking standard Spanish and Puerto Rican Spanish has implications for identification of disorders (Goldstein & Iglesias, 2001).

SEMANTICS

Principles of Early Lexical Development

Children follow a developmental path in acquiring and expanding their lexicon. To trace this course of development, a theoretical model is needed that accounts for the developmental underpinnings of this process. The framework for such a theoretical model is grounded in the principles of reference, extendability, object scope, categorical scope, novel name–nameless category (N$_3$C), and conventionality. The principles of this model are divided into two tiers. Tier one encompasses a set of principles that initiate the development of the lexicon. These principles do not necessitate the use of complex cognitive-linguistic processes to begin word learning; rather, information about words and their referents can be accessed through signals during social interactions (beginning at approximately 12 months of age). The principles applied in this tier include reference, extendibility, and object scope. Tier two principles facilitate rapid word learning (approximately from 18 to 24 months of age) and include the application of categorical scope, novel name–nameless category (N$_3$C), and conventionality (Golinkoff, Mervis, & Hirsch-Pasek, 1994).

Tier One Principles

The **principle of reference** proposes that very young children, on hearing a new word, make the assumption that the word should be mapped onto something that is in their immediate environment (i.e., a referent). The word may be mapped onto an object, action, attribute, or ongoing event (Golinkoff, Mervis, & Hirsch-Pasek, 1994).

When children learn a word, they apply the word to other instances of the initial referent by utilizing a rudimentary skill, that is, the **principle of extendibility**. Lexical extensions are typically based on a perceived similarity between the initial referent and a new instance that is encountered. For example, a child may learn that some balls are bouncy (the new encounter) and add this to her or his knowledge of balls; hence, "bouncy ball" is the new extension. Typically, this similarity is based on perceptual characteristics that the two referents have in common, often that of shape (Golinkoff, Mervis, & Hirsch-Pasek, 1994; Golinkoff, Shuff-Bailey, Olguin, & Ruan, 1995).

Object scope is another principle used in lexical development. There are two components to this principle. First, children apply a new label to an object rather than to the action associated with it. Second, they assume that the new, unique word that they labeled is the name of the whole referent rather than a name for a portion of it. (Golinkoff, Mervis, & Hirsch-Pasek, 1994). For example, labeling "chocolate chip cookies" as the whole rather than learning and labeling "chocolate chip."

Tier Two Principles

Unlike tier one, in which the children access information from environmental cues and social interactions, tier two word learning hinges on the use of syntax and language knowledge. Whereas tier one sets the groundwork for learning words, the principles of tier two are more advanced and assist the child in learning words quickly. Using syntax and language knowledge principles, word learning occurs more rapidly and the lexicon expands at an accelerated rate (Golinkoff, Mervis, & Hirsch-Pasek, 1994).

The **principle of categorical scope** represents a shift in word learning. Children now assign names based on basic categorical similarities rather than the perceptual similarities used in tier one extendability (Golinkoff, Mervis, & Hirsch-Pasek, 1994; Golinkoff, Shuff-Bailey, Olguin, & Ruan, 1995). Golinkoff et al. (1994) demonstrate this contrast through the use of a piggy bank. When children apply the principle of extendability, they call the piggy bank a ball because of its perceptual quality of roundness; whereas when they apply the principle of categorical scope, they assign the object to the bank category.

The principle of **novel name–nameless category** (N_3C) assumes that children assign a novel name to an object and/or category that does not already have a name. Children use novel or new names of objects to label unknown objects; that is, the child uses novel names for unknown or nameless objects (Golinkoff, Mervis, & Hirsch-Pasek, 1994; Mervis & Bertrand, 1994). N_3C is the principle that accounts for the process of fast-mapping. **Fast-mapping** is the manner by which children use the linguistic and nonlinguistic context to determine the quick meaning of an unknown word. Children as young as two use the fast-mapping N_3C strategy to add new words to their lexicon (Heibeck & Markman, 1987).

As children develop words, it is not unusual for them to use words that are not conventional or that do not align with the word typically used by the communication community (see the discussion of overextension and underextension later in this chapter). The **principle of conventionality** requires that the use of nonstandard or unconventional words ceases and in its place are words that are accepted names for objects, actions, and the like. (Golinkoff, Mervis, & Hirsch-Pasek, 1994).

Nature of the Early Lexicon

From the point at which first words are acquired, lexical development continues to expand through the preschool years and beyond. Lexical development can be tracked from the point at which first words are produced by monitoring the increase in the numbers of words or rate of acquisition with respect to the child's age. A phase characterized as a vocabulary spurt—the point at which there is a sizeable expansion in the amount of words used—can yield insight into lexical development. Development of the lexicon can also be measured by the relationship between the number of words used in utterances, as measured by a mean length of utterance (MLU). Another aspect of word learning is the distribution of words used according to word categories (e.g., nominals, actions words).

The number of words acquired at a certain age has been a long-established method of tracking lexicon development. It is agreed that prior to 12 months of age, children display minimal word use (Nelson, 1973; Fenson et al., 1993; Bates et al., 1994; Fenson et al., 1994). There is also great variability among children of the same age regarding the numbers of words that they use (Bates et al., 1994). At 12 months, the median number of words that children use is six, although the actual range in the productive lexicon may be as few as zero words and up to as many 52. Initially, vocabulary grows at a steady pace after a child's first birthday. Children's vocabulary grows to a median of 15 words at 13 months, 30 words at 14 months, and 46 words at 15 months. By 16 months, the median number of words that children use is 40. Again, great variability has been observed and must be taken into account when gauging lexical development. It should be considered that the lowest 10% of 16-month-olds may produce only 8 words, where as the upper 10% may produce as many as 179 words (Bates et al., 1994). By 20 months, children's vocabulary increases to a median of 170, with the lowest 10% using only 3 and the highest 10% using 544 words (Bates et al., 1994). By 24 months, vocabulary reaches an average of 250 to 300 words (Fenson, et al., 1993), with a range of 57 to 534. Children 30 months of age use a median of 574 words. As is indicated, there is a substantial change in the number of words produced once a child reaches a vocabulary of approximately 50 to 100 words.

Most children exhibit this rapid expansion in vocabulary when their productive vocabulary reaches approximately 50 words (Goldfield & Reznick, 1990). Prior to the spurt, children acquire new words at a rate of one to three per week. During the vocabulary growth, the rate of new words increases to eight or more words per week (Barrett, 1995). Most of the words added during this period of growth are nouns. Prior to the vocabulary expansion, children's vocabularies are comprised of approximately 48% nouns, while during the spurt, the percentage increases to 75% (Mervis & Bertrand, 1995).

Although the existence of the vocabulary growth is well documented, it is not without controversy. Some suggest that there is more variability across children in terms of both when this increase occurs and the very nature of the surge (Mervis & Bertrand, 1995; Bates et al., 1994; Goldfield & Reznick, 1990). Some question its authenticity as a consistent occurrence across all children (Ganger & Brent, 2004).

Two patterns of vocabulary spurt have been observed. There are those children who are termed early spurters and those who are termed late spurters (Mervis & Bertrand, 1995). These variations indicate that all children do indeed go through a vocabulary increase, but they display a different course of events that hinges on the number of words in their vocabulary at the onset of the spurt. Early spurters begin their spurt when they have a vocabulary of 50 words, whereas the late spurters begin at approximately 100 words. The groups resemble each other because they both add primarily nouns during the period of vocabulary expansion (Mervis & Bertand, 1995). A third group of children has been identified who do not experience any significant vocabulary increase of any kind (Goldfield & Reznick, 1990). These children demonstrate a more gradual and steady rate of vocabulary acquisition. They may have some moderate spurts, but their vocabulary development might also decline at times or remain steady (Goldfield & Reznick, 1990). These children do not show a differentiation in word class development. They use a balance of nouns in relation to other word types.

Any discussion of vocabulary development should not center only on the numbers of words acquired but also on the distribution of words across word classes. Overwhelmingly, early vocabularies are comprised of a majority of labels for things in the environment, that is, nominals (Nelson, 1973; Bates et al., 1994; Rescorla, Alley, & Christine, 2001). Nominals can be further divided into general nominals and specific nominals. Children use general nominals to refer to all members of a category, such as "kitty" for all cats or "puppy" for all dogs. Specific nominals refer to only one instance of that category; for example, "puppy" is a young dog. General nominals make up the largest proportion of children's first 50 words, and this is followed early by the use of specific nominals (Nelson, 1973). Action words or predicates are the next most common word class that are evident in early vocabularies (Bates et al., 1994; Nelson, 1973). The action/predicate categories include verbs and descriptive terms (adjectives) (Bates et al., 1994; Nelson, 1973). The next sets of words, in sequence, represent a small proportion of the first 50 word vocabulary words: modifiers, personal-social words, and function or closed-class words. **Modifiers** are any words that describe the attributes of a thing or event. **Personal-social words** are those words used for social purposes or that convey affective feelings (Nelson, 1973). **Function or closed-class words** include pronouns, determiners, conjunctions, and prepositions. Once vocabulary expands beyond 50 words, some change in lexical composition appears. When children's vocabularies reach approximately 100 to 200 words, noun use reaches 55.2% of the total lexicon. At that point, the proportions of other word categories begin to increase. For example, while noun class decreases to 41.9% of the total vocabulary, predicate class words increase from 7.6% to 25.2% (Bates et al., 1994). The one category that does not demonstrate a linear increase is the closed-class word.

Referential Versus Expressive Style

As with many developmental patterns, variability is evident in the semantic growth used by children (Bates, 1974; Nelson, 1973). One notable difference is the use of a referential style versus an expressive style (Nelson, 1973). The primary marker that defines the difference between these two styles is the number of object names present in children's early lexicon, in contrast to the number of self-oriented terms. Barrett (1995) indicated that even though stylistic differences do occur, children do not typically fall at one extreme of these styles; rather, a continuum of styles is used.

Children characterized as using a **referential style** have lexicons comprised of at least 50% nominals. Children using a referential style tend to talk about things in their environment (Nelson, 1973), and their vocabularies are comprised largely of object names (Barrett, 1995). Children whose language is best described as an **expressive style** use a greater number of person-social words, action names, state names, and personal names when their vocabularies are at 50 words (Nelson, 1973; Barrett, 1995). Their communication conveys information about their feelings and needs. Their language includes the use of more phrases such as "I want it" and "I do it." In sum, they tend to use this type of language to accomplish various functions (Nelson, 1973).

Overextension, Underextension, Overlap, and Mismatch

As children's lexicons develop and expand, their word references do not always align with conventional word meanings. One example of this process is overextension, which occurs frequently in children's lexical use between the ages of 1;0 and 2;6 (Clark, 2001). Children do not overextend when first learning a new word. In fact, children usually exhibit accurate word use initially for a few weeks and then overextensions might appear. **Overextensions** (evidenced in children's lexicons up to 2;0 or 2;6) (Clark, 1993) consist of labels also given to other objects, attributes, or actions that are not designated by that word (Barrett, 1995). For example, children may use the word *tub* not only for the container that holds their bath water but for any body of water. If children see a lake, they may call it "tub."

Children do not typically overextend in comprehension, but they may overextend in production (Clark, 1993; Naigles & Gelman, 1995). When overextensions do occur, they are used for communicative purposes; for example, children have not yet expressively acquired the range of vocabulary they need to convey their ideas (Clark, 1995). Other reasons may be that they are either not able to say the words (Clark, 1995) or they are unable to retrieve the appropriate word (Clark, 1995; Naigles & Gelman, 1995).

While overextension is frequently observed, children may also produce **underextensions** (Anglin, 1977; Clark, 1993; Barrett, 1995). The combination of overextensions and underextensions may appear in up to one-third of young children's productive vocabulary (Clark, 1993). Unlike overextensions, children's underextensions reflect more narrow, restricted word use (Barrett, 1995). When children underextend, they use a word to represent only a portion of the potential referents. For example, given the word *cup*, a child may use that word only when referring to glasses that are similar to the cup they use. A glass would be called a cup. A factor that influences underextension is the degree to which the word is a more central or peripheral word choice (Anglin, 1977). Peripheral words or less common words tend to be underextended. These concepts are based on the concept of prototype theory. More central words are considered to be good examples of or good fits for the referent. The further away a word is from the best example, the less similar the word is and the more peripheral it becomes. Hence, for underextensions, the more central the instance it is, the less likely it is to be underextended, while the more peripheral it is, the greater is likelihood that it will underextended (Anglin, 1977).

Children's words may also be overlapped, mismatched, or identical or in concordance with adult productions (Anglin, 1977; Barrett, 1995). What is important is that all types of words can be affected by these processes, that is, objects, actions, attributes, or states (Barrett, 1995). When children **overlap** words, they use a word to designate some of the adult referents but also to refer to some referents not referred to by adults (Anglin, 1977). With a **mismatch**, children's use of a word bears no resemblance to the adult use (Barrett, 1995). This type of relationship is rarely observed (Clark, 1993). With concordance (Anglin, 1977), children use the same word as the adult to label a referent.

Relational Terms

A growing lexicon is not the only measure of semantic development in young children. Once children begin to combine words, their semantic abilities can be described by relational meaning (Chapman, 1981). Referential meaning refers to words that children use in conjunction with their associated referents. In contrast, relational meaning goes beyond discrete word meaning. It describes the meaning conveyed through the relationship that links one word to another (Leonard, Bolders, & Miller, 1975). Relational meanings reflect children's understanding of relationships in the environment and are best understood within the context in which they are said (Leonard, 1976). These combinations have also been termed semantic-syntactic relationships because they not only address meaning but also involve the grammatical purpose expressed through the semantic role (Bloom, Lightbown, & Hood, 1975; Bloom, 1973). For example, agents are one semantic category that are usually the grammatical subject of an utterance. Action and states are usually the verbs of a sentence. Thus, there is an interconnection between the semantic relations and the various syntactic categories (Chapman, 1981).

Bloom, Lightbown, and Hood (1975) have noted the developmental progression of semantic relations as children's mean length of utterance (MLU) increases from 1.0 to 2.5 morphemes. The first relations to develop are of a functional category, that is, existence, negation, and recurrence. **Existence** calls attention to or provides the name of an object (e.g., "That ball"). **Negation** expresses the nonexistence, disappearance, or rejection of an object or action (e.g., "No ball"). **Recurrence** communicates the concept of more of a given object or action (e.g., "More ball"). These functional categories emerge before utterances that include verb relations (Bloom, Lightbown, & Hood, 1975). Once verb relations emerge, children begin by using action events before they use stative events. **Stative** events represent a state of being or a static relationship such as being happy, being hungry, or being sad. These events are static because the person will not perpetually be happy, hungry, or sad. Action verbs are used when agents cause an effect on an object with no change in location (e.g., "Daddy hold doggy"). At least two of the components need to be present with action verbs, that is, agent + action, agent + object, or action + object (e.g., "Daddy hold," "Daddy doggy," "Hold doggy"). A second type of utterance is where the action actually describes the movements of the agent but no object was affected, that is, agent + action (e.g., "Bobby run"). Another category of action verbs are locative action where the place or target of the action is added. Locative action utterances must have at least two of the following components: agent + action + object + place (e.g., "Mommy put book table," "Mommy book," or "put book," or "book table"). The minimum form of these utterances consists of (1) agent + action, (2) action + object, (3) agent + object, or (4) action + locative (Freedman & Carpenter, 1976).

With regard to verb relations, action generally emerges before locative action. State relationships, which emerge after action relationships, refer to internal states of either people or something animate (e.g., "Andy want cookie") (Bloom, Lightbown, & Hood, 1975). State relationships that describe the location or qualities of an object occur in both entity + locative and entity + attribute utterances (Freedman & Carpenter, 1976). States also refer to an external state, as in "It's cold." Additional categories appear once verb relations are in place: (1) instrument, (2) recipient/beneficiary, and (3) wh- questions. The categories of possession and attribution develop, but not in a consistent order (Bloom, Lightbown, & Hood, 1975). Refer to Table 2–1 for definitions of semantic roles.

Parental Input and Lexical Development

To best understand semantic development, it is necessary to be familiar with the context in which it occurs and the transaction that occurs between the child and the environment. Exposure to words should occur within a range of rich contexts that includes mealtime, play, and book-reading interactions. Adults use various support strategies to assist in the child's word learning. Children's exposure to these support strategies has been shown to be predictive of children's vocabulary in kindergarten (Tabors, Beals, & Weizman, 2001). Adults use physical context by referring to objects or actions in the immediate environment. They may use prior knowledge by making statements about past experiences or they may refer to social context highlighting social expectations. Last, adults may use semantic support by providing verbal discussion and descriptions about word meanings (Tabors, Beals, & Weizman, 2001). Children who are more socially competent may be engaged in more situations

TABLE 2–1
Semantic Role Definitions

Major Noun Roles	Definition
Agent	The person/object that produces an action
Object	The person or object that receives an action or internal feeling
Entity	A person/object that exists and is not acted upon
Recipient/beneficiary	The person/animate object that benefits from an action

Major Verb Roles	Definition
Action	An external action produced by an agent
Process	An internal feeling or experience
State	An expression of a state of being

Modifier/Adverbial	Definition
Attribute	A quality or characteristic of an entity
Locative	Place where an action occurs or location of an entity

where language is used and thus have greater opportunities for exposure to vocabulary (Bornstein, Haynes, & Painter, 1998).

Joint book reading provides a prime opportunity to stimulate vocabulary learning (Hall, Burns, & Pawluski, 2003; Tabors, Beals, & Weizman, 2001). Words can be learned from the book and/or the adult's vocabulary in conversation. During book reading adults (1) refer to illustrations, (2) define words and offer synonyms, (3) encourage inference and comparison, and (4) provide words-to-life examples (Tabors, Beals, & Weizman, 2001).

Exposure to rare words has been documented as a strong predictor of children's vocabulary skills when they reach kindergarten (Tabors, Beals, & Weizman, 2001; Beals, 1997). Rare words are defined as atypical new words that preschool children may encounter in their interactions with others. Adults use rare words during toy play, book reading, mealtime, and other activities (Tabors, Beals, & Weizman, 2001). The density of rare words used in the environment aids in vocabulary development.

Cross-Linguistic Considerations

Comparisons have been made between the patterns of vocabulary growth of monolingual children and bilingual children across different languages such as Spanish-English, German-English, and Hmong-English (Pearson & Fernandez, 1994; Patterson, 1998; Junker & Stockman, 2002; Kan & Kohnert, 2005). Pearson and Fernandez (1994) followed bilingual Spanish-English-speaking children across 2- to 4-month intervals from the time they were 8 months of age through 30 months of age. The overall total growth in vocabulary began slowly and then increased at the middle or end of the second year. A vocabulary spurt was evident in many but not all of the children, similar to that seen with monolingual English-speaking children. Three patterns emerged: (1) some children had an equivalent of a full vocabulary spurt, (2) others' vocabulary had spurt-like growth, and (3) some did not spurt at all. This is commensurate with the patterns found in monolingual English-speaking children (Goldfield & Reznick, 1990).

Children who did demonstrate a spurt did so in one language or the other but not in both languages simultaneously. Vocabulary growth was not parallel for the two different languages. Similar patterns to those described for monolingual English language development were noted for bilingual children. That is, initial lexicons were comprised primarily of nominals, with an increase in verbs once children had a substantial overall lexicon and also social words (Pearson & Fernandez, 1994). Comparing German-English-speaking toddlers (24 to 27 months of age) to monolingual German- and English-speaking peers, it was found that once vocabulary was pooled across German and English, the respective vocabularies were similar for the bilingual and monolingual children. The bilingual group used a slightly greater number of lexical forms, but the number of verbs or event words and conceptual vocabulary was equivalent (Junker & Stockman, 2002). This was also noted with bilingual children learning English and Mandarin Chinese who also used a preponderance of nouns. Overall, children produced more words in Chinese than English, leading to a Chinese lexicon that contained a greater number of nouns than the English lexicon. Further, although nouns were used in both languages, verbs emerged only in Chinese (Levey & Cruz, 2003). The results from this study need to be replicated.

Patterson combined Spanish and English vocabularies of bilingual toddlers (21 to 22 months) and found that there was considerable variability in the size of the young toddlers' lexicons, with a decrease in variability in the two languages as the toddlers got older. Similar to monolingual children, by 23 to 25 months of age most toddlers' lexicons consisted of at least 50 words, while 100% of children 26 to 27 months had 50-word lexicons. Of the younger group, 21 to 22 months, only 45% had 50-word lexicons (Patterson, 1998).

The age at which bilingual children combine words has also been studied (Patterson, 1998; Junker & Stockman, 2002). The milestone for word combinations of both Spanish-English and German-English bilingual children was 50+ words (Patterson, 1998; Junker & Stockman, 2002), which is comparable to monolingual children. Ninety percent of Spanish-English children with lexicons of at least 50 words had begun to use word combinations. Eighty-one percent of children with fewer than 50 words had not yet begun to use word combinations. Therefore, word combinations in bilingual and monolingual children appear to emerge after acquiring a 50-word vocabulary.

The use of translation equivalents or doublets can provide insight into bilingual children's language use. Translation equivalents are words that are produced and/or recognized in both languages. Although there is a range in the use of translation equivalents in children's vocabularies (Junker & Stockman, 2002), typically younger children have fewer in their lexicons than do older children (Kan & Kohnert, 2005; Peña, Bedore, & Zlatic-Giunta, 2002). Younger children learning English (with either Spanish, German, or Hmong as their first language) all seem to demonstrate the same pattern. It is proposed that young bilingual children initially add words through translation to their weaker language (Brice & Wertheim, 2004/2005). There is a shift in development toward the use of translation equivalents as a function of age or number of words in the lexicon. Children whose lexicons were comprised of over five hundred words use more translation equivalents. In addition, as children become more balanced in their bilingual abilities, their use of translation equivalents also increases (Brice & Wertheim, 2004/2005). It is suggested that the language environment might influence the use of translation equivalents. The greatest number are used by children who are learning the languages from speakers who are both monolingual and bilingual in the same setting (Pearson & Fernandez, 1994).

CASE STUDY PERSPECTIVES

Case Study One Background: Chad

Chad is a young 3- year 4-month-old boy who is enrolled in a preschool enrichment program 5 days a week for 4 hours per day. He is experiencing some articulation difficulties, some vocabulary issues, and some problems in playing with others.

Chad has been "hard to understand" by his teacher and his playmates. For example, he deletes the initial /s/ in an /st/ blend (e.g., "top" for "stop"), resulting in consonant blend reduction. He also substitutes /t/ for /k/, resulting in fronting (e.g., "tat" for "cat" or "tar" for "car"). Chad also omits syllables in words; for example, he says, "elphant" and "raffe" for "elephant" and "giraffe."

Chad still has difficulty with word categories because he overextends words and concepts. He calls all small animals cats and all large animals horses. In addition, his father noted that he names a "saw" a "knife."

Chad seems to have difficulty initiating play with others, sustaining conversations, and maintaining play with others. The other children seem to enjoy playing with Chad because he is social despite his communication deficits.

Case Study One Comments: Chad

Chad appears to have some articulation and phonological difficulties and expressive language delays. His articulation and expressive vocabulary should be targeted because he is difficult to understand by others. In addition, his articulation/phonology and vocabulary deficits may be impeding his ability to interact with others in social and play environments. It is recommended that Chad receive speech and language therapy to address his communication delays.

Case Study Two Background: Tess

Tess is a 3-year 7-month-old girl enrolled in a preschool program. Tess enjoys circle time and having stories read to the group. Tess starts conversations very readily, retells events accurately, and possesses good vocabulary and syntactic skills. She has been heard by the teacher to comment "This is the apple the caterpillar ate" in response to having heard the story about the very hungry caterpillar.

Tess initiates and maintains conversations and play activities with her peers. She enjoys playing in the dramatic play area and dressing up in costumes. She tells other children what is occurring during her imaginative activities. Tess's pragmatic skills appear to be developing appropriately.

Case Study Two Comments: Tess

Tess appears to be normally developing her language and social skills. She does not demonstrate any articulation errors. She also possesses good vocabulary, syntax, and pragmatic skills. In contrast, Chad seems to be delayed in these areas.

SYNTAX AND MORPHOLOGY

Sentence Constituents

Children's sentences are typically made up of (1) noun phrases (NP), (2) verb phrases (VP), and (3) adjectives and adverbs. Noun phrases consist of the main noun and can include articles or adjectives. Verb phrases include a main verb and can include auxiliaries and modals. Combinations of these constituents form the five basic syntactic sentence types: (1) NP + VP + (Adv), (2) NP^1 + VP + NP^2 + (Adv), (3) NP + V_L + Adj, (4) NP^1 + V_L + NP^1 + (Adv), and (5) NP + V_L + Adv (Heidinger, 1984). Please note that the subscript L represents a linking verb (Heidinger, 1984) that often takes the form of the copula. Brown (1973) identified basic constituent combinations in children's utterances during the early stages of development using semantic case relationships to describe them. Semantic constituents can be converted to syntactic constituents to illustrate the relationship between the two. Children may combine two words using agent + action for agent + action+ object, utterances omitting the object. The syntactic description of this utterance is NP[1] + VP with NP[2] omitted. Agent + object with action omitted would be NP[1] + NP[2] with VP omitted. Agent + locative with action omitted would be NP + Adv with VP omitted. Action + dative with agent and object omitted would be VP + indirect object. Action + locative with agent and object omitted would be VP + Adv with the initial and final NPs omitted. These are but some of the potential combinations. Therefore, the underpinnings are set for children's early syntactic growth as they incorporate the syntactic forms into their earliest word combinations.

Mean Length of Utterance

Mean length of utterance is one measure for determining the stage of a child's syntactic development and the length of her or his utterances. Brown (1973) described utterances in morphemes; therefore, most speech-language pathologists and linguists view MLU to be calculated in morphemes. However, mean length of utterance can be calculated in words (MLU-W) or in morphemes (MLU-M). **Morphemes** are the smallest meaningful syntactic unit of language. There are two types of morphemes: free morphemes and bound morphemes. **Free morphemes** stand alone and convey meaning by themselves. **Bound morphemes** are affixed to free morphemes and modify the meaning of the free morpheme in two ways. One way is to change the grammatical class of the free morpheme. This type of bound morpheme is termed a derivational morpheme. For example, if the free morpheme is *rapid* (an adjective) and the bound morpheme *-ly* is added, the word becomes *rapidly*. The word class changes from adjective to adverb by virtue of adding the bound *-ly* morpheme. In addition, **inflectional morphemes** attach to the free morpheme but do not change its grammatical class. Rather, the inflectional morpheme adds additional grammatical meaning. For example, if the word is *cat* and the inflectional morpheme *-s* is added to make it *cats*, the word remains a noun but the notion of plural is added to it.

To calculate MLU, it is first necessary to collect a representative language sample of the child's utterances. Brown based his calculations on a 100-utterance sample, although calculations can also be generated from 50- or 75-utterance samples (Chapman, 1981). Utterances that are unintelligible or even partially unintelligible are not included in the calculation (Brown, 1973; Chapman, 1981). Morpheme counts are performed following a uniform set of rules.

Brown (1973) calculated the MLU-M for his utterance sample and created five developmental stages. These stages were refined by deVilliers & deVilliers (1978) into more discrete stages. MLU-M increases at a rate of approximately 1.2 morphemes per year (Miller & Chapman, 1981). This increase in MLU-M and the range in development between stages demonstrate the extent to which the child's language expands during this time period. Further, age can be assigned to the MLU-M to provide a developmental and normative milestone perspective (deVilliers & deVilliers, 1978). If MLU-M is known, then age predictions can be made, and vice versa (Miller & Chapman, 1981). Table 2–2 provides a comparison of the systems by Brown (1973) and deVilliers and deVilliers (1978).

TABLE 2–2
Mean Length of Utterance Comparisons

Brown (1973)		deVilliers and deVilliers (1973)		
Stages	MLU-M	Stage	MLU-M	Age in Months
Stage I	1.0–2.0	Early Stage I	1.10–1.49	19.1–23
Stage II	2.0–2.5	Late Stage I	1.50–1.99	23.8–26.9
Stage III	2.5–3.0	Stage II	2.00–2.49	27.7–30.8
Stage IV	3.0–3.75	Stage III	2.50–2.99	31.6–34.8
Stage V	3.75–4.5	Early Stage IV	3.00–3.49	35.6–38.7
		Late Stage IV/ Early Stage V	3.50–3.99	39.6–42.6
		Late Stage V	4.00–4.49	43.4–46.6
		Post Stage V	4.50+	47.3–58.3

Brown tracked the emergence of fourteen morphemes and noted a sequence of development across syntactic stages II to V. It should be noted that no morphemes were observed in Stage I. They did not begin to emerge until children moved into Stage II. The criterion for emergence of a morpheme was three successive language samples where the morpheme was observed to be used 90% of the time. The following is a list of morphemes according to the stages by which they appear: (1) Stage II presents progressive -*ing* (He is runn*ing*), *in* (The ball is *in* the bag), *on* (The bowl is *on* the table), regular plural (Two cat*s* are running.); (2) Stage III presents past irregular (She *ate* her cereal), possessive (It's Bobby'*s* car), uncontractible copula (*Is* it mine?); (3) Stage IV presents articles (*A* cat ran in *the* garage), past regular (She jump*ed* high), third person regular of the present tense (He eat*s* popcorn every day), third person irregular (He *has* a dog); and (4) Stage V presents uncontractible auxiliary (*Is* she coming?), contractible copula (She'*s* happy), and contractible auxiliary (I'*m* sitting in this chair). DeVilliers and deVilliers (1978) analyzed the order of emergence of these morphemes by stage and identified a different sequence. They observed that the present progressive -*ing*, the plural, and the preposition *in* were produced during Stage II. The preposition *on* and the possessive were observed in Stage III. The regular and irregular past, the third person singular of the present tense, articles *the* and *a*, and the contractible copula were observed in Stage V. Stage V+ children produced the contractible auxiliary *be*, the uncontractible copula and auxiliary *be*, and the irregular third person of the present tense (deVilliers & deVilliers, 1973). These variations highlight differences that can occur across children and underscores the need for flexibility in judging children across the developmental continuum.

The stages not only delineate the MLU-M at each point but also represent major advances in sentence structure. From his studies, Brown (1973) identified five aspects of sentence construction that correspond to the five stages of MLU-M. They are characterized by the following sentence constructions: (1) Stage I: relations or roles within simple sentences, (2) Stage II: modulations of meaning within simple sentences, (3) Stage III: modalities of simple sentences, (4) Stage IV: embedding one sentence within another, and (5) Stage V: coordination of simple sentences and propositional relationships.

Stage I: Relations is best described by the use of semantic-syntactic relationships. The words children use reflect semantic concepts such as agents, actions, patients, and locatives, while representing such syntactic constituents as subjects, verbs, and objects. These components are expressed in a linear order. Stage II: Modulations of Meanings refers to the beginning of the use of noun and verb infections. Further, the emergence of the use of definite and indefinite articles, the copula, and prepositions *in* and *on* appear at this stage. Use of modalities of the simple sentence, which characterizes Stage III, includes the appearance of interrogatives such as yes/no and wh-questions. Yes/no questions require the listener to confirm or deny the information conveyed in the question. By contrast, wh- questions require that the listener respond with specific content that is elicited through the question word. Wh- questions include who, whose, what, where, when, why, and how questions, although all these questions types do not emerge at this stage. The wh- word is in the initial position for all wh- questions, but the rest of the sentence varies in structure based on the grammatical constituent requested.

Negatives are yet another modality to appear in Stage II. Nonexistence, rejection, and denial are the most frequent negative meanings to be expressed at this stage. Children begin to use imperatives at Stage II; they serve to regulate pragmatically the behavior of their listeners. When children reach Stage IV, they begin embedding one sentence in another, where one sentence serves as a sentence constituent, such as its subject or object. Embedding is achieved through the use of grammatical forms such as object noun phrase complements, embedded wh- questions, or relative clauses.

Stage V is characterized by coordination of simple sentences and propositional relationships. Coordination is typified by the use of coordinating conjunctions. Two complete sentences can be conjoined or sentence constituents can be conjoined, such as subjects, predicates, subjects and verbs, direct objects, and adverbials (Brown, 1973). By the time children reach Late Stage V, or approximately 46.6 months of age, their utterances should reflect a range of different modalities, modulations, and embedded and coordinated structures, which reflects sophisticated language use.

Interrogative Forms

The development of question forms can best be traced through the sequence of the emergence of the question by type and the growth in syntactic structure. The question type conveys the content or information being requested through the question, while the syntactic structure entails the appropriate use of inversion of auxiliaries and modals. The use of inversion is indicative of the most highly developed interrogative structure. Although yes/no questions predominate across the preschool years (Tyack & Ingram, 1977), children also begin to use wh- questions during this time. The emergence of wh- questions appears in the following sequence: (1) where and what questions emerge at approximately 26 months; (2) who questions, at approximately 28 months; (3) how questions, at approximately 33 months; and (4) when questions, at approximately 36 months (Bloom, Merkin, & Wooten, 1982; Rowlan, Pine, Lieven, & Theakston, 2003). The order of acquisition seems to be linked to structural similarity between the questions types. Wh- pronominals (where, what, who, and which) emerge first. Where questions request location information, what questions request object information, and who questions request person information. Using the sentence "Cheri is putting the book on the chair," the constituent "on the chair" would answer the where question, "book" would answer the what question, and "Cheri" would answer the who question. Wh- sententials—why, how, and when—are more difficult question types because rather than asking for a constituent, these question words request information about the relationship among the constituents. The answers to these questions provide reasons, manner, or time (Bloom, Merkin, & Wooten, 1982). The use of why and how questions increases as children reach 3 years of age (Tyack & Ingram, 1977).

Question development is not only characterized by the content it encodes but also by its syntactic structure, most notably the pattern of noun-verb inversion. Inversion refers to reversing the order of the noun and the auxiliary, modal, or copula in the question form. In the sentence "What are the boys doing?" the auxiliary *are* is inverted. In the sentence "Is the dog big?" the copula *is* is inverted. In the sentences "Can I go with you?" and "Where would you find it?" the modals *can* and *would* are inverted. A single, consistent developmental pattern of inversion has not been documented (O'Grady, 1997). One reason for the later emergence of inversion is because it does, indeed, necessitate that children use auxiliaries, or modals, and copulas, in their utterances. The copula first appears in Stage III (2;5–3;0), while the uncontracted form of the auxiliary is not incorporated into children's utterances until Stage V (3.75–4.5). One perspective on inversion suggests that as children begin to produce questions, they use the noninverted form of the auxiliary first (O'Grady, 1997). Yet another perspective suggests that there is a relationship between the use of inversion and the type of the question word. Who, what, where, and which questions tend to be used with inversion prior to why, how (Erreich, 1984; Kuczaj & Brannick, 1979), how come, and how long (Kuczaj & Brannick, 1979). Further, children seem to demonstrate two patterns of emergence. Some children produce yes/no questions and wh- questions in both inverted and noninverted forms; others produce yes/no questions in noninverted forms while producing wh- question in both inverted and noninverted forms (Erreich, 1984). While these patterns of inversion have been noted, it has also been observed that children use inversion more consistently than not using inversion. Thus, a single clear pattern of inversion has not been identified as children begin to use the syntactic structure associated with fully developed yes/no and wh- question forms.

Negation

Three stages of sentential negation have been identified (Klima & Bellugi, 1966). In Stage I, the negative marker, usually *no*, is placed at the beginning of the utterance. Although utterances using this structure are well documented, the meaning of the negative conveyed by the structure is controversial and has been interpreted from various perspectives. Some researchers have stated that the negative word negated the verb phrase of the utterance (O'Grady, 1997; Bloom, 1991). Thus, if a child sees his or her mother eating cookies and says, "No mommy eat," then the typical meaning conveyed is to negate the message of eating cookies. Two other possible interpretations of initial utterance negatives have been described (O'Grady, 1997). One possible explanation is that the no conveys "I don't want" with respect to the message conveyed in the utterance. Another explanation is that, rather than conveying denial of the verb, it conveys an objection to the message conveyed in the utterance.

Whereas there are numerous interpretations of the negative for Stage I, the use of the negative in Stages II and III is more clear-cut. In Stage II, the negative word is placed within the utterance before the verb (as is described by Bloom as a negative utterance). In Stage III, the negative utterance is similar to the adult form, with the use of auxiliaries, modals, and the like.

Compound and Complex Sentences

The use of complex and compound sentences signals children's entrance into Stages IV and V and appears between the ages of 2 and 4 (Bowerman, 1979). A steady increase in the use of complex sentences from 6% of the utterances children use (MLU-M of 2.0 to 2.49) to 25.9% of children's utterances (MLU-M of 5.0 to 5.99) has been observed (Tyack & Gottsleben, 1986). Compound sentences are characterized by the merging of two independent clauses (e.g., "Annie ran and fell"), while complex sentences are characterized by the combination of an independent and dependent clause (e.g., "Sara left because she was tired"). Various categories of compound and complex sentences have been noted in children's sentences at these stages, including the use of infinitives, coordination, complementation, and relativization. Conjunctions are acquired first, followed by complementation; last to be acquired is relativization (Bloom, Lahey, Hood, Lifter, & Fiess, 1980).

Very few compound or complex sentences are used by children until they reach an MLU-M of 2.99. From 3.0 to 3.99, the earliest type of complex sentence incorporates modal infinitives (words such as *gonna, wanna, hafta, hasta, want*) (Tyack & Gottsleben, 1986). Infinitive sentences using "Let's" appear at this time (e.g., "Let's go"). Infinitival sentences using *to* ("I want to eat") increase steadily across MLUs of 4.0 to 4.99 and 5.0 to 5.99 (Tyack & Gottsleben, 1986).

Children's early use of coordination is marked by the use of *and* where two propositions are conjoined. Coordination with the conjunction *and* appears around an MLU-M of 3.0 to 3.99 but is used more consistently once children reach an MLU-M of 4.0 to 5.99. *And* is by far the most frequently used conjunction across the MLU-M span of 3.0 to 5.99 (Tyack & Gottsleben, 1986). Sentence coordination can include both sentential and phrasal coordination. In sentential coordination, complete sentences are conjoined by *and*. In phrasal coordination, sentences are conjoined while redundant information is not included. Phrasal coordination includes conjoining sentence constituents such as noun phrases (e.g., "Sue and Mark ate dinner"; "Henry ate apples and pears") or verb phrases (e.g., "Mary did her homework and went to bed"). Tager-Flusberg (1999) suggests that sentential and phrasal coordination emerge at the same time. This simultaneous appearance of sentential and phrasal coordination implies that phrasal coordination is not the outcome of deleting redundant information; rather, it is the product of direct coordination of phrase constituents. The use of *and* conveys a range of semantic meanings, including additive, temporal, causal, and adversative. When *and* expresses an additive meaning, the two events or states in an utterance are just added together. One event or state is not dependent on the other (e.g., "Todd played and Maya ate"). *And* can be used to convey a temporal relationship when one event or state is juxtaposed in time with respect to another event or state (e.g., "I got up and went to school"). *And* expresses a causal relationship when one action or state is the reason for another action or state (e.g., "I was hungry and I ate a snack"). When one action or state is in contrast to the other, *and* conveys an adversative relationship ("I am big and you are little"). Additive meanings are acquired first, then temporal meaning, followed by causal, with adversative meanings last to appear (Bloom, Lahey, Hood, Lifter, & Fiess, 1980).

Although *and* is clearly the earliest occurring and most prevalent connective, other connectives also emerge during the preschool years. The other frequent and early emerging connectives are *because, what, when,* and *so.* These emerge between 27 months and 35 months, 28 months and 37 months, 29 months and 35 months, and 29 months and older, respectively (Bloom, Lahey, Hood, Lifter, & Fiess, 1980). With respect to *because*, it appears first and more frequently as a fragment (e.g., "Cause I want it") than in full sentence form used in the medial position of a sentence (e.g., "I'm going to sleep because I'm tired") (Tyack & Gottsleben, 1986).

Relativization is the process of embedding one sentence within another sentence. Two types of relative clause utterances can be produced: (1) a right-branching relative clause, where the relative clause modifies the object of the sentence ("He's the boy that I saw"); and (2) a center-embedded relative clause, where the relative clause modifies the subject (e.g., "The boy that I met is coming to play") (Bowerman, 1979). Relative clauses are late in development (Bloom, Lahey, Hood, Lifter, & Fiess, 1980; Tyack & Gottsleben, 1986; Tager-Flusberg, 1999). The relative pronoun *that* is used with great frequency (e.g., "I want the doll that I saw") (Tyack & Gottsleben, 1986). Children at this age use the *that* relative pronoun structure primarily to modify the object of the sentence (Bloom, Lahey, Hood, Lifter, & Fiess, 1980; Tyack & Gottsleben, 1986; Tager-Flusberg, 1999).

Passive sentences are produced by reordering the components of a sentence, for example, "The dog was touched by Josie." Passives are not fully acquired until far into the preschool years (O'Grady, 1997). By the time children reach 5;0 they are able to understand passive sentences with active verbs but still have difficulty with those that incorporate nonaction verbs (Tager-Flusberg, 1999). Thus by 5 years of age, children are able to understand "The dog was touched by Josie" but they are more challenged by the sentence "The dog was liked by Josie" because this verb describes an internal state rather than an action.

Cross-Linguistic Considerations

The use of compound and complex syntax provides a way for children to express relationships among events, people, and objects. The use of syntactic forms by children speaking African American English (AAE) has been studied for preschool children ages 3, 4, and 5 (Craig & Washington, 1994; Jackson & Roberts, 2001). A set of syntactic forms showed a marked increase in the percentage of children using compound and complex sentences across 3, 4, and 5 years of age: noninfinitive wh-clauses (3 years old, 15%; 4 years old, 38%; 5 years old, 58%), the conjunction *and* (3 years old, 35%; 4 years old, 51%; 5 years old, 58%), noun phrase complements (3 years old, 18%; 4 years old, 31%; 5 years old, 44%), unmarked infinitives (3 years old, 6%; 4 years old, 22%; 5 years old, 27%), relative clause (3 years old, 6%; 4 years old, 4%; 5 years old, 31%) and tag questions (3 years old, 0%; 4 years old, 2.4%; 5 years old, 7%). Other forms acquired between 3 and 5 years of age are infinitives with the same subject (3 years old, 63%; 4 years old, 66%; 5 years old, 64%), let's/lemme (3 years old, 31%; 4 years old, 44%; 5 years old, 36%), infinitives with different subjects (3 years old, 18%; 4 years old, 31%; 5 years old, 29%), and wh- infinitive clauses (3 years old, 5%; 4 years old, 21%; 5 years old, 22%) (Craig & Washington, 1994; Jackson & Roberts, 2001). The increase in use of compound and complex sentences gives children complex sentence forms that provide a foundation for school language as they enter school.

While children develop in the area of complex language, they also may incorporate aspects of AAE syntax in their utterances. For those children ages 3 to 4, the AAE forms that were used more than 25% include zero copula, subject-verb agreement, zero past tense, undifferentiated pronoun, multiple negation, and zero possessive (Jackson & Roberts, 2001). Wyatt (1995) cautions that there is diversity and variability in the use of AAE speech, and this needs to be taken into account when determining age-appropriate language use.

PRAGMATICS

Joint Attention and Joint Action Routines

Purposeful communication begins when infants are quite young and is based in social interactions with others. These interactions lead to the development of intentionality. The origin of intentional communication lies in **joint attention**. Joint attention is "an attentional state during which the child and a partner share a site of interest such as an object or an event, in their immediate surrounding." (Adamson & Chance, 1998, p 16). Three phases of joint attention have been identified. During the first phase, infants attend to someone who is doing something that attracts their interest; however, there is no mutual attention between infants and their partners. The hallmark of the second phase is a shared focus of attention between infants and the communication partner. Infants can maintain coordinated attention among individuals, objects, and actions. This phase begins as young as 6 months and is evidenced through 18 months of age (Adamson & Chance, 1998). By 6 months, infants shift their gaze between their partner and an object, while at 13 months they can do a 3-point gaze shift (e.g., object-person-object or person-object-person (Bakeman & Adamson, 1984). The final phase, called the transition phase, occurs when young children understand that symbols can represent objects and events; i.e., they are able to use language as the basis of joint attention (Adamson & Chance, 1998).

Once infants establish the ability to engage in joint attention, they have the skill to participate in **joint action routines**. A joint action routine embeds predictable, routine conversation into an interactive activity (McLean & Snyder-McLean, 1999). Bruner (1981) describes joint action routines as occurring within a format. Bruner defines a **format** as "a constrained and segregated transaction between a child and an adult that undergoes an elaboration. A format provides a familiar locus and familiar routine in which communicative intentions can be conventionalized and interpreted" (p. 162). Thus, formats form the foundation for joint action routines. By virtue of their familiarity and predictability, children can learn about both the form and function of language within the context of an interaction. Joint action routines follow a pattern. It begins with the adult establishing joint attention with the infant (Bruner, 1975; Bruner, 1981; McLean & Snyder-McClean, 1999). Adults may begin by using an attentional vocative (e.g., "Look") (Bruner, 1981). This action ensures that the infant is attending to the adult, something the adult is holding, or something in the environment that both the child and adult can see (McLean & Snyder-McLean, 1999). The adult then engages the child in the routine. The adult takes a turn and waits for the infant to respond with a turn (McLean & Snyder-McLean, 1999). During his turn, the adult uses the language that is associated with the specific routine. He or she may ask questions or provide labels. He or she also provides the infant with feedback on his or her turn (Bruner, 1981).

Infants' involvement in joint engagement increases steadily over time. Between the ages of 9 and 15 months, joint engagement increases in average time spent in each joint engagement opportunity, in the number of episodes of joint engagement, and in the duration of each joint engagement episode. The changes, particularly for infants between 9 and 12 months, are attributed to the fact that infants take part in more joint engagement episodes over considerable time periods (Carpenter, Nagell, & Tomasello, 1998).

Nonverbal Communication and Gestures

A review of children's use of communicative acts would not be complete without addressing nonverbal communication. **Communicative** refers to the manner in which children communicate, including gestural, vocal, gestural + vocal, or verbal means. Children's use of gestures on a consistent basis is an action that signals intent to communicate. Communicative gestures are produced by using hands, fingers, and arms as well as facial gestures and body language (Crais, Douglas, & Campbell, 2004; Iverson & Thal 1998).

Crais, Douglas, and Campbell (2004) classify gestures as deictic and representational. Deictic gestures, such as points and reaches, are used by children to call attention to objects or actions that are grounded in context. In other words, the object or event needs to be in the environment for the listener to be able to comprehend its meaning. In contrast, representational gestures function in two ways. They both refer to an object or action and symbolize the actual object or action (Iverson & Thal, 1998). Within the representational category are those gestures that are labeled as conventional. These gestures are culturally accepted, not related to a specific object, and used in a given manner in conversation. These gestures are exemplified by a gesture such as waving or nodding. Another type of representational gesture is the object-related gesture. This gesture type actually mimes the object or action it is referring to.

Within the gestural framework, there is yet one more distinction: the difference between contact and distal gestures (Crais, Douglas, & Campbell, 2004; McLean & Snyder-McLean, 1999). Gestures where there is actual physical contact between children and either an object or person are labeled as contact gestures. Children use a contact gesture when they hold a ball up to the listener with the purpose of showing it. Conversely, a distal gesture is one where children use a gesture without touching an object or a person (e.g., pointing with a finger) (McLean & Snyder-McClean,

1999). Children use a distal gesture when they point to an object and open and close their fingers to request the item.

The course of development of the use of gestures, vocalizations, and verbalizations individually and in conjunction with each other has been well documented (Carpenter, Mastergeorge, & Coggins, 1983; Wetherby et al., 1988; Crais & Day, 2000; Crais, Douglas, & Campbell, 2004). Developmental progression indicates that for the prelinguistic stage, coordination of gestures and vocalizations are key components. This progression increases at the one-word stage and decreases at the multiword stage (Wetherby et al., 1988). From 8 to 12 months of age, children primarily use gestures, and gestures with vocalizations, with some use of vocalizations occurring alone. By the time children reach 10 months of age, few vocalization-only communications are noted, although there is an increase of vocalizations in conjunction with gestures. By the time children reach 12 months, they begin to produce sounds that are phonetically recognizable, and these are combined with ritualized gestures. Once children reach 13 months, verbal behaviors emerge with gestures, although gestures plus vocalizations are still evidenced through 15 months (Carpenter, Mastergeorge, & Coggins, 1983).

Gestures continue to play a role in children's communication as they begin to use words. Iverson and Thal (1998) describe gestures and words as being one system of communication because (1) words and gestures convey the same communicative intents, (2) words and gestures can be used to convey similar semantic notions, and (3) gestures are used in a complementary way with words rather than overlapping with them. Once children reach the multiword stage, there is a decrease in use of gestures and vocalizations and an increase the use of words alone or words and gestures (Wetherby et al., 1988). The overall use of gestures decreases between 16 and 20 months as children's overall lexicon increases (Iverson & Thal, 1998). Prior to the two-word stage, children combine a single word with a gesture. They then move from using a single word and a gesture to combining two words together. Children first use complementary gestures with their words and then use supplementary gestures. From 14 to 16 months, children use primarily complementary gestures, which are gestures that express similar information to that conveyed by words. From 16 to 18 months, supplementary gestures are used. With supplementary gestures, the word expresses one type of information and the gestures express another. Children begin to use two-word combinations once they have moved from using complementary to supplementary gestures (Iverson & Thal, 1998).

The developmental progression of the use of gestures culminates with children using gestures in a similar fashion as adults. Prior to the two-word stage, children use a gesture either before they utter a word or after they utter a word. Once they begin to use two-word combinations, the timing of their gesture is simultaneous with the production of words. This timing parallels the adult use of gestures and words (Iverson & Thal, 1998).

Conversation and Discourse: Protoconversations

The very foundation of conversation resides in the early interactions between adults and infants. These early interactions have been termed protoconversations. **Protoconversations** are interactions between adults and infants that involve reciprocity between the adult and the infant. Protoconversations usually begin when infants demonstrate social behaviors, such as social smiling, vocalizing, gazing, and facial expressions, while the adults engage in these exchanges based on the child's behaviors (Reddy, 1999). Adults' responses are selective and coordinated (McTear, 1985). Adults select which behaviors to respond to, while coordination of communication is reflected in the timing of adult communication with the infant behavior. Adults respond to infant behaviors that appear to be communicative in nature, even though there may not be communicative intent on the part of the infant. Adults time their communications to take turns with the infant's behavior, inserting pause time at the appropriate moment (McTear, 1985). Sensitivity to the structure of protoconversations has been observed in infants as young as 4 months of age (Rochat, Querido, & Striano, 1999).

Topic Initiation and Responses

To engage others in conversation, infants and young children need to expand their skills in topic initiation. Initiations begin conversations and consist of utterances that carry the expectation of a response (McTear, 1985). **Topic initiation** begins with attention getting and attention directing through verbal or nonverbal means (Foster, 1986; McTear, 1985). Attention getting recruits the partner's attention, while attention directing focuses the partner's attention (i.e., joint attention) on the object, action, or event of the topic (i.e., joint reference) (McTear, 1985). Children as young as 9 months of age can procure a listener's attention by giving and showing objects, sometimes coupled with vocalizations (Crais, Douglas, & Campbell, 2004). As children get older, attention getting includes pointing, looking at objects, making eye contact with the listener, gesturing, and verbalizing (Crais, Douglas & Campbell, 2004; McTear 1985). Once the listener's attention is gained, then it must be directed to the topic of the conversation. This is accomplished through behaviors such as pointing and showing, attention-directing words such as *see*, or combinations of both strategies. Children as young as 14 months can direct the listener's attention to a topic. They usually do so through nonverbal pointing or showing. By 20 months the use of nonverbal means decreases, and by 32 months, most attention directing becomes verbal (Ninio & Snow, 1996). By 4 years of age, children use gaze direction, leaning over and facing conversational partners, vocatives, and attention-getting words (e.g., *hey*) to signal the impending topic initiation.

Once the listener's attention is directed to the topic, then children can initiate the topic. Topic initiation is accomplished through questions, requests for actions, and/or statements (McTear, 1985). The earliest topic initiation expressed by infants occurs through object manipulation (Ninio & Snow, 1996). The means by which children initiate topics evolves over time. Initially, children use primarily nonverbal means of focusing the listener's attention on the topic, through pointing or showing. The number of nonverbal initiations decreases as the number of verbal initiations increases.

Types of topics initiated by infants and children vary by age. Children's conversational topics include self-topics, environmental topics, and intangible topics. Self-topics are those where children direct the listener to some aspect of themselves. Environmental topics focus on some object, action, or event in the environment. Environmental topics focus on either physical or social aspects of the environment. Intangible topics refer to objects, actions, or events that are not present in the here and now or features of objects that are not readily perceivable (Foster, 1986). Use of these topics shows developmental trends. Self-topics predominate in the interactions of youngest children. As children reach 1;0 they begin to include environmental topics, although self-topics continue to be evident. Intangible topics emerge as children get closer to 3 years of age, although they still do not occur with great frequency (Foster, 1986; Ninio & Snow, 1996). Ninio and Snow suggest that children must be able to use words to talk about objects and events that are removed from the immediate environment.

Early conversations are often focused on the here and now. Topics typically center on play, and the actions and objects involve play activities. Contextual support at this stage is so important that the quality of conversations has been noted to decline when context is not available. Young children can engage in a shared topic by using joint attention and joint action but not entirely through conversation (Ninio & Snow, 1996).

Ninio and Snow (1996) noted that children begin to talk about objects, actions, and events that are not present as young as 14 months. These conversations include topics such as story telling (about past events) and talking about future events. It was observed that 27% of 20-month-old children and 51% of 32-month-old children were able to talk about present events. This age range is consistent with Eisenberg's (1985) observations of two young Spanish-speaking girls. She noted that one of the girls included past events in her conversation at 21 months of age and the other at 33 to 34 months. Eisenberg (1985) identified three phases of development of talking about past events based on her case study observations. Phase One, which was noted as young as 23 or 24 months, is where the adult partner contributed most of the content of the conversation and asked many questions. Children answered with yes or no responses or single-word responses. Children typically did not initiate the topic and contributed only one to two utterances to the topic. During Phase Two, which emerged at 27 to 29 months, half of the children's utterances that were self-initiated contained past information and were in response to adults' questions. The focus of the topics was highly familiar to the participants. Familiar topics could be either those that were general knowledge or those that reflected events that had been previously discussed. In Phase Three, which was observed in children as young as 27 to 29 months, few topics were elicited or context-dependent. The children remembered past events and talked without support from the ongoing discourse. They also included new information to the topic, that is, up to 75% of the time. Conversations remained somewhat disorganized and often did not include contextualizing information needed by the listener initially to interpret the topic.

Turn Taking and Topic Maintenance

Once topics are initiated, turns must follow that add new information. **Conversational turns** can be described in terms of their **adjacency** and **contingency** to a previous turn. For a turn to be adjacent, it needs to be produced after a previous utterance. A turn is considered to be nonadjacent if there is no previous utterance by a conversational partner or if there is an extended pause between the two turns. Adjacent turns consistently exceed nonadjacent speech for children at Brown's Stage I through to Brown's Stage V. Even for children at Stage I, adjacent turns outnumber nonadjacent turns (Bloom, Rocissano, & Hood, 1976).

A contingent turn shares the topic of a previous utterance and adds additional topic-based information. Contingent turns show a steady increase as children progress from Brown's Stage I to Brown's Stage V. At Stage I, contingent turns comprise 31% of turns produced, whereas at Stage V, 73% of turns are contingent (Bloom, Rocissano, & Hood, 1976). Turn contingency can be linguistic or contextually based. Linguistic contingency refers to turns that are related semantically and through similar grammatical clause structure. Contextually contingent turns relate to a situation or action. They do not share the clause structure of the previous turn. Contextual contingency occurs to a greater extent in young children and decreases as children move from Stage I to Stage V. Linguistic contingency occurs as children incorporate syntactic aspects of adult utterances in their turns (Bloom, Rocissano, & Hood, 1976).

Preschool children's verbal interactions in natural contexts provide insight into the factors that contribute to successful topic maintenance and also the nature of their interactions (Mueller, 1972; Garvey & Hogan, 1973; Ninio & Snow, 1996). One way to describe children's conversations is through the time the child spends interacting. Garvey and Hogan (1973) explored the rate of utterance units used by children 3;6 to 5 years of age. An utterance unit was defined as a set of utterances that were bounded by a pause of greater than one second or bounded by another person's turn. The dyads produced one utterance unit every 4.6 seconds. As children got older, they also produced more words per utterance unit, with the younger children producing 4.73 words and the older children producing 6.04 words. Mueller (1972) judged turns as successful if the listener responded with a verbal or nonverbal contingent response. Of a group of 3;6- to 5-year-olds, 62% of their turns were successful, 15% were failures, and 23.5% were indeterminable. Turns were successful if the speaker had the listener's attention and the response by the listener was contingent to what the speaker said. Turns were not successful if the speaker's utterance was not clear or was a sentence fragment and was not syntactically understandable.

Another important aspect of children's conversation is **balance**, which refers to the relative number of contributions produced by each partner. Garvey and Hogan (1973) suggest that conversations are balanced if partner participation doesn't vary by more than 5%. Of the dyads they observed, most were balanced while some varied between 16% and 18%. Focus (i.e., staying on topic) is another aspect of conversation that entails mutual engagement during the conversation. They noted that children were focused approximately 66% of the time, with only brief periods when they were not focused.

Clarification and Repair Strategies

Communication breakdowns sometimes occur in conversation. When this happens, the listener must determine where the breakdown has occurred and repair the conversation, for example, asking for clarification (McTear, 1985). To be able to maintain topics and the conversation flow, the speaker needs to be able to repair disruptions in communication. Typically, conversational repairs occur in response to a partner's signal that there has been a misunderstanding. Repairs allow turn-taking flow to be maintained (Ninio & Snow, 1986).

Adults direct clarification requests for a variety of reasons. The utterance may not have been heard or may have been misunderstood. The adult may also use a clarification request to indicate acknowledgment or surprise (Corsaro, 1976).

Children's repair responses can be repetitions, revisions, additions, or term definitions, or they can provide background context (Briton, Fujiki, Loeb, & Winkler, 1986). A repair is a repetition when the response is a complete or partial repetition with no addition of new information. A revision contains no change in semantic content or syntactic adjustments. Additions encompass repairs where supplementary information is incorporated into the original utterance. Word definitions from the original message are given when children employ a defining terms strategy. Children provide additional contextual information when replying with a background repair. For 3-year-olds, the greatest number of repairs were repetitions. Three-year-olds used some revisions and additions, but they did not define terms or repair background information. Five-year-olds primarily used repetitions, but they used more additions than 3-year-olds did. As with the 3-year-olds, the 5-year-olds did not define terms or provide background repairs. It is noteworthy that young children are able to use strategies that sustain a conversation and maintain the topic (Briton, Fujiki, Loeb & Winkler, 1986).

Children differentiate their responses according to clarification types requested of them. If a neutral request (e.g., "Huh?") is made, then the typical response is to repeat what was previously said. When a clarification requests specific information, children are likely to respond with a specific repair strategy. For example, children may respond with the specific information requested. Children may also reformulate their responses to specific requests. When children reformulate their responses, they may add new information, change words, or expand the content. Children functioning in Brown's Stage II to Brown's Stage V use these types of responses. Children also initiate requests for clarification. Clarification requests emerge around 20 months of age. The earliest requests, such as "Huh" or "What," are not highly developed. Requests occur more consistently when children reach 32 months of age. These requests are in the form of "Huh," "What," or a repetition (Ninio & Snow, 1996).

Development of Communicative Intents

Communicative intents encompass two aspects of communication, that is, speaker goal and listener effect (Wetherby, Cain, Yonclas, & Walker, 1988). The speaker has an intention or communication goal; therefore, the imparted message has an effect on the listener. Intentions are the reasons behind every communication. They can be best described through their perlocutions, illocutions, and locutions (Austin, 1962).

A **perlocution** the impact that a message or signal has on a listener. The impact can be intentional or unintentional (Bates, Camaioni, & Volterra, 1979). For example, a speaker might say to a listener, "Close the door." The speaker has an effect on the listener, who gets up and closes the door. This is an intentional effect because the speaker conveyed what she or he wanted to be done. On the other hand, an infant is lying in a crib and he or she starts to cry. The parent comes over and changes the baby's diaper. This is an unintentional effect because the baby did not cry to convey that he or she wanted the diaper changed. Rather, the discomfort caused him or her to cry, which then had an effect on the parent.

Illocution is the intention behind the communication. This intention can be conveyed through verbal or nonverbal means and corresponds to a specific communicative function or goal (Bates, Camaioni, & Volterra, 1979). For example, a young child is sitting in a high chair and sees his or her cup on the table close by. The child reaches out toward the cup, opening and closing his or her hand. His or her father gives him or her the cup. The child's intention, or illocution, was that he or she wanted to be given the cup.

As children get older, they are able to add a locution to their communication. The **locution** consists of the words, utterances, and nonverbal communication in the message; hence, locution equals the message. The message may contain verbal and nonverbal information. Using the previous example of the cup, if a child adds the words *cup*, *Want cup*, and/or points to the cup, these verbal and nonverbal messages would be the locutionary component of the communication.

McLean and Snyder-McLean (1978) summarize the pragmatic model in four steps:

1. Language is acquired if and only if the child has an intent or reason to communicate. The child has learned (or not learned) that he can influence his environment through nonverbal and verbal communication.

2. Language supplements and replaces existing and less precise communication methods.

3. Language is learned in dynamic and interactive social interactions involving the child and an older, mature language user, for example, an adult.

4. The child is an active participant in the communication-exchange process and must contribute to it so that he or she benefits from the interaction.

As children develop, so does their repertoire of communicative intents. The earliest intent that is used is protesting, which is observed between 8 and 9 months of age (Carpenter, Mastergeorge, & Coggins, 1983). When children protest, they are conveying displeasure at another person's actions or utterances (Coggins & Carpenter, 1981) or refusal of an object or other person's action (Wetherby et al., 1988). The next set of intentions to emerge is requests, both requests for actions and requests for objects. Children's use of requests emerges between 9 and 10 months of age (Carpenter, Mastergeorge, & Coggins, 1983). Requests include communications that demand or command the listener to either perform an action (e.g., extending the arms to be picked up) or get a desired object and give it to the child (Coggins & Carpenter, 1981; Wetherby et al., 1988). Comments on objects and comments on actions emerge between 9 and 13 months of age (e.g., pointing to an object) (Carpenter, Mastergeorge, & Coggins, 1983). Comments involve directing someone else's attention to something or someone in the environment, or to an action that is immediately observable (Coggins & Carpenter, 1981; Wetherby et al., 1988). The final intent to appear is answering, which was not observed until 13 to 15 months of age (Carpenter, Mastergeorge, & Coggins, 1983). Answering necessitates that a child provide information in response to a request for information by another person (Coggins & Carpenter, 1981).

Additional communicative acts have been documented in children from the prelinguistic stage to the multiword stage. Requests for social routines emerge at the prelinguistic stage and peak at the one-word stage. When children request a social routine, they are directing another person to engage with them in an interaction that is gamelike (Wetherby et al., 1988). Greetings also appear during the prelinguistic stage and continue through the multiword stage. Showing off, where children call attention to themselves, is present in the prelinguistic and single-word stage but diminishes in the multiword stage (Wetherby et al., 1988). One type of act, requesting information, is consistently noted as a later developing act (Carpenter, Mastergeorge, & Coggins, 1983; Wetherby et al., 1988). Children are not observed using this act until the multiword stage (Wetherby et al., 1988).

The communicative intents or acts that young children use can be classified into three different categories based on the perlocutionary effect they have on the listener. These categories consist of behavior regulation, social interaction, and joint attention (Bruner, 1981; Wetherby et al., 1988; Crais, Douglas, & Campbell, 2004). Children use acts within the behavior regulation function when their goal is to enlist someone else's help in achieving their goal by controlling the other person's actions (Bruner, 1981; Wetherby et al., 1988). Thus, communicative acts such as requesting and protesting fall within this category. The social interaction category affects someone else's behavior by drawing that person's attention to oneself. The communicative acts of requesting social routine, showing off, greeting, calling, acknowledging, and requesting permission are included in this category (Wetherby et al., 1988). The third category, joint attention, affects the listener by drawing his or her attention to create mutual focus on an object or action (Bruner, 1981; Wetherby et al., 1988). Communicative acts that achieve joint attention include commenting and requesting information (Wetherby et al., 1988).

Wetherby et al. (1988) monitored children through the prelinguistic, one-word, and multiword stages with respect to communicative functions and acts used within and across each stage. Notably, they found that children used some acts that fell within all three categories across each of the stages. However, most of the acts fell into the categories of behavior regulation and social interaction. The most common pragmatic functions used in these categories were requests for action and comments. Further, the number of acts used was comparatively stable from the prelinguistic to one-word stages, but showed a marked increase at the multiword stage. The rate of use of communicative functions also increased steadily from one language stage to another.

Cross-Linguistic Considerations

Classroom interactions between preschool children and their peers and/or teachers provide a window into their communicative competence. Tabors (1997) observed 15 children in a Head Start classroom with a broad range of different languages. Tabors (1997) found that children learning English as a second language used many nonverbal means to facilitate communication, including getting attention, requesting objects or actions, protesting, and/or joking. These strategies can be mixed because they can be ambiguous and/or not understood by the listener, resulting in a communication failure. Tabors noted that if communicative attempts were not successful, then children would either persist or cease in their attempts (Tabors, 1997).

Saenz, Iglesias, Huer, and Parette (1999) studied children making requests of peers in a Head Start classroom. The children in this classroom were from Puerto Rican and African American backgrounds. The children from Puerto Rican backgrounds spoke Spanish and English. Most spoke English during their classroom interactions. Some types of requesting behaviors were more successful than others. The most successful requests involved moving toward the desired objects coupled with a verbal request, statement, or claim. Those request strategies that were less successful were verbal requests not accompanied by gestures or movement actions.

These findings emphasize the need for culturally and linguistically diverse preschool children to acquire successful communication strategies that will enable them to communicate effectively in the preschool environment.

The importance of classroom routines cannot be overemphasized (Tabors, 1997). As with young nonverbal children, routines provide a context in which consistent language is paired with consistent activities.

CONCLUDING REMARKS

Language is a complex interaction of phonological, morphological, semantic, syntactic, and pragmatic skills. Early in life, infants show a sensitivity to language and soon differentiate the language in their environment from other languages. Each language component follows a specific development course that must be considered when determining the appropriateness of a child's productions. Early in development, a child's language may appear different from mature forms, but as the child progresses, his or her language will most likely mirror the adult model. These components are neither learned in a vacuum nor function well alone. Rather, it is the cumulative development of the components that forms complete communication.

In sum, language is learned developmentally. It emerges through various stages of growth and is learned in interaction with others. Language is a complex and dynamic process. Speech-language pathologists and special education teachers should always be aware of the complexity of language in teaching students.

INSTRUCTIONAL STRATEGIES

Dialogic Book Reading

1. Ask what questions.
2. Follow answers with a question.
3. Repeat what a child says.
4. Help the child where needed.
5. Offer praise and encouragement.
6. Follow the child's interests.
7. Ask open-ended questions.
8. Expand on what the child has said.
9. Use a completion prompt.

(Zevengergen & Whitehurst, 2003)

Vocabulary Stimulation Strategies Using Dialogic Book Reading

1. Select 8 to 10 words or phrases ahead of time to review before reading.
2. Identify and point to possibly unknown words.

(continued)

3. Define unknown words.
4. Provide a similar word.
5. Point to pictures.
6. Ask or make a text-to-life question or comment.

Language Stimulation Techniques

1. Modeling
2. Expanding
3. Extending
4. Using open-ended questions
5. Prompting
6. Eventcasting
7. Observing, waiting, listening, turn-taking
8. Scaffolding; talking about present, past, habitual, and future events

Language-Rich Preschool Environment

Centers: Literacy, Dramatic Play, Blocks, Creative Arts, Math, Science

REFLECTION QUESTIONS

1. Explain the phonological patterns that Chad is using.
2. Explain Chad's word use and the semantic relations he uses.
3. What would you say to Chad's teacher and Chad's mother about his phonological patterns, his word use, and the semantic relations?
4. From what Tess's teacher said, what are the syntactic and pragmatic skills that Tess is using?
5. How do these skills match what is expected for a child of Tess's age?
6. Tess's skills are age appropriate. Cite the information in the text and relate it to her language skills.
7. What emerging book and listening skills can Tess learn prior to entering kindergarten and how can these skills be reinforced at home?

REFERENCES

Adamson, L. B., & Chance, S. E. (1998). Coordinating attention to peoples, objects, and language. In A. M. Wetherby, S. F. Warren, & J. Reichle (Eds.), *Transitions in prelinguistic communication* (pp. 59–86). Baltimore, MD: Paul H. Brookes.

Anglin, J. M. (1977). *Word, object and conceptual development*. New York: W. W. Norton & Company.

Austin, J. (1962). *How to do things with words.* Cambridge, MA: Harvard University Press.

Bakeman, R., & Adamson, L. B. (1984). Coordinating attention to people and objects in mother–infant and peer–infant interaction. *Child Development, 55,* 1278–1289.

Barrett, M. (1995). Early lexical development. In P. Fletcher & B. MacWhinney (Eds.), *The handbook of child language* (pp. 362–392). Malden, MA: Blackwell.

Bates, E. (1974). The acquisition of pragmatic competence. *Journal of Child Language, 1*(2), 277–282.

Bates, E., Camaioni, L., & Volterra, V. (1979). The acquisition of performatives prior to speech. In E. Ochs & B. Scheifflin (Eds.), *Developmental pragmatics* (pp. 111–129). New York: Academic Press.

Bates, E., Marchman, V., Thal, D., Fenson, L., Dale, P., Reznick, J. S., Reilly, J., & Hartung, J. (1994). Developmental and stylistic variations in the composition of early vocabulary. *Journal of Child Language, 21*, 85–123.

Beals, D. (1997). Sources of support for learning new words in conversation: Evidence from mealtimes. *Journal of Child Language, 24*, 673–694.

Becker, M. C. (1982). *Phonological analysis of speech samples of monolingual Mexican four-year-olds.* Unpublished master's thesis, San Diego State University, San Diego, CA.

Bland-Stewart, L. (2003). Phonetic inventories of patterns of African American two-year-olds: A preliminary investigation. *Communication Disorders Quarterly, 24*(3), 109–120.

Bloom, L. (1973). *One word at a time: The use of single word utterances before syntax.* The Hague, The Netherlands: Mouton.

Bloom, L. (1991). *Language development from two to three.* New York: Cambridge University Press.

Bloom, L., Lahey, M., Hood, L., Lifter, K., & Fiess, K. (1980). Complex sentences: Acquisition of syntactic connectives and the semantic relations they encode. *Journal of Child Language, 7*, 235–261.

Bloom, L, Lightbown, P., & Hood, L. (1975). Structure and variation in child language. *Monographs of the Society for Research in Child Development, 40*(2), 1–97.

Bloom, L., Merkin, S., Wootten, J. (1982). Wh- questions: Linguistic factors that contribute to the sequence of acquisition. *Child Development, 53*, 1084–1092.

Bloom, L., Rocissano, L., & Hood, L. (1976). Adult-child discourse: Developmental interaction between information processing and linguistic knowledge. *Cognitive Psychology, 8*, 521–552.

Bornstein, M. H., Haynes, M. O., & Painter, K. M. (1998). Sources of child vocabulary competence: A multivariate approach. *Journal of Child Language, 25*, 367–391.

Bowerman, M. (1979). The acquisition of complex sentences. In P. Fletcher & M. Garman (Eds.), *Language acquisition* (pp. 285–305). Cambridge, UK: Cambridge University Press.

Brice, A. (1996). Spanish phonology: A review of the literature. *The Florida Journal of Communication Disorders, 16*, 14–17.

Brice, A., & de la Paz, A. (1997). Disordered Cuban Spanish and American English phonology. *Florida Journal of Communication Disorders, 17*, 20–24.

Brice, A., & Wertheim, E. (2004/2005). Language differentiation in young bilingual children. *Tejas. Texas Journal of Audiology and Speech Language Pathology, 28*, 24–31.

Brinton, B., Fujiki, M., Loeb, D. F., & Winkler, E. (1986). Development of conversational repair strategies in response to requests for clarification. *Journal of Speech and Hearing Research, 29*, 5–81.

Brown, R. (1973). *A first language: The early stages.* Cambridge, MA: Harvard University Press.

Bruner, J. (1975). The ontogenesis of speech acts. *Journal of Child Language, 2*, 1–19.

Bruner, J. (1981). The social context of language acquisition. *Language and Communication, 1*, 155–178.

Carpenter, R., Mastergeorge, A., & Coggins, T. (1983). The acquisition of communicative intentions in infants eight to fifteen months of age. *Language and Speech, 26*, 101–116.

Carpenter, M., Nagell, K., Tomasello, M. (1998). Social cognition, joint attention, and communicative competence from nine to fifteen months of age. *Monographs of the Society for Research in Child Development*, Serial 255, *63*(4), 1–179.

Chapman, R. S. (1981). Procedures for analyzing free-speech samples: Syntax and semantics. In J. F. Miller (Ed.), *Assessing language production in children: Experimental procedures* (pp. 21–72). Baltimore, MD: University Park Press.

Clark, E. (1993). *The lexicon in acquisition.* Cambridge, UK: Cambridge University Press.

Clark, E. (1995). Language acquisition: The lexicon and syntax. In J. L. Miller & P. D. Eimas (Eds.), *Speech, language, and communication* (pp. 303–338). San Diego, CA: Academic Press.

Clark, E. (2001). Emergent categories in first language acquisition. In M. Bowermann & S. C. Levinson (Eds.), *Language acquisition and conceptual development* (pp. 379–405). Cambridge, UK: Cambridge University Press.

Coggins, T. E., & Carpenter, R. L. (1981). The communicative intentions inventory: A system for observing and coding children's early intentional communication. *Applied Psycholinguistics 2*, 235–251.

Corsaro, W. A. (1976). The clarification request as a feature of adult interactive styles with young children. *Language in Society, 6*, 183–207.

Cotton, F., & Sharp, J. (1988). *Spanish in the Americas.* Washington, DC: Georgetown University Press.

Craig, H. K., & Washington, J. A. (1994). The complex syntax skill of poor, urban African-American preschoolers at school entry. *Language, Speech, and Hearing Services in the Schools, 25*, 181–190.

Crais, E., & Day, D. (2000, November). *Gesture development from six to twenty-four months.* ASHA Annual Convention, Washington, DC.

Crais, E., Douglas, D. D., & Campbell, C. C. (2004). The intersection of the development of gestures and intentionality. *Journal of Speech, Language, and Hearing Research, 47*, 678–694.

deVilliers, J., & deVilliers, P. (1973). A cross-sectional study of the acquisition of grammatical morphemes in child speech. *Journal of Psycholinguistic Research, 2*, 267–268.

deVilliers, J. G., & deVilliers, P. A. (1978). *Language acquisition.* Cambridge, MA: Harvard University Press.

Dore, J., Franklin, M. B., Miller, R. T., & Ramer, A. L. (1976). Transitional phenomena in early language acquisition. *Journal of Child Language, 3*, 13–28.

Eisenberg, A. (1985). Learning to describe past experience in conversation. *Discourse Processes, 8*, 177–204.

Elbers, L., & Wijnen, F. (1992). Effort, production skill, and language learning. In C. A. Ferguson, L. Menn, S. Stoel-Gammon (Eds.), *Phonologicial development: Models, research, & implications* (pp. 337–368). Timonium, MD: York Press.

Erreich, A. (1984). Learning how to ask: Patterns of inversion in yes-no and wh- questions. *Journal of Child Language, 20*, 579–592.

Fenson, L., Dale, P. S., Reznick, J. S., Bates, E., & Thal, D. (1994). Variability in early communicative development. *Monographs of the Society for Research in Child Development, 59*(5), 1–185.

Fenson, L., Dale, P. S., Reznick, J. S., Thal, D., Bates, E., Hartung, J. P., Thethick, S., & Reilly, J. S. (1993). *MacArthur communicative development inventories.* San Diego: Singular.

Foster, S. H. (1986). Learning discourse topic management in the preschool years. *Journal of Child Language, 13*, 231–250.

Freedman, P., & Carpenter, R. (1976). Semantic relations used by normal and language-impaired children at Stage I. *Journal of Speech and Hearing Research, 19*, 784–795.

Garvey, C., & Hogan, R. (1973). Social speech and social interaction: Egocentrism revisited. *Child Development, 44*, 562–568.

Goldfield, B. A., & Reznick, J. S. (1990). Early lexical acquisition: Rate, content, and vocabulary spurt. *Journal of Child Language, 17*, 171–183.

Goldstein, B. A., & Iglesias, A. (1996). Phonological patterns in normally developing Spanish-speaking 3- and 4-year-olds of Puerto Rican descent. *Language, Speech, and Hearing Services in the Schools, 27*, 82–90.

Goldstein, B., & Iglesias, A. (1998). Phonological production in Spanish-speaking preschoolers. ERIC ED424935.

Goldstein, B. A., & Iglesias, A. (2001). The effect of dialect on phonological analysis: Evidence from Spanish-speaking children. *American Journal of Speech-Language Pathology, 10*, 394–406.

Golinkoff, R., Mervis, C., & Hirsch-Pasek, K. (1994). Early object labels: The case for a developmental lexical principles framework. *Journal of Child Language, 21*, 125–155.

Grunwell, P. (1982). *Clinical phonology.* Beckenham, UK: Broom Helm.

Haelsig, P. C., & Madison, C. L. (1986). A study of phonological processes exhibited by 3-, 4-, and 5-year-old children. *Language, Speech, and Hearing Services in Schools, 17*, 107–114.

Hall, D. H., Burns, T. C., & Pawluski, J. L. (2003). Input and word learning: Caregiver sensitivity to lexical category distinctions. *Journal of Child Language 30*, 711–729.

Heibeck, T. H., & Markman, E. M. (1987). Word learning in children: An examination of fast mapping. *Child Development, 58*, 1021–1034.

Heidinger, V. A. (1984). *Analyzing syntax and semantics.* Washington, DC: Gallaudet College Press.

Ingram, D. (1974). Phonological rules in young children. *Journal of Child Language, 1*, 49–64.

Iverson, J. M., & Thal, D. J. (1998). Communicative transitions: There's more to the hand than meets the eye. In A. M. Wetherby, S. F. Warren, & J. Reichle (Eds.), *Transitions in prelinguistic communication* (pp. 59–86). Baltimore, MD: Paul H. Brookes.

Jackson, S. C., & Roberts, J. E. (2001). Complex syntax productions of African American preschoolers. *Journal of Speech, Language, and Hearing Research, 44*, 1083–1096.

Jimenez, B. C. (1987). Acquisition of Spanish consonants in children aged 3–5 years, 7 months. *Language, Speech, and Hearing Services in Schools, 18*, 357–363.

Junker, D. A., & Stockman, I. J. (2002). Expressive vocabulary of German-English bilingual toddlers. *American Journal of Speech-Language Pathology, 11*, 381–394.

Justice, L. M., & Ezell, H. K. (2002). *The syntax handbook: Everything you learned about syntax but forgot.* Eau Claire, WI: Thinking Publications.

Kan, P. F., & Kohnert, K. (2005). Preschoolers learning Hmong and English: Lexical-semantic skills in L1 and L2. *Journal of Speech, Language, and Hearing Research, 48*, 372–383.

Kent, R. (1992). The biology of phonological development. In C. A. Ferguson, L. Menn, C. Stoel-Gammon (Eds.), *Phonological development: Models, research, implications* (pp. 65–90). Timonium, MD: York Press.

Kent, R. D., & Bauer, H. R. (1985). Vocalizations of one-year-olds. *Journal of Child Language, 12*, 491–526.

Kent, R. D., & Miolo, G. (1995). Phonetic abilities in the first year of life. In P. Fletcher & B. MacWhinney (Eds.), *The handbook of child language* (pp. 303–334). Malden, MA: Blackwell.

Khan, L. M. L. (1982). A review of 16 major phonological processes. *Language, Speech, and Hearing Services in Schools, 13*, 77–85.

Klima, E., & Bellugi, U. (1966). Syntactic regularities in the speech of children. In J. Lyons & R. Wells (Eds.), *Psycholinguistic papers*. Edinburgh, Scotland: Edinburgh University Press.

Kuczaj, S. A., & Brannick, N. (1979). Children's use of the wh- question modal auxiliary placement rule. *Journal of Experimental Child Psychology, 28*, 43–67.

Lahey, M. (1988). *Language disorders and language development*. New York: Macmillan.

Leonard, L. B. (1976). *Meaning in child language*. New York: Grune & Stratton.

Leonard, L. B., Bolders, J. G., & Miller, J. A. (1975). An examination of the semantic relations reflected in the language usage of normal and language-disordered children. *Journal of Child Language, 19*, 371–392.

Levey, S., & Cruz, D. (2003). The first words produced by children in bilingual English/Mandarin Chinese environments. *Communication Disorders Quarterly, 24*(3), 129–136.

Mann, D., & Hodson, B. (1994). Spanish-speaking children's phonologies: Assessment and remediation of disorders. *Seminars in Speech and Language, 15*(2), 137–147.

Martinez, R. (1986). *Phonological analysis of Spanish utterances of normally developing Mexican-American Spanish speaking 3-year-olds*. Unpublished master's project. San Diego State University, San Diego, CA.

McLean, J., & Snyder-McLean, L. (1978). *A transactional approach to early language training*. Columbus, OH: Merrill.

McLean, J., & Snyder-McLean, L. (1999). *How children learn language*. San Diego, CA: Singular Publishing.

McTear, M. (1985). Pragmatic disorders: A case study of conversational disability. *British Journal of Disorders of Communication, 20*, 119–128.

Menyuk, P., & Menn, L. (1979). Early strategies for perception and production of words and sounds. In P. Fletcher & M. Garman (Eds.), *Language acquisition* (pp. 49–70). London, UK: Cambridge University Press.

Mervis, C. B., & Bertrand, J. (1994). Acquisition of novel name–nameless category (N_3C) principle. *Child Development, 65*, 1646–1662.

Mervis, C. B., & Bertrand, J. (1995). Early lexical acquisition and vocabulary spurt: A response to Goldfield and Reznick. *Journal of Child Language, 22*, 461–468.

Miller, J. F., & Chapman, R. S. (1981). Research note: The relation between age and mean length of utterance in morphemes. *Journal of Speech and Hearing Research, 24*, 154–161.

Mitchell, P. R., & Kent, R. D. (1990). Phonetic variation in mutisyllabic babbling. *Journal of Child Language, 17*, 247–265.

Mueller, E. (1972). The maintenance of verbal exchanges between young children. *Child Development, 43*, 930–938.

Naigles, L. G., & Gelman, S. A. (1995). Overextensions in comprehension and production revisited: Preferential-looking in a study of dog, cat, and cow. *Journal of Child Language, 22*, 19–46.

Nelson, K. (1973). Structures and strategies in learning to talk. *Monographs of the Society for Research in Child Language, 38*, 1–135.

Ninio, A., & Snow, C. E. (1996). *Pragmatic development*. Boulder, CO: Westview.

O'Grady, W. (1997). *Syntactic development*. Chicago, IL: University of Chicago Press.

Oller, D. K. (1980). The emergence of sounds of speech in infancy. In G. H. Yeni-Komishian, J. F. Kavanaugh, & C. A. Ferguson (Eds.), *Child phonology, volume I* (pp. 93–112). New York: Academic Press.

Oller, D. K. (2000). *The emergence of the speech capacity*. Mahway, NJ: Lawrence Erlbaum.

Oller, D. K., & Eilers, R. E. (1983). Speech identification in Spanish- and English-learning two-year-olds. *Journal of Speech and Hearing Research, 26*, 50–53.

Oller, D. K., Eilers, R. E., Neal, A. R., & Schwartz, H. K. (1999). Precursors to speech in infancy: The predictors of speech and language disorders. *Journal of Communication Disorders, 2*(4), 223–245.

Patterson, J. L. (1998). Expressive vocabulary development and word combinations of Spanish-English bilingual toddlers. *American Journal of Speech-Language Pathology, 7*, 46–56.

Pearson, B. Z., & Fernandez, S. C. (1994). Patterns of intersection in the lexical growth of two languages of bilingual infants and toddlers. *Language Learning, 44*(4), 617–652.

Peña, E. D., Bedore, L. M., & Zlatic-Giunta, R. (2002). Category-generation performance of bilingual children: The influence of condition, category, and language. *Journal of Speech, Language and Hearing Research, 45*, 938–947.

Prater, R. J., & Swift, R. W. (1982). Phonological process development with MLU-referenced guidelines. *Journal of Communication Disorders, 15*, 395–410.

Reddy, V. (1999). Prelinguistic communication. In M. Barrett (Ed.), *The development of language,* (pp. 229–250). Sussex, UK: Psychology Press.

Rescorla, L., Alley, A., & Christine, J. B. (2001). Word frequencies in toddlers' lexicons. *Journal of Speech, Language, and Hearing Research, 44*, 598–609.

Roberts, J. E., Burchinal, M., & Footo, M. M. (1990). Phonological process decline from 2 to 8 years. *Journal of Communication Disorders, 23*, 205–217.

Rochat, P., Querido, J. G., & Striano, T. (1999). Emerging sensitivity to the timing and structure of protoconversation in early infancy. *Developmental Psychology, 35*(4), 950–957.

Rowlan, C. E., Pine, J. M., Lieven, E. V., & Theakston, A. L. (2003). Determinants of acquisition order in wh- questions: Re-evaluating the role of caregiver speech. *Journal of Child Language, 30*(3), 609–635.

Saenz, T. I., Iglesias, A., Huer, M. B., & Parette, H. P. (1999). Culturally and linguistically diverse preschoolers' verbal and nonverbal requests. *Communication Disorders Quarterly, 21*(1), 39–49.

Stark, R. E. (1979). Prespeech segmental feature development. In P. Fletcher & M. Garman (Eds.), *Language acquisition* (pp. 285–305). Cambridge, UK: Cambridge University Press.

Stockwell, R. P., & Bowen, J. D. (1965). *The sounds of English and Spanish.* Chicago, IL: University of Chicago Press.

Stoel-Gammon, C. (1992). Research on phonological development: Recent advances. In C. A. Ferguson, L. Menn, S. Stoel-Gammon (Eds.), *Phonologicial development: Models, research, & implications* (pp. 273–282). Timonium, MD: York Press.

Stoel-Gammon, C. (1998). Role of babbling and phonology in early linguistic development. In M. Wetherby, S. F. Warren, & J. Reichle (Eds.), *Transitions in prelinguistic communication* (pp. 87–110). Baltimore, MD: Paul H. Brookes.

Tabors, P. O. (1997). *One child, two languages: A guide for preschool educators of children learning English as a second language.* Baltimore, MD: Paul H. Brookes.

Tabors, P. O., Beals, D. E., & Weizman, Z. O. (2001). "You know what oxygen is?" In D. K. Dickenson & P. O. Tabors (Eds.), *Beginning literacy with language* (pp. 93–110). Baltimore, MD: Paul H. Brookes.

Tager-Flusberg, H. (1999). Acquisition of grammar. In F. Fabbro & R. E. Asher (Eds.), *Concise encyclopedia of language pathology* (pp. 112–119). Oxford, UK: Elsevier.

Tyack, D. L., & Gottsleben, R. H. (1986). Acquisition of complex sentences. *Language, Speech, and Hearing Services in the Schools, 17*, 160–174.

Tyack, D., & Ingram, D. (1977). Children's production and comprehension of questions. *Journal of Child Language, 4*, 211–224.

Vihman, M. M. (1988). Words and babble at the threshold of language acquisition. In M. D. Smith & J. L. Locke (Eds.), *The emergent lexicon: The child's development of a linguistic vocabulary* (pp. 151–184). San Diego, CA: Academic Press.

Vihman, M. M. (1992). Early syllables and the construction of phonology. In C. A. Ferguson, L. Menn, S. Stoel-Gammon (Eds.), *Phonologicial development: Models, research, & implications* (pp. 393–422). Timonium, MD: York Press.

Vihman, M. M. (2004). Early phonological development In J. E. Bernthal & N. W. Bankson (Eds.), *Articulation and phonological disorders* (pp. 63–104). Boston, MA: Pearson Allyn and Bacon.

Vihman, M. M., Ferguson, C. A., & Elbert, M. (1986). Phonological development from babbling to speech: Common tendencies and individual differences. *Applied Psycholinguistics, 7*, 3–40.

Wells, G. (1985). *Language development in the preschool years.* Cambridge, UK: Cambridge University Press.

Wetherby, A. M., Cain, D. H., Yonclas, D. G., & Walker, V. G. (1988). Analysis of intentional communication of normal children from the prelinguistic to the multiword stage. *Journal of Speech and Hearing Research, 31*, 240–252.

Wyatt, T. A. (1995). Language development in African American English child speech. *Linguistics and Education, 7*, 7–22.

Zevenbergen, A. A., & Whithurst, G. J. (2003). Dialogic book reading: A shared picture book reading intervention for preschoolers. In S. A. Stahl, A. van Kleeck, & E. B. Bauer (Eds.), *On reading books to children* (pp. 177–202). Mahwah, NJ: Lawrence Erlbaum.

Chapter **3**

First-Language Development

Toya A. Wyatt and Terry Irvine Saenz

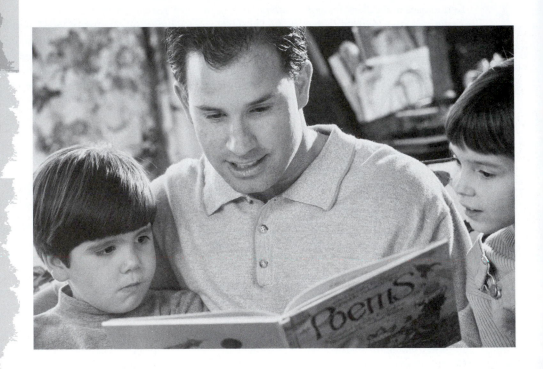

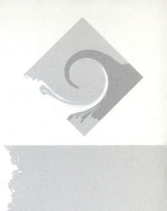

CHAPTER OUTLINE

ACQUISITION OF PHONOLOGY

Preschool-Age Years

By 3 years of age, most English-speaking children have mastered (are able to correctly produce) the following consonant sounds in at least two word positions, most typically the beginnings and ends of words: /n/, /m/, /p/, /b/, /h/, /k/, /g/, /f/, /w/, /j/, /t/, /d/. Children are also improving in their ability to produce words using more adult pronunciation patterns; therefore, some of the early developing phonological processes begin to disappear. By the end of the preschool years, most English-speaking children have mastered the /s/, /z/, /l/, /r/, /ʃ/, /tʃ/ sounds. Other sounds, such as /v/, /ð, θ/, and /dʒ/, continue to be difficult to produce into the early school-age years with the entire speech/sound repertoire not fully mastered until sometime around 8 years of age (Peña-Brooks & Hedge, 2000).

For children who are speakers of languages other than English, the sequence of speech/sound development can differ from that of English-speaking children even when they are acquiring sounds that occur in both languages. For example, according to data reported by Amayreh and Dyson (1998), the /h/ sound, which is found in both Arabic and English, is not acquired by Arabic-speaking children (used correctly at least 75% of the time in all word positions) until 5 years of age. According to data reported by Prather and Hedrick (1975) and Sander (1972), 90% of English-speaking children have mastered the /h/ sound between 28 to 36 months of age. In addition, there are obviously different speech/sound development norms for sounds that are language-specific. For example, there are no norms for when English-speaking children acquire the trilled /R/ sound because it does not exist in English. There are developmental norms, however, for acquisition of the trilled /R/ for Spanish-speaking children.

There can also be cross-linguistic differences in the timetable for when certain phonological processes are likely to be suppressed. The deletion of initial unstressed syllables, for example, is typically suppressed by the age of 4 years according to data reported by Bernthal and Bankson (1998). The process of initial unstressed syllable deletion, however, can persist into the later preschool-age years in typically developing Spanish-speaking children (Iglesias & Goldstein, 1998). Similar types of differences have been noted for children from differing English-language backgrounds. For example, according to the research of Haynes and Moran (1989), the devoicing and deletion of certain final sounds has been found to persist far longer in the speech of children who are speakers of African American English (AAE) than for children who are speakers of Mainstream American English (MAE). In addition, substitutions of /d/ for the voiced "th," /ð/, sound and /f/ for the voiceless "th," /θ/, sound are likely to continue into adulthood for individuals who are predominant speakers of AAE associated with normal dialectal variations, while it typically disappears by about 8 years of age in children who are MAE speakers.

School-Age Years

Children's **morphophonemic** knowledge, or knowledge of changes in sound production that result in changes of meaning, expands during the elementary school years (Guasti, 2002; Miller, 1991; Owens, 2005). Children learn the plural rule for /s/ and /z/, but not for "es," by the first grade and may continue to have difficulty with the plural endings of nouns ending in *-sk* and *-st* as late as third grade. Children also learn rules for the shifting of vowels during the school years, in which root words' vowels change with the addition of a suffix (e.g., /eI/ to /æ/ in *vain* to *vanity*, /aI/ to /I/ in *divide* to *division*, and /i/ to "eh") (Owens, 2005). This process continues through high school.

Through the age of 12, children are learning that stress is used to indicate the grammatical function of a word as well as other ways in which stress is used (Guasti, 2002; Owens, 2005; Vogel & Raimy, 2002). For example, stress differs when two words form a phrase or a compound word, as in *side walk* compared to a *side* walk. In addition, the stress in words also differs depending on whether the word is used as a noun or a verb. When used as a noun, stress may be on the first syllable of a word; when used as a verb, stress may be on the last syllable (e.g., a *per* mit compared to per*mit*).

Adolescence

As is evident from the previous section on school-age phonological development, the phonological inventory of an individual's native language has been mastered by adolescence. As a result, there should not be any persisting speech/sound error patterns like those found during early preschool years unless an individual has an underlying speech disorder. This applies to speakers of all languages and dialects. Typically developing adolescent speakers should be producing all of the sounds of the native language and/or dialect to which they have been exposed. It is possible, however, for those speakers who have been exposed to and are in the process of acquiring the phonological system of a second language to display patterns of normal first-language interference in their production of sounds in the less proficient language that differ from those found in their most proficient language (refer to Chapter 4 for further discussion of second-language learning issues). For those speakers who do not begin to acquire the speech/sound system of a second language until adolescence, normal first-language influences can persist into adulthood and become stabilized as "accents" that are detectable to native speakers of the other language.

ACQUISITION OF MORPHOLOGY

Preschool-Age Years: Key Morphological Developments

During the first two years of life, the primary language developments that occur in children's emerging language skills are the use of single-word utterances to express meaning. Around 18 months of age, however, children begin to produce two-word utterances that gradually increase in length and complexity. These changes begin during the later toddler years but occur most significantly during the preschool-age years.

Developmental changes that occur in the length and complexity of monolingual English-speaking children's utterances can be measured through the use of **mean length of utterance (MLU),** a linguistic measure that is calculated by dividing the total number of morphemes present in a child's spontaneous language productions by the total number of utterances within that same sample. Morphemes represent the small parts of words that carry linguistic meaning and constitute the smallest linguistic unit of meaning that cannot be broken into smaller components without destroying meaning (Guasti, 2002; Miller, 1991; Owens, 2005). When one analyzes the internal structure of a word like *cats* for example, one finds two morphemes: the **free morpheme** *cat* (a free morpheme is one that can independently convey meaning) as well as the **bound morpheme** *-s* (a bound morpheme is one that must be attached to another to convey meaning, in this case plurality). Other types of common bound morphemes found in English speaking children's earliest words include the past tense *-ed* morpheme and third person singular *-s* morpheme.

Changes in MLU have also been associated with differing stages of language development based on the original research of Roger Brown (1973), who conducted a longitudinal study of three children's preschool language development. Brown studied the language development of these three children over an 18-month period as they progressed from a single-word stage of development to a multiword stage of development. Brown observed similar patterns of language development across the three children and proposed a sequence of language development that is still used by child language researchers and speech-language professionals today to profile the individual stages of children's language development. Children tend to overgeneralize rules in their early language acquisition. For example, "runned" and "goed" are common errors that demonstrate general rule knowledge without knowledge of the irregular morphological exceptions. The child is still in the acquisition phase and has not quite mastered the rule. Such examples are to be seen as typical errors among all children acquiring the English language. It should also be noted that children may undergo a **U-shape learning effect**. That is, a child may produce correct morpheme usage, followed by incorrect usage, and then produce the correct usage again. This phenomenon may also apply to other language features being acquired (e.g., phonology). The child may initially learn the feature through rote learning, learn the rule and incorrectly overgeneralize the production, followed by correct rule usage and correct generalization usage. For example, the child may correctly say "two feet," then learn the plural "s" marker and say "two foots," and then relearn the correct irregular plural production of "two feet."

Stages of Acquisition

Based on findings from his research, Brown (1973) postulated five different stages of language development, with each stage characterized by a new linguistic achievement:

Stage I is characterized by the emerging use of single-word utterances that express early emerging semantic knowledge.
Stage II is characterized by the appearance of the first English grammatical morphemes.
Stage III is characterized by the beginning use of simple sentence forms.
Stage IV is characterized by the emergence of more complex sentences with embedded phrases and clauses.
Stage V is characterized by the emerging use of complex sentences containing conjoined clauses (Miller, 1991; Owens, 2005).

TABLE 3–1
Brown' Stages, MLU Range, Predicted Age Range, and Ages Within One Standard Deviation of Predictions

Brown's Stage	MLU Range	Age Range[a]	Age Range Within 1 SD of Predicted Values[b]
Early I	1.01–1.49	19–22 months	16–26
Late I	1.50–1.99	23–26 months	18–31
II	2.0–2.49	27–30 months	21–35
III	2.50–2.99	31–34 months	24–41
Early IV	3.0–3.49	35–38 months	28–45
Late IV/Early V	3.50–3.99	39–42 months	31–50
Late V	4.0–4.49	43–46 months	37–52
Post V	4.50+	47+ months	41–

[a]Predicted from the linear regression equation: Age = 11.199 + 7.857 (MLU).
[b]Computed from obtained standard deviations.
Source: Reprinted with permission from Miller, J. F., & Chapman, R. S. (1981). The relationship between age and mean length of utterance in Morphemes. *Journal of Speech and Hearing Research, 14,* 154–161. Copyright © 1981 by American Speech-Language-Hearing Association. All rights reserved.

Each stage can also be distinguished by an approximate MLU and age range. Table 3–1 provides a summary of the MLU ranges and approximate ages associated with each stage of Brown's stages of development, based on research conducted by Miller and Chapman (1981). In their study, Miller and Chapman examined the relationship among MLU, stage of development, and age in a group of 123 children from a middle- to upper-middle-class community in the Midwest. While findings may differ slightly for other child language populations, the MLU ranges, stages of development, and age ranges reported in Table 3–1 should provide a fairly good estimate of general language expectations for all English-speaking children.

Sequence of Acquisition

In addition to studying the changes in utterance length and complexity associated with each stage, Brown also studied the emergence of 14 different grammatical morphemes that began to emerge during these early stages of language development. The earliest developing morphemes, such as present progressive *-ing* and plural *-s,* began to emerge at some point during Brown's Stage II, somewhere between the ages of 27 and 30 months. While some of the grammatical morphemes that emerged during these early stages of development were mastered by one or more of the children sometime between Stages II and V, others such as copula and auxiliary *be* were not mastered until after Stage V (Miller, 1991; Owens, 2005). Since Brown's early research study, a number of other child language scholars (deVilliers & deVilliers, 1973; Kuczaj, 1979) have observed similar patterns of language development in other English-speaking child populations, although the specific order and stages of acquisition for some grammatical forms have been found to vary across these studies. Research findings from each of these studies have all revealed, however, that individual children vary with respect to the exact age at which certain forms emerge and are mastered. As a result, it is important to realize that age ranges rather than specific developmental language milestones, as for other aspects of language development, are most appropriate for capturing early children's language development patterns.

As with the development of phonology, there will be language-specific differences in morphological development of speakers from differing language backgrounds. For example, in Spanish-speaking children, the plural -s marker and copula verb forms (of *ser* and *estar*) are acquired by age 3 years (Anderson, 1995), which is earlier than the age at which the equivalent forms are mastered by English-speaking children. There also will be some morphological forms that exist in other languages but not in English that must be acquired by child speakers of that language. In these cases, the norms for acquisition of these forms will be language-specific, that is, relevant to that language but not others. In addition, it is important to recognize that many of the English grammatical morphemes, such as past tense -ed, plural -s, and copula *be*, that are produced 100% of the time by typically developing MAE-speaking children, once mastered, in obligatory (required) sentence contexts occur more variably in the sentences of children who are emerging and established African American English (AAE) speakers. This is because these forms are not required to occur to the same extent according to the rules of AAE grammar and can be variably absent in some of the contexts considered obligatory for Mainstream American English (MAE). There are some sentence contexts in AAE, however, where these forms are obligated to occur 100% of the time, as in MAE. For example in AAE, the **copula** or main verb form of *is* must occur in the final positions of sentences and clauses, as in the sentence "Yes, he *is*" and as well as after *it, that,* and *what* subjects, as in "It's a cat."

School-Age Years

During the school years, there is considerable development of **inflectional** prefixes (e.g., *non-, dis-*) and **derivational** suffixes (e.g., *-ment, -hood*), as well as some development of inflectional suffixes (Nagy, Diakidoy, & Anderson, 1991, cited in Owens, 2005). Inflectional suffixes and prefixes change the meaning of the word but not the word class of the word (e.g., *responsible* and *irresponsible* are both adjectives). In contrast, derivational suffixes usually change the word class of the base word (e.g., *love*, a noun, becomes *lovely*, an adjective) (Miller, 1991). Among others, derivational suffixes include the following, listed in the order of acquisition: *-er, -y*, noun compounds, and *-ly*. At age six, children understand the suffixes of *-man* and *-er* and use many plural nouns (Miller, 1991; Owens, 2005). Eight-year-olds use *-er* to indicate someone who initiates an action (e.g., *baker*), and 11-year-olds use *er* to indicate an instrument (e.g., *eraser*) (Miller, 1991; Owens, 2005). The *-y* used to form adjectives (e.g., *soapy*) is acquired at age 11, and the *-ly* used to form adverbs (e.g., *jokingly*) at adolescence (Owens, 2005). Children also learn to use their growing knowledge of derivational suffixes to expand their vocabulary (Lewis & Windsor, 1996).

The school years also are a time when children learn to use **comparatives** (e.g., long*er, more* intelligent) correctly (Graziano-King & Cairns, 2005). Before age 6, children tend to show few preferences for using the suffix *-er* or the adjective *more* to express a comparison. However, between ages 6 and 8, children appear to overgeneralize the suffix *-er* to form comparatives, frequently using it incorrectly (e.g., *wronger*). Finally, at age 9 and older, children's production of comparatives become more adultlike.

Children refine their understanding of count nouns and mass nouns during the elementary school years. **Count nouns** occur as distinct countable units (e.g., *chairs* or *desks*), whereas **mass nouns** occur as indivisible quantities (e.g., *corn* or *soap*) (McLaughlin, 2006). *Many* and *few* occur with count nouns, while *much* and *little* are used to modify mass nouns. Children's use of mass and count nouns and their modifiers continues to develop throughout the school years.

Adolescence

During the adolescent years, there are few differences from the morphological developments that take place during the school-age years, with adolescent students continuing to refine their use and comprehension of later developing morphological inflections that begin to emerge during the school-age years. These refinements take place in both spoken and written discourse and reflect growing **metalinguistic knowledge**, the ability to analyze language.

ACQUISITION OF SEMANTIC KNOWLEDGE

Preschool-Age Years: New Vocabulary Words and Meanings

As children move past the 18- to 24-month mark of language development, their vocabulary begins to expand rapidly. According to Owens (2005), the vocabulary of toddlers expands from 50 words to 200 to 300 words between 2 and 3 years of age. Their vocabulary triples to 900 to 1,000 words around 3 years of age. From 3 to 5 years of age, their vocabulary more than doubles to 2,100 to 2,200 words.

As discussed in McLaughlin (2006) and Owens (2005), preschooler word learning involves two stages. The first stage, known as the **fast mapping** stage, is where children begin to form an initial impression of what a word means and make a temporary association between a word that they have heard used with a given meaning or referent after their first exposure to a word. At this point in word learning, children generally understand only a small portion of the meaning associated with a word. In essence, they have only a tentative definition of the word. During the next stage of vocabulary development, the **extended mapping phase**, children gradually expand, refine, and modify their meanings of a word with additional experience and exposure, eventually arriving at a correct interpretation of the word.

When children are trying to figure out the underlying meaning of a new unfamiliar word and/or to select the most appropriate label for an unfamiliar object or other referent, they may use any one of a variety of strategies. Several different hypotheses attempt to explain how children figure out the meaning of or the label for a new word. Some of these hypotheses suggest that children use perceptually based strategies and criteria for labeling unfamiliar referents (the **semantic feature hypothesis**). Others suggest that children use functional criteria, such as how an object is used, for labeling a newly observed item (the **functional core hypothesis**). Under the **associative complex hypothesis**, children may use shifting criteria for labeling unfamiliar referents; under the prototypic complex hypothesis, they may choose a label for an unfamiliar referent based on how closely it matches the children's prototype of a given word category.

Preschool-Age Years: Conceptual Category Knowledge and Terms

During children's preschool years (which represent one of the most important stages of vocabulary development), several different key semantic concepts and word categories emerge and/or are mastered in children's expressive (produced) as well as receptive (understood) vocabulary (McLaughlin, 2006). Some of the key semantic concept categories that emerge and are established during the preschool-age years are dimensional terms (e.g., *big, little, wide, narrow, tall, short, deep, shallow*), color terms (e.g., *yellow, blue, red*), spatial terms (e.g., *in, on, under, behind*), kinship terms (e.g., *mother, father, brother, aunt, grandfather*), and temporal terms (e.g., *after, before, since, until*).

Dimensional terms. There are general trends in how these conceptual word categories emerge and are mastered in children's speech. For example, when children begin to acquire dimensional words, such as *big* and *little*, to reference the varied dimensions of objects, those words are associated with the positive member of the dimensional pair. The term that denotes the presence of a given dimension, such as *big* versus *little* and *tall* versus *short*, is typically learned first. In addition those concepts that are experienced more frequently in a child's daily encounters with the world, such as *big* and *little*, tend to be mastered earlier than those experienced less frequently such as *deep* and *shallow*.

Color terms. Color terms that are definitely associated with academic language learning in preschool and kindergarten classroom settings are typically acquired by 4 to 5 years of age. Children's mastery of these terms is greatly influenced by the emphasis placed on the use of these terms in early educational settings. It is important to recognize, however, that children's familiarity with certain academic vocabulary like color terms is also influenced by the emphasis that parents place on these words in the home environment and on the conscious teaching of such terms. For example, in some cultural communities, parents may not place as much emphasis on the direct teaching of these terms prior to children's entry into the school environment. This can play a role in the age at which such color terms are mastered.

Evidence of cross-cultural differences in language socialization practices can be seen when one examines the age at which certain vocabulary terms, such as color words, are expected to be mastered by children from Spanish- versus English-speaking backgrounds on a commonly used preschool speech and language test called the *Preschool Language Scale-4,* which has a Spanish as well as an English version. These two test versions, while similar, were actually normed on two different language populations. As a result, some items that are found in the English version are not found in the Spanish version, and vice versa. There are also differences between the two tests with regard to the ages at which differing language concepts are expected to be acquired and mastered. On the *Preschool Language Scale, Fourth Edition—English* (Zimmerman, Steiner, & Pond, 2002a) the authors test an item, assessing children's color identification skills, found at the 3;6 to 3;11 year level. The same item occurs at the 4;6 to 4;11 age level on the *Preschool Language Scale, Fourth Edition—Spanish* (Zimmerman, Steiner, & Pond, 2002b). The differences in children's mastery of these concepts do not reflect differences in cognitive or language potential, but rather they reflect the differences in the cross-cultural language socialization and exposure experiences of children from differing cultural and linguistic backgrounds.

Spatial terms. Within certain concept category vocabularies, there can also be differences in the order or sequence with which certain terms are acquired and mastered. For example, by the age of 4 years, most children have mastered the spatial terms of *in, on,* and *under.* Other spatial terms such as *in front of* and *behind* are not mastered until about one year later (McLaughlin, 2006). Before these terms are fully mastered, children may also show a bias in their interpretation of these terms. For example, regardless of the spatial word used, children are likely to follow the principles that objects should always go *inside* a container and that objects should always go *on* an item with a supporting surface (Miller, 1991; Owens, 2005). As a result, it would not be unusual for younger children or older children with cognitive delays to show a bias toward putting a block on top of a table when presented with the command "Put the block under the table" or to put a block inside a box when presented with two boxes and given the spoken command of "Put the block on the box" (one box is standing upright and the other box is placed upside down). Movement terms are also often interpreted as meaning "toward." As a result, *from* can be incorrectly interpreted as meaning "to," *out of* can be incorrectly interpreted as meaning "into," and *off* can be incorrectly interpreted as meaning "onto."

Kinship terms. With respect to kinship terms, preschoolers are more likely to understand first those kinship terms that relate directly to their lives and what they experience in their home. According to McLaughlin (2006) and Owens (2005), most children are therefore likely to develop first an understanding of kinship terms such as *mother, father, sister,* and *brother* which are first-generation family members, with second- and third-generation family member terms such as *grandfather, aunt, niece,* and *cousin* developing later. It is important to realize, again, that cross-cultural variations that can potentially occur in children's understanding and use of kinship terms are based on the family unit structures and networks existing in their home and local community environments.

Communities vary considerably with respect to how families and households are structured. In some cultural communities, extended families and extended family members are likely to have more direct and frequent contact with nuclear family members than in other communities, sometimes because extended family members are residing in the same household as are nuclear family members. In addition, the nature of the relationships can differ cross-culturally. For example, in some cultural communities, cousins may be viewed and treated in the same manner as brothers and sisters. In other communities, nonkin adults who reside in the community may have the same rights and privileges as kin in the raising and disciplining of children. Each of these differences could potentially play a factor in the degree of familiarity that children have with differing kinship relationships, with degree of familiarity with a given kinship relationship not necessarily being equivalent across communities.

Temporal terms. There is also a developmental sequence in children's acquisition of temporal terms, with those words indicating the general order of events and activities often being mastered first (e.g., *after* and *before*) and those words indicating duration being mastered later (e.g., *since* and *until*). Temporal words used to indicate simultaneously occurring events, such as *while* and *at the same time,* are generally understood last but typically still acquired by 5 years of age (McLaughlin, 2006). Children's comprehension of these terms is also highly influenced by factors such as linguistic context and/or order of mention within sentences. For example, until children fully master an understanding of the temporal terms *before* and *after,* they are likely to interpret each of the following sentences as meaning the same:

"Before you go to school, stop at the store."
"Go to school before you stop at the store."
"After you go to school, stop at the store."
"Go to school after you stop at the store." (Owens, 2005, pp. 280–281)

For each of the statements above, children are likely to rely on order of mention for interpretation, assuming that, regardless of the sentence spoken, the first action to be performed is to go to school.

School-Age Years

An important aspect of semantic development is the ability to produce definitions. Definitions of objects in the early elementary school years often involve descriptions of the physical properties of the objects and their functions (Benelli, Arcuri, & Marchesini, 1988; McGregor, Friedman, Reilly, & Newman, 2002). As children grow older, definitions are less based on personal experience and more based on socially shared information that others associate with the word (McLaughlin, 2006). By age 11, children have all of the elements of conventional adult definitions and can create abstract definitions (Owens, 2005). They become more effective in producing **Aristotelian, formal, or dictionary definitions** (Marinellie & Johnson, 2003; Nippold, 1995). Definitions like these include a category accompanied by specific characteristics (e.g., "A desk is a *piece of furniture* [category] *that you write on*" [characteristic]). Formal definition development includes both changes in content with the use of categorical terms and changes in grammatical form (e.g., "A is a type of B that is C") (Marinellie & Johnson, 2003; Nippold, Hegel, Sohlberg, & Schwarz, 1999).

In a process called **horizontal vocabulary development,** children add features to each definition that are part of the adult definition of the word (McLaughlin, 2006; Owens, 2005). For example, a child may have a narrow understanding of the word *dog* that includes only a few types of breeds in a limited size range. As a child's definition of *dog* expands, it includes different breeds and sizes of dogs. In addition, children gather together all of the definitions that fit one word in **vertical vocabulary development** (McLaughlin, 2006). In this case, a child learns that *rule* means having dominion over others as well as a requirement. During the school years, students also grow in their ability to identify synonyms, or words that mean the same (Botting & Adams, 2005).

Especially after the fourth grade, many words are added from context, often from children's reading (Owens, 2005). Children grow in their ability to make inferences, or to abstract information that is not directly presented (Botting & Adams, 2005). They also use inferencing in conjunction with their reading comprehension skills to learn the meanings of new words from context during reading (Cain, Oakhill, & Elbro, 2003).

Around the age of 7, children undergo a syntagmatic-paradigmatic shift, in which their word associations change (Miller, 1991). Prior to that age, a child makes syntagmatic word associations based on syntax, so that a child may associate the word *man* with *sit*. Later, paradigmatic associations are based on semantic relationships, so that *man* is associated with *woman*. The shift begins in preschool and continues into adulthood, although the most rapid rate of change occurs between the ages of 5 and 9. The shift in word associations appears to be related to children's growing reading abilities (Cronin, 2002), and also is reflected in children's greater use of superordinate terms, or categorical terms, in their definitions (Guasti, 2002).

The number of vocabulary words grows during this time period. It is estimated that 5- to 6-year-olds know between 2,500 and 5,000 words (Beck & McKeown, 1991). It is also estimated that children learn approximately 9 or 10 new words each day (Carey, 1978), or 3,000 words per year (Beck & McKeown, 1991). Children's comprehension is even higher than expressive language. First graders comprehend about 20,000 words, while sixth graders understand approximately 50,000 words (McLaughlin, 2006).

Adolescence

Upon graduation from high school, it is estimated that the average adolescent has learned the meaning of at least 80,000 words (Larson & McKinley, 2003). As adolescents move into adulthood and begin to pursue some form of occupation, vocation, or career, they begin to acquire the specialized technical words or jargon associated with their chosen occupation, vocation, or career (Munro, 2002). Adolescence is also a period where older learners are beginning to master the slang vocabulary spoken within their affiliated peer groups. The slang that is used by adolescents from different language communities can vary as a function of ethnic-cultural background and identity (Green, 2002; Munro, 2002).

ACQUISITION OF SYNTAX

Preschool-Age Years: Early Sentence Development

As children move closer to the age of 3 years, they begin to produce simple three-word subject + verb + object or agent-action-object **declarative** sentences like "daddy kick ball" and "doggie eat cake" (Brown, 1973; Owens, 2005). This stage of sentence development occurs around Brown's Stage III level of language development. Once they have mastered simple sentence forms, they begin to produce more elaborate sentences containing expanded noun and verb phrases (Miller, 1991; Owens, 2005).

Children initially expand and elaborate the noun phrases in their sentences through the use of articles (e.g., "doggie eat the cake"), possessive pronouns (e.g., "doggie eat my cake"), adjectives (e.g., "doggie eat big cake"), demonstratives (e.g., "doggie eat that cake"), and quantifier words such as *two* (e.g., "doggie eat two cake"). Noun phrase expansions typically occur first at the ends of sentences. This is known as **objective case expansions**. Objective case expansions involve the expansion of nouns occurring in the object position of a sentence, as in each of the examples given above. Subjective noun phrase expansions, which involve the expansion of noun phrases in the beginnings of sentences, as in "The doggie eat cake" and "My doggie eat cake," typically occur later.

Children also begin to expand the verb phrases in their sentences by adding morphological inflections such as past tense *-ed* (e.g., "boy kicked ball"), present progressive *-ing* (e.g., "boy kicking ball"), third person singular *-s* (e.g., "boy kicks ball"), auxiliary verbs (e.g., "boy is kicking ball"), modals (e.g., "boy can kick ball"), and adverbs (e.g., "boy kick ball hard").

The next stage of sentence development involves the production of sentences that contain more than one of the previously described modifying elements, as in "Doggie eating that big cake." As children move into a more complex stage of sentence development, they also begin to produce sentences that are expanded through the use of postnoun modifiers, as in "The doggie that is over there is eating my cake." These postnoun modifiers involve the use of complex embedded sentence elements such as relative clauses.

In addition to expanding the basic noun and verb phrase structure of declarative sentences, children are also learning how to produce other sentence types, such as those containing negatives and interrogative (question) forms. The development of sentences containing negatives proceeds from the early emerging use of single and simple multiword utterances containing the negatives *no, not, don't,* and *can't,* as in "no bed" and "no, not sleepy," to more complete sentences with the negative appearing after auxiliary verb forms like *is,* as in "The dog is not eating," to sentences containing later developing negatives such as *isn't, aren't, doesn't, didn't, wouldn't, couldn't* and *shouldn't.*

Questions follow a similar path of development, from early question forms involving the use of simple single-word questions like "Book?" to two- and three-word questions like "What that?" and "Where Daddy?" to more complicated questions involving the use of noninverted **auxiliary (helping) verbs,** as in "Where Daddy is going?" More complicated question forms follow in which the subject and auxiliary verb are inverted or switch in sentence position, as in "Where is Daddy going?" Later question form developments include the emerging use of *how, when,* and *why* questions, as well as tag questions such as "He's going to store, isn't he?"

Preschool-Age Years: Later Sentence Development

Another aspect of sentence development that occurs during the preschool-age years, primarily during Brown's Stage IV, is the development of sentences containing embedded or conjoined phrases and clauses. **Embedded phrases** are sentence elements that either modify or serve as part of a main clause of a sentence but do not include a subject and predicate. For example, in a sentence like "The boy kicked the ball with his foot," the embedded phrase "with his foot," which is actually a prepositional phrase, is used to describe how the ball was kicked. In this example, the embedded phrase ("with his foot") is serving as a postnoun modifier. In contrast, in a sentence like "I love to swim," the embedded phrase "to swim," which is also known as an infinitive phrase, occurs as the object of the sentence rather than as a modifier of the object phrase. Infinitive phrases like the example above include a primary verb ("love") followed by the word *to* and a secondary verb *swim.* The *to* that separates these two verbs is different from the preposition word *to* as in "I'm going to the store," where the word *to* refers to movement in the direction of the store. A list and examples of various embedded phrases that can occur in English-speaking children's sentences can be found in Table 3–2.

In addition to producing sentences that contain embedded phrases, preschoolers are also beginning, during more complex stages of sentence development, to produce sentences that contain embedded clauses. **Embedded clauses**, like embedded phrases, can either modify a portion of the main clause in a sentence or serve as the object of the subject of a sentence. For example, in the sentence "She is the girl that we met last week," the clause "that we met last week" describes the girl identified in the object position of the main clause. In contrast, in the sentence "I know that you can do it," the "that you can do it" portion of the sentence serves as the object of the main clause ("I know"). Clauses do differ from phrases, however, because they contain an underlying or understood subject and predicate. For example, both the main clause and the modifying relative clause in the sentence "She is the girl that we met last week" contain an underlying subject and **predicate** (the part of the sentence that contains the verb and any following object phrase). In the main portion of the sentence, or main clause ("She is the girl"), the word *She* represents the subject and

TABLE 3–2
Bloom and Lahey's (1978) Content Categories with Initial Phase of Emergence

Content Category	Example	Initial Phase
Existence	"That a baby"	Phase 1
Non-existence/disappearance	"daddy gone," "no doggie"	Phase 1
Recurrence	"another cookie"	Phase 1
Rejection	"no bed!"	Phase 1
Denial	"not a girl!"	Phase 1
Attribution	"big yellow ball"	Phase 1
Possession	"my shoe"	Phase 1
Action	"I make a cake"	Phase 1
Locative action	"playing down here"	Phase 1
Locative state	"on chair"	Phase 3
State	"cup broken"	Phase 3
Quantity	"two kitties"	Phase 3
Notice	"look at birdie!"	Phase 4
Temporal	"Now it's done"	Phase 4
Additive	"He going to school and she going home"	Phase 5
Causal	"I hurt my knee cause I fell"	Phase 5
Specification	"I take this one. You take that one"	
Dative	"this for you"	Phase 5
Epistemic	"I think it's gonna be good"	Phase 7
Adversative	"She's happy but he isn't"	Phase 7
Communication	"Tell me how to do it"	Phase 8

Source: From Lahey, M. (1988). *Language disorders and language development.* Boston, MA: Allyn and Bacon. Copyright © 1988 by Pearson Education. Adapted by permission of the publisher.

the phrase "is the girl" represents the predicate. In the modifying portion of the sentence ("that we met last week"), which is also considered to be a relative clause, the word *we* serves as the subject of the sentence and the verb phrase "met last week" serves as the predicate.

Conjoined clauses represent another type of clause found in the sentences of older preschoolers. While embedded clauses serve to support some aspect of the main clause in a sentence, as in the examples given before (e.g., "She is the girl *that we met last week*" and "I know *that you can do it*"), conjoined clauses are independent of each other. For example, in the sentence "I like to skate and Jamie likes to swim," there are two independent clauses that each have an underlying or expressed subject and predicate. In the first independent clause, "I like to skate," the word *I* serves as the subject of the sentence and the phrase "like to skate" represents the predicate. In the second independent clause, "Jamie likes to swim," the word *Jamie* serves as the subject of the sentence and the phrase "likes to swim" represents the predicate. Both of these clauses are connected through the use of a linking word also known as a **conjunction**.

Other conjunctions often used to link two or more independent clauses in a sentence include words such as *but* (e.g., "Carrie likes the beach but she is afraid of crabs"), *because* (e.g., "He hit me because he is mean"), and *or* (e.g., "I want to go to the movie or the shopping center"). In some sentences that contain two or more conjoined clauses, the subject and predicate of the second clause is the same as the first but is not directly expressed (e.g., "I want to go to the movie or [I want to go to] the shopping center"). In other cases, the subjects and/or predicates of the two clauses can differ, as in "I like to skate and Jamie likes to swim," where the subjects and predicates of the two clauses do differ. In the sentence "Carrie likes the beach but she is afraid of crabs," the subject of both clauses is the same, as represented by the use of the pronoun *she* to refer to *Carrie*. The predicate of the two clauses, however, is different. The predicate in the first clause is "likes the beach" while the predicate in the second clause is "is afraid of crabs."

As children move out of Stage IV into Stage V, they begin to produce sentences that contain both embedded and conjoined clauses and/or phrases, as in "I saw Spider Man *and* Clarita saw the movie *that had the other guy in it.*" The word *and* links two independent clauses, while the phrase "that had the other guy in it" modifies or describes the movie seen. Children also begin to produce sentences with multiple embeddings, as in "I think [that] we gotta go home now," which contains the embedded relative clause beginning with the word *that* as well as the embedded phrase "gotta go home now," which represents an infinitive phrase.

School-Age Years

During the elementary years, children's noun phrases undergo important developments. Less than 50% of children in first grade can use correct pronouns (Owens, 2005). With age, children are better able to distinguish between subject pronouns, such as *we*, *they*, *he*, *she*, and *I*, and object pronouns, such as *us*, *them*, *him*, *her*, and *me*. Children also begin to use reflexives, such as *himself, herself, myself,* and *ourselves*.

Children aged 6 to 8 demonstrate some understanding and use of more advanced verb forms, including present perfect (e.g., "She *has eaten*"), past progressive (e.g., "He *was eating*"), and perfect progressive (e.g., "He *has been eating*") (Sutter & Johnson, 1990). Children also increase their use of modal auxiliaries such as *could, might,* and *should* (e.g., "He *could* hit the ball") (Owens, 2005; Scott & Stokes, 1995).

Sentence length and clausal density, or subordination index, are two measures of older children's syntactic development (Nippold, Hesketh, Duthie, & Mansfield, 2005). During the school years children's sentence length is often measured in terms of **terminable units**, or **T-units**, (Scott, 1988b), which consist of a main clause and any attached or embedded subordinate clauses or nonclausal structures (Hunt, 1970). **Communication units**, or **C-units**, are another measure of sentence length; they include all T-units as well as responses to questions that do not include an independent clause (Loban, 1976). Sentence length includes mean number of words per T-unit, which is obtained by adding the number of words in a language sample and dividing the sum by the number of T-units. Clausal density is defined as the mean number of clauses, including independent and dependent clauses, per T-unit (Nippold et al., 2005). It is obtained by adding the number of clauses in a language sample, both main and subordinate, and dividing by the number of C-units or T-units (Nippold et al., 2005). Some measures of words per C-unit and number of dependent clauses per C-unit are presented in Table 3–3 (Loban, 1976). In addition, 35% of third graders', 36% of fourth graders', and 50% of fifth graders' sentences include at least three clauses (e.g., "The boy *who was running quickly* fell down *where the road curved*") (Marinellie, 2004).

Children who speak African American English demonstrate a similar increase during the school years in the number of morphemes per communication unit (Craig, Washington, & Thompson, 2005). During the middle elementary years, they may produce longer sentences than children who speak Mainstream American English (Smith, Lee, & McDade, 2001).

Children additionally produce a variety of types of dependent clauses in elementary school. Children aged 5 to 8 are most likely to correctly produce subordinate clauses used as direct objects (e.g., "Sara forgot *that Joshua fed the dog,*") and adjectives

TABLE 3–3

Mean Number of Words per Communication Unit and Dependent Clauses per Unit for School-Age Children

Grade	Mean Number of Words per Communication Unit	Mean Number of Dependent Clauses per Communication Unit
1	6.88	0.16
2	7.56	0.21
3	7.62	0.22
4	9.00	0.30
5	8.82	0.29
6	9.82	0.37
7	9.75	0.35
8	10.71	0.39

Source: Adapted from Loban, W. (1976). *Language development: Kindergarten through grade twelve.* (pp. 27, 37). Research Report No. 18. Urbana, IL: National Council of Teachers of English. Copyright © 1976 by the National Council of Teachers of English. Reprinted with permission.

(e.g., "Sara told Juan *that Joshua fed the dog*") (Owen & Leonard, 2006), but from first through eighth grade, the proportions of specific types of noun, adjectival, and adverbial clauses fluctuate (Loban, 1976). By third through fifth grade, children rarely make errors in their use of subordinate clauses (Marinellie, 2004). Children in the middle elementary years who speak African American English may also produce more complex sentence structures than children who speak Mainstream American English (Smith et al., 2001).

As children advance through the school years, they increase their use of passives in verb phrases. By school age, children can consistently use the *-ed* of the past participle in producing short passive sentences (e.g., "The cake *was baked*") (Redmond, 2003). About 80% of students between 7 and 8 produce full passive sentences, which include *be* or *got* with a past tense marker and a preposition followed by a noun phrase (e.g., "The cake *was baked by the girl*") (Owens, 2005).

Passives are also divided into different types. There are **reversible passives,** in which the actor and object of the action logically may be switched (e.g., "The boy *was chased by the girl*" makes sense if changed to "The girl *was chased by the boy*") (Owens, 2005). There also are **nonreversible passives,** in which the two roles cannot be interchanged. In instrumental nonreversible passives (e.g., "The window *was hit by the ball*"), the action is performed by an inanimate object, and in agentive nonreversible passives (e.g., "The window *was hit by the girl*"), the action is performed by a human or an animal (Miller, 1991). Children produce only reversible and instrumental nonreversible passives until age 9, when agentive nonreversible passives appear. However, children between the ages of 11 and 23 continue to use instrumental nonreversible passives more than agentive nonreversible passives (Miller, 1991; Owens, 2005).

The types of *wh-* questions asked by children increase during the school years. By age 8, students can consistently produce *how, when,* and *why* questions (Wallach, 1984).

In terms of conjunctions, the **coordinating conjunction** *and* remains the most common conjunction into adulthood (Scott, 1984, cited in Scott, 1988a) and is used in 50% to 80% of compound sentences (Scott, 1988a). However, the use of **subordinating conjunctions**, such as *because* or *if,* which connect the clauses of complex sentences, increases (e.g., "She is happy *because* she had a birthday") (Verhoeven et al., 2002). At ages 6 to 7, *if* begins to be used in dependent clauses (e.g., "*If* you are ready, we can leave") (Loban, 1976). Between ages 8 and 10, children begin to relate specific concepts to ideas and use conjunctions like *unless* and *even if* (e.g., "Unless you are famished, I don't need to eat") (Loban, 1976). In addition, *because* and *when* are used most often to join clauses up to age 12, with *in order to* and *if* used frequently as well (e.g., "*In order to have time*, we will have to hurry") (Nippold, 1998). However, children may not consistently comprehend the meaning of *because* until age 10, *if* and *though* until age 11 (Owens, 2005), and *unless* until age 15 (McLaughlin, 2006).

Finally, children use adverbial conjuncts as connective devices (Miller, 1991; Owens, 2005). Children use the adverbial conjuncts of *now, though,* and *then* by age 6 (Miller, 1991; Owens, 2005) and include adverbial conjuncts such as *however, therefore,* and *otherwise* in their sentences by age 12 (e.g., "Don't think twice; *otherwise,* you will regret it") (Scott, 1988a; Owens, 2005).

Children also use relative pronouns to produce relative clauses (e.g., "The boy *who* jumped fell down"). Additional relative pronouns acquired during the school years include *whose, whom,* and *in which* (e.g., "This is the story *in which* the prince gets his three wishes granted") (Scott, 1988a).

Adolescence

As children progress from the school-age into the adolescent years, they continue to exhibit small but regular increases in sentence length and complexity that can still be described in terms of increases in C-unit and/or T-unit length. Increases in average T-unit length were first documented in both oral and written discourse by Loban (1976). The types of increases observed in written discourse have been found to vary as a function of written discourse mode, such as whether the writing genre is persuasive, narrative, or descriptive. For example, according to a research study of written compositions from older adolescent students, Crowhurst and Piche (as cited in Nippold, 1998) found a greater number of words per T-unit in written language samples where students were asked to take and defend a position on a given controversy (e.g., persuasive mode). The number of words was lower in descriptive writing samples where students were asked to describe a picture, and it was lowest in narrative writing samples where students were asked to write a story.

During the adolescent years, children are also beginning to master a variety of later developing conjunctions that begin to emerge during the school-age years: subordinating conjunctions such as *after, although, before, if, unless,* and *when* that introduce dependent clauses, and correlative conjunctions, such as *both/and, either/or,* and *neither/nor,* that express symmetrical relationships between ideas, individuals, or events. Adolescents are also beginning to master the use of adverbial conjuncts such as *fortunately, furthermore, consequently,* and *therefore.* Some adverbial conjunct phrases such as "by the way" and "on the other hand" are used to signal the transition to a new or related topic.

ACQUISITION OF PRAGMATIC SKILLS AND ABILITIES

Preschool-Age Years: Communicative Speech Acts and Functions

During the preschool-age years, children are refining their earlier use of developing pragmatic functions and speech acts to control and regulate the behaviors of others, state their own needs and desires, and gain the attention of adults (Miller, 1991; Owens, 2005). For example, during the first few years of preschool development, children tend to use fairly direct requests for desired objects and activities with phrases like "I want." Toward the end of the preschool years, there is a sharp increase in children's use of indirect requests, such as "That doll would look really good in my room, mommy" along with the use of more explanations and justifications for requests, such as "I want a bigger bike so I can be like Jason" or "I think I should have two candies too, daddy, because you gave Tanisha two candies." By 5 years of age, children are also beginning to comprehend indirect requests such as "Can you give me a cookie?" as requests for actions versus simple yes/no questions to be answered. Indirect requests may not be fully mastered, however, until 10 to 11 years of age (Brice, Miller, & Brice, 2006). Children are also becoming more adept at selecting the most socially polite and appropriate form for certain social communication situations based on important dynamics such as listener age, status, and/or background. Again, there are a number of pragmatic taxonomies, such as Dore's (1978) conversational speech acts, that can be used for describing the primary functions of language expressed during the preschool-age period (see Table 3–4).

During the preschool-age years, in addition to refining their use of communicative speech acts and functions emerging during the early stages of development, children from differing cultural backgrounds also begin to acquire some of the culture-specific speech acts associated with their cultural community. Examples from the African American community include the beginning of culture-specific language use patterns such as rapping, playing the dozens (a verbal game where individuals joke about members of one's family, more commonly referred to as "Yo Mama" jokes), and signifying (an indirect way of putting others down). These examples are part of some of the oral traditions. Examples of emerging preschooler knowledge and execution of these culture-specific acts can be found in Wyatt (1991, 1999).

Conversational Discourse

Other key pragmatic developments during the preschool-age years include the growth of important conversational skills such as knowing how to initiate conversation and topics, as well as knowing how to change and maintain topics. Adults typically take the role in initiating conversation with younger preschoolers, even though children are aware of how to initiate conversation. Younger children can initiate conversation, but they are limited in the topics that they can discuss. Repetition without elaboration or modification is the most frequently used strategy for

TABLE 3–4
Dore's (1978) Conversational Speech Acts

Pragmatic Category	Specific Conversational Acts
Requests	Yes/no, wh-, clarification, and rhetorical questions; action and permission requests.
Reponses	Answers to yes/no and wh- questions; clarifications; compliances; qualifications; repetitions.
Descriptions	Identifications; described events, actions, and processes; described properties, traits, conditions; expressed locations/directions; reported times.
Statements	Rules; evaluations; internal reports; attributions; explanations.
Acknowledgments	Verbal acceptances; approval/agreements; disapproval/disagreements; returns that acknowledge rhetorical questions/requests.
Organization	Boundary markers; calling; speaker selections that label speaker of next turn; politeness markers; accompaniments.
Performatives	Protests; jokes; claims; warnings; teasing.
Miscellaneous	No answer; uninterpretable, incomplete, or anomalous utterances; exclamations.

Source: Adapted from Dore, J. (1979). Conversational acts and the acquisition of language. In E. Ochs and B. Schieffelin (Eds.), *Developmental pragmatics* (pp. 339–361). New York: Academic Press. Copyright © 1979 by Elsevier.

maintaining conversation and topics. At the age of 2 years, most children can sustain topics for only approximately one to two turns. The length of sustained turn-taking increases to as many as 12 turns in at least 50% of children by age 5 years. Children also improve in their ability to take alternating turns during conversation, with fewer interruptions of their conversational partner, as they get older. Another key pragmatic ability that develops during the preschool years is the ability to repair conversational breakdowns through the use of contingent queries (e.g., questions such as "huh?" and "what?") whenever children do not understand all or part of something that has been said to them. They learn how to respond to others' queries as well, although their responding is inconsistent. Children are also learning how to use verbal acknowledgments such as "yeah" and "uh-huh" to keep conversation going (Miller, 1991; Owens, 2005).

Cross-culturally, there can be differences in how children are socialized to initiate conversation, maintain conversation, and engage in turn-taking interactions. For example, in some cultural communities, diverted instead of sustained eye gaze, with or without ongoing verbal acknowledgments, is the conversational strategy used for sustaining discourse. In addition, in some communities, simultaneous, overlapping turn-taking versus alternating, nonoverlapping turn-taking is the style used for engaging in conversation. In some cultural communities, there is considerably more silence and pause typically used between turns than in others. All of these represent just some of the culture-specific conversational rules that must be acquired by children in accordance with the communication standards of the community in which they reside and/or are affiliated.

Other key developments include understanding how much information or what kind of information a listener needs to follow conversation, also known as **listener presupposition**. One of the key developments associated with the development of listener presupposition skills is the increased use of **deitic terms** (referencing terms that shift in reference depending on the perspective of the listener). This includes terms such as *this* to refer to an object close to the speaker but away from the listener and *that* to refer to an object close to the listener but more distant from the speaker. Other shifting terms of reference that children are learning to use include pronouns like *I* and *you*. **Ellipsis** or the omission of presupposed shared information is also a key aspect of pragmatic development during these early years of development. During their preschool years, children are learning how and when they can leave out redundant information already stated in a previous statement and already understood by the speaker. English-speaking children also learn how to use the definite and indefinite articles *a* and *the* accurately the majority of the time by about age 3 years. During earlier stages of development, children often overuse the definite article *the*, which assumes previously shared and/or understood information, for *a*, which is typically used to indicate new information or information that has not been previously shared (Owens, 2005). One additional aspect of pragmatic competence that is acquired during the preschool years is learning how to adjust conversation based on perceived listener language background, level of language ability, and language exposure. For children who are bilingual, there is evidence that as early as the early preschool years, they are learning to switch the language that they use with their listeners based on their perceptions of the listener's language needs, ability, and exposure (Langdon & Merino, 1992). Even with children who are exposed to more than one dialect of English, there is evidence of early emerging linguistic competence in the ability to code-switch between dialects based on factors such as the primary purpose of communication, topic of focus, and the dialect background of the speaker (Wyatt & Seymour, 1990; Wyatt, 2001).

Narratives

One aspect of pragmatic competence that begins to emerge during the preschool years is the development of **narratives** or stories. Once again, several theoretical frameworks have been proposed for analyzing children's narratives. According to Lahey (1988), for example, the early developing narratives of children can be described in terms of additive, temporal, or causal chain narratives.

Additive chain narratives, which are the earliest to develop in child speech, are simple narratives where there is no temporal or time-ordered/related association between events within the stories. These types of narratives generally contain a simple listing or description of events that occur within the story, with no clear reference as to when events in the story occurred. The following is an example of an additive chain narrative:

> Once there was a horse
> and a little farm
> and some pigs were there
> and once there was a apple tree
> and there was a banana tree
> there was a little farmer who gave hay to the horse
> and there was a little pond with little fish in it
> and a little house
> that's it. (Sutton-Smith, 1981, cited in Lahey, 1988, p. 269)

Temporal chain narratives, the next type of narrative to emerge in preschoolers' speech, differ from additive chain narratives because there is some delineation of the time relationship between events occurring within the story. As a result, these types of narratives begin to include time words like *when*, *then*, and *after*, as well as time phrases like "the next day" and "last night." However, these types of narratives continue to lack an expression of causality between events within the story (why or what caused certain events to happen). The following is an example of a temporal chain narrative.

> When I was at home I looked in the closet and I saw a big giant bear. I treated him like a nice little bear. We went to the park a lot. We slept together and also we ate together. Next morning we looked at a book together and then we helped our father paint the house. Next winter it was Christmas and I got a new jacket. My teddy bear got a baby teddy bear, and they lived happily together. The end. (Sutton-Smith, 1981, as cited in Lahey, 1988, p. 270)

The final type of narrative chain to emerge in preschooler speech, toward the end of the preschool years as children are beginning to enter the early school years, is the **causal chain narrative.** The primary distinction between causal chain narratives and the other two earlier developing narratives is that causal chain narratives also include some expression of the causal relationship between events within stories.

The earliest developing causal chain narratives contain a simple delineation of a problem situation and a resolution to that problem, as in the following:

> Once upon a time there lived a zebra
> and the zebra he went to the park
> and he got lost
> and he didn't know his way home
> so he had to try both ways
> and he had to tell the police which way to go
> that's the end
> he had to tell him what house was like
> the zebra telled the police
> and that's the end. (Sutton-Smith, 1981, as cited in Lahey, 1988, p. 270)

Once children begin to produce their earliest causal chain narratives, the internal structure of their narratives can be defined in terms of episodes, which are smaller units within causal chain narratives that can be defined in terms of six different **story grammar components**, according to Stein and Glenn (1979). A brief description of each component, along with an example of each, can be found in Table 3–5. For episodes within children's narratives to be considered complete, they must contain, at minimum, the following three story grammar components or units: (1) setting or initiating event, (2) attempt, and (3) direct consequence.

TABLE 3–5
Stein and Glenn's (1979) Narrative Frameworks

Story Grammar Components

Setting: Provides information, usually at the beginning of the story, about where a story is taking place, the key characters, and the relationships between characters (e.g., "Once upon a time, there was this wicked old witch who lived in a forest far away")

Initiating event: Provides information about key events that lead up to the start of the main story (e.g., "One day the witch went looking in the forest for frogs that she could put in her stew")

Internal response: Provides information about what one or more characters are thinking, (e.g., "She saw one big fat frog on a log and she thought to herself, 'Hmm, that frog looks nice and delicious' ")

Internal plan: References any mental planning by a character in the story (e.g., "She began to think of a way to trick the frog into her home")

Attempt: Represents some action or attempt on the part of a character to execute a plan or attain a given goal (e.g., "She said to the frog, 'Hello, Mr. Frog, you look mighty nice today. Would you like to dine with me in my home tonight?' ")

Direct consequence: Refers to the outcome of any attempts or actions (e.g., "The frog, who was flattered, puffed up his chest and said, 'Thank you so kindly. I would love it!' and he followed the witch to her house")

Reaction: References a character's emotional response to or thoughts about the outcome of previous actions and attempts (e.g., "The witch smiled to herself, saying 'I am so, so, so smart,' and she chuckled.")

Source: Adapted from An analysis of story comprehension in elementary school children. In R. O. Freedle (Ed.) *New directions in discourse processing* (Vol. 2) westport, CT: Greenwood Publishing Group, Inc. Copyright © 1979 by Ablex Publishing Corporation. Reproduced with permission of Greenwood Publishing Group.

The structure of children's early developing personal event narratives (stories about things that happen in their personal lives) have also been described using a scheme proposed by Peterson and McCabe (1983, as presented in McCabe and Rollins, 1994). Under this organizational framework, children progress from a stage of simple one-event narratives to narratives with more expressed events that are logically and causally sequenced, to high-point narratives where the story ends in a climax of events without resolution, to more classic narratives where a resolution to a problem situation after the climax event is included. Research by McCabe and Peterson (as reported in McCabe and Rollins, 1994) reveals the predominant use of each of these differing types of narratives produced by North American Caucasian English-speaking children at different ages. For examples, **two-event narratives** (narratives containing more than two past events) were the most common type of narrative produced by 3-and-a-half-year-olds. **Leap-frog narratives** (narratives that have more than two events and a causal sequence but that do not mirror the logical sequence in which the events are likely to have occurred) were produced most often by 4-year-olds. **End at high-point narratives** (narratives that end prematurely) were produced most often by 5-year-olds. Classic narratives (well-formed and ordered narratives) were the most commonly used in younger school-age children: 6 years of age and older.

Additional frameworks that have been used to describe the developmental changes in children's narratives include that proposed by Labov (1972) and Labov and Waletzky (1967, as cited in Lahey, 1988), which focuses on the degree of informativeness within children's narratives. Under this framework, children's narratives can be analyzed with respect to their use of (1) **orientations** that provide information about who the participants are in the narrative as well as where, when, and why the events took place, (2) **evaluations** (the narrator's expressed feelings about the events within the stories), and (3) **appendages** (the ways in which the narrator indicates that a story is about to begin or end). In their earliest narratives, children tend to produce only a limited amount of information about the characters in their story and where a story takes place. With age, they begin to include more information about character relationships, actions, and traits, as well as character names and locations of events within the story. As they develop, children also begin to include an increased number and variety of evaluations, with evaluations being stated more explicitly. They also begin to use an increasing number of appendages that become more sophisticated in nature (e.g., "And they rode into the sunset, never to be seen again" versus "And that's the end").

Children's stories also become cohesive (flowing and better organized), with the links between elements within their stories, characters, and events being more clearly referenced through the use of pronouns, **demonstrative** words like *this* and *that*, articles, conjunctions, ellipsis, and **lexical cohesion** (e.g., where previously mentioned elements are mentioned again by name).

Although the general path of narrative development is likely to be fairly familiar and similar across different cultural communities, there are also a number of cross-cultural differences in how stories are organized and structured, the type of information typically contained within stories, the perceived purpose of stories, how stories are told (e.g., individually or collectively), and the channels of communication that are used for conveying certain types of story information (Champion, 2003;

Gutierrez-Clellen & Quinn, 1993; Hyter & Westby, 1996; Westby, 1994). It is not clear when children begin to display these culture-specific differences in storytelling (e.g., during preschool or the early school-age years), but it is clear that as children learn to tell stories, they eventually learn to tell them according to the narrative expectations of their home community.

School-Age Years

Children's presuppositional skills mature during the school years. By age 7, children understand and use most deictic terms correctly (Owens, 2005). Another aspect of presuppositional skills is **perspective taking**. There are three aspects of perspective taking (McLaughlin, 2006). **Linguistic perspective taking** is the ability to adjust the level of one's language to that of the listener. **Perceptual perspective taking** is the ability to comprehend what one's listener perceives. For example, a child learns that another person can see an object that is not visible to the child. Finally, **cognitive perspective taking** is the ability to infer others' thoughts, intentions, and feelings (McLaughlin, 2006; Westby, 1998). Children's ability to do so is associated with more positive interactions with peers (Garner, 1996).

Both linguistic and perceptual perspective taking begin during the preschool years (Westby, 1998). However, cognitive perspective taking develops during the school years (Westby, 1998) and is an important aspect of pragmatics because children's ability to identify others' thoughts and feelings make them more effective communicators. By around age 6, children become more adept in their ability to identify and understand others' feelings and to demonstrate empathy toward the feelings of other individuals (McLaughlin, 2006), although children continue to improve their ability to understand feelings throughout elementary school (Spackman, Fujiki, & Brinton, 2006). By the middle to end of elementary school, students can tell stories from multiple characters' perspectives (Westby, 1998). Children additionally learn to characterize people based on their responses to a social situation between ages 9 and 11 and to analyze and integrate the information they have obtained from more than one social situation between ages 11 and 13 (Westby, 1998).

In addition, children's requests become progressively more polite, or indirect. At age 7, students become more successful in producing indirect requests (e.g., "Can I have a cookie?") (Owens, 2005). At age 8, children can respond to indirect hints (e.g., "It's really cold in here"). Eight-year-olds additionally vary the politeness of their requests. They are more polite when requesting something difficult to do, when they are not from the peer group of the listener, and when they are interrupting the listener's activities (Owens, 2005). However, comprehension of indirect requests may continue to be difficult until later elementary and adolescence (Brice, Miller, & Brice, 2006; Owens, 2005. There also appears to be a developmental hierarchy of indirect request comprehension (Owens, 2005). Requests formed as questions (e.g., "Could you help me?") are more difficult than requests formed as statements (e.g., "You could help me"), and negative requests (e.g., "You should not take that") are more difficult than positive requests (e.g., "You should leave that").

Children's responsiveness to questions improves during the early school years (Bishop, Chan, Adams, Hartley, & Weir, 2000). Children increase their verbal responsiveness to questions, relying less on nonverbal gestures such as head nods or shakes. They also grow in their comprehension of questions and in the specificity of their answers (Bishop et al., 2000). In addition, children become more apt to answer peers' questions in conversation, with only half of the questions in second graders' conversations with peers receiving answers (Dorval & Eckerman, 1984).

School-age children's conversational abilities generally improve with age, although their conversation already resembles adult conversation in many respects (Dorval & Eckerman, 1984). Approximately 90% of second graders' talk is related to others' talk or nonverbal events occurring with the conversation. By comparison, 98% to 99% of fifth graders' verbalizations are related to their conversation. Second graders appear to engage in conversation less to exchange information than to participate in conversation itself, while fifth graders make fewer tangential and unrelated contributions to conversations and are more skilled at returning to topics. However, 8-year-olds tend to discuss concrete topics in conversation, whereas 11-year-olds are able to have sustained, abstract discussions (Miller, 1991; Owens, 2005).

During the school-age years, children also become more proficient in specifying individuals and objects while conversing. They learn to rely more on nouns and less on pronouns to introduce individuals and objects in conversation (Schelletter & Leinonen, 2003).

Second graders include a number of repetitions and insults in their conversations (Dorval & Eckerman, 1984). Second and fifth graders also use minimally related disagreements, storytelling, and directives that do not add additional information to conversation more often than adolescents.

Children's **turn-taking skills** rapidly increase between second and fifth grade. Over half of second graders' dialogues are of 10 turns or less, in comparison to the 65% of fifth graders' dialogues that are over 30 turns (Dorval & Eckerman, 1984).

Children also improve in their ability to make **conversational repairs** when their utterances are misunderstood by listeners (Brinton, Fujiki, Loeb, & Winkler, 1986). Elementary school children typically respond to an initial request for repair with a repetition of their own response. Seven-year-old children usually respond to all requests for clarification appropriately and provide additional specific information on the third request for clarification (e.g., "The girl is swimming in the water" after clarification is requested for "The girl is swimming"). Finally, 9-year-old children often respond to a third request for clarification by defining terms (e.g., "A sleigh is something you sit on to slide on snow"), providing additional background context (e.g., "The boy in the picture is sitting on a chair and eating a muffin"), or talking about the process of repairing their utterance (e.g., "I can't say it better") (Brinton et al., 1986). Children also mature in their ability to consistently detect ambiguous messages (Lloyd, Camaioni, & Ercolani, 1995) from 16% at age 6 to 38% at age 9.

Students' comprehension of figurative language improves during the school years. Both **similes** and **metaphors** involve a comparison of an actual object to a description of an image (Owens, 2005). Similes involve an explicit comparison that usually includes *like* or *as*, as in "He is *as fast as* a speeding bullet." Metaphors have implied comparisons, such as "She is a real *rocket scientist*." As a result, children understand similes more easily than metaphors (Lane & Molyneaux, 1992). Students also grow in their comprehension of **idioms**, or figurative expressions that cannot be analyzed grammatically, such as "Don't pull my leg" or "He really flipped his wig" (Nippold, Moran, & Schwarz, 2001; Owens, 2005). Young school-age children typically interpret **proverbs**, or sayings that state a generally accepted thought or advice, literally, as in "Don't count your chickens before they are hatched" (Owens, 2005).

In general, children have difficulty with figurative language in the early elementary years (van Kleeck, 1994), although some children as young as 5 years of age understand simple similes and metaphors (Nippold & Sullivan, 1987). There is steady improvement between ages 5 and 7 (Lane & Molyneaux, 1992), and older school-age children are more skilled in their use (Owens, 2005). First graders find explaining idioms difficult (Johnson & Anglin, 1995), but fifth graders are more proficient in doing so (Nippold & Rudzinski, 1993). Proverbs are usually the most difficult type of figurative language for elementary school children to comprehend, and their comprehension is literal until adolescence, especially when proverbs are presented out of context (Lane & Molyneaux, 1992).

Another type of nonliteral language is **irony** (Dews & Winner, 1997), in which the speaker intends the opposite of what he or she says. For example, a speaker can say, "He's really fast," to describe a runner who is running slowly. To detect irony, the hearer must infer that the speaker believes the opposite of what he or she is saying. In this example, the hearer must know that the speaker thinks that the runner is slow. In addition, the hearer must understand that the speaker thinks that the hearer believes the opposite of what the speaker is saying. In this case, the hearer must comprehend that the speaker believes that the hearer also thinks that the runner is slow. The complex ability to detect irony begins to appear at about the age of 6.

As children mature, differences in language use emerge between boys and girls (McLaughlin, 2006; Owens, 2005). Kindergarten girls may talk about traditional female roles, while boys converse about a variety of topics. Boys' groups are often larger than girls' groups (Blatchford, Baines, & Pellegrini, 2003), their roles in groups are more hierarchical, and a large part of their relationships is based on actions (Owens, 2005). Games and activities are often the focus that brings them together (Blatchford et al., 2003). In addition, boys often use their conversation and actions to assert themselves (Owens, 2005), especially in their use of directives (Leaper & Smith, 2004), and are often less willing to negotiate (Francis, 1997).

In contrast, girls frequently play in pairs and share in their play (Blatchford et al., 2003). Girls are also more likely to engage in solitary behavior and parallel behavior during play, in which they are engaged in the same activity as another person but do not interact (Blatchford et al., 2003). Girls often come together to converse independently of a game (Blatchford et al., 2003). They confide their personal problems and concerns to their friends and make frequent use of the words *we* and *let's* (Owens, 2005). In addition, they frequently use humor to defuse situations (Francis, 1997). Girls are more likely to use positively responsive language, as in elaborating on a peer's comment, although they can be as assertive as boys when playing in a mixed-gender group (Leaper & Smith, 2004).

Boys and girls may also use different styles to problem-solve with peers (Leman, Ahmed, & Ozarow, 2005). Girls use more collaborative and obliging acts than do boys, who use more controlling acts. In problem solving with children of the opposite gender, girls may attempt to use persuasion to coax boys into agreement, and boys may rely more on negative interruptions. However, as children reach pre-adolescence, both genders generally become more competitive in their conversations, using insults, put-downs, and practical jokes to gain the attention of others and to assert themselves (Owens, 2005).

Care must be taken not to overgeneralize gender differences to children of other socioeconomic classes, races, or ethnicities. In studies done of school-age girls of different cultures and/or socioeconomic backgrounds (Goodwin, 2002; Goodwin, Goodwin, & Yaeger-Dror, 2002), girls have exhibited a highly assertive interactive style with their female peers.

Children also continue in their development of different **conversational registers** or styles. Some conversational rules are explicitly taught, such as the need to say *please* and *thank you*, while others are implicitly learned (van Kleeck, 1994). Children learn to acknowledge a listener's probable interpretation of an event (Pan & Snow, 1999), developing the use of more formal and polite language with teachers and other adults than with peers. In addition, they come to acknowledge an opponent's perspective in an argument and to predict a listener's probable response to a request or a joke (Pan & Snow, 1999). Their knowledge of style shifting is evidenced by an increasing use of modal auxiliaries (e.g., *could you, may I*) (McLaughlin, 2006).

As children progress through elementary and middle school, teachers increasingly use a formal, **expository style** in the classroom, in which information is structured and presented in a logical manner (McLaughlin, 2006). With the exception of language arts, all of the curriculum uses an expository format by junior high school (Westby, 1998). In addition, teacher language in the classroom includes more imperatives for obtaining attention and questions for ascertaining comprehension than less formal speech, which involves the frequent use of declaratives (McLaughlin, 2006).

The use of expository patterns in school texts increases by grade, and texts challenge students to make logical inferences (Westby, 1998). There are different expository patterns in textbooks. **Descriptive patterns** describe something (often signaled by *is similar to* or *refers to*), and **collection patterns** are used to list items that are related (often introduced by *including* and *such as*) (Westby, 1994, cited in McLaughlin, 2006). **Sequence patterns** delineate a sequence of steps or events (often signaled by *first* or *next*), while **comparison patterns** may compare or contrast concepts (often introduced by *although* or *similarly*) (Westby, 1994, cited in McLaughlin, 2006). Finally, **cause-effect patterns** describe the reasons for an occurrence and are often introduced by *therefore* or *because* (Westby, 1994, cited in McLaughlin, 2006). Comparison and sequential patterns may be easier to remember than description and collection patterns, while cause-effect patterns may not be identified until adolescence (Westby, 1998).

Narrative discourse is an important part of elementary school children's experiences. In class, students learn to use narratives in the activity of Show and Tell or sharing (Lane & Molyneaux, 1992). Narratives become an increasingly important type of discourse during the school years in the classroom, which mark important developments in narrative production.

Plots emerge between 5 and 7 years of age and become increasingly clear after age 8 (Stein & Glenn, 1979). By age 9, students produce **focused chains**, in which the sequence of events in a narrative are more focused on a central character, but the character's intentions or internal plans are not included (McLaughlin, 2006). Children at age 9, however, are able to produce all elements of a story grammar, although they continue to use the conjunction *and* as frequently as preschoolers in their narratives (Stein & Glenn, 1979). **Complete narratives** include reciprocal relationships between a character's characteristics, events, and achievement of a goal (McLaughlin, 2006). Not until adolescence can students produce **complex narratives,** in which there are several subplots or embedded episodes (McLaughlin, 2006).

Adolescence: Conversational Discourse

As children move into adolescence, their social and conversational interactions dramatically increase. As a result, several new conversational refinements take place. These include learning how to use strategies such as persuasion and interpersonal negotiation to get listeners to comply with stated requests, reach a stage of mutual agreement, and/or resolve conflict. The development of these conversational skills involves learning how to provide listeners with possible advantages and/or benefits for complying with requests, adjusting persuasion strategies to match listener background, generating varied arguments to support requests, anticipating and replying to counterarguments, using strategies such as politeness and bargaining to persuade, and being able to reason with words (Nippold, 1998). As with other aspects of pragmatics, the skills and means for accomplishing these acts can be culture-specific, depending on the community, settings, individuals, and situations where they are used. As a result, it is important for adolescents to acquire the culture-specific rules, knowledge, and skills associated with each to use these verbal skills.

Communicative Speech Acts and Functions

With respect to language use and function, communicators in their adolescent years are refining their understanding and use of figurative language expressions such as metaphors, similes, idioms, and proverbs. They are becoming increasingly exposed to new, varied forms of academic expository language (e.g., informing, explaining, and debating) that are important to success in the classroom setting. Adolescents are also refining their use of *social registers* (differing styles of speaking used for different communicative partners, speaking situations, and settings). Specifically, they are learning how to effectively use polite versus impolite registers, social group-related registers, intimate versus nonintimate, and gender-based registers (Brice & Montgomery, 1996; McLaughlin, 1998; Munro, 2002; Owens, 2005).

Brice (1992) developed a pragmatics scale (see Chapter 5) for investigating student pragmatics performance in various classroom contexts at a pre-evaluation or screening level. He used this scale to study the pragmatics performance of students from three adolescent groups: monolingual language-disordered, bilingual (Spanish-English-speaking), and monolingual English-speaking general-education students. The findings of his study indicated that the adolescent language-learning-disabled students had difficulties expressing themselves, establishing greetings, initiating and maintaining conversations, and listening to a speaker. These difficulties placed the language-learning-disabled students at risk for following and completing classroom lessons and participating in classroom discussions. The language-learning-disabled students displayed difficulties with spoken language particularly when it involved more grammatical and semantic aspects of language (e.g., describing personal feelings in an acceptable manner).

The bilingual (non-language-learning-disabled) students also displayed difficulties, particularly in making requests of others and in listening to a speaker. Speech-language pathologists (SLPs) and exceptional-education teachers should not provide direct services to normally developing bilingual students (that is, nondisordered). The bilingual students' difficulties placed them at risk for cooperative learning situations in the classroom. Brice (1992) recommended that the teacher coach, model, and possibly instruct the behaviors of making requests and actively listening (to increase listening comprehension and follow-through on tasks). The school professional may offer suggestions about focusing on listening actively. This knowledge may assist in learning the behaviors of making requests. Since many of the behaviors may be affected by an inadequate control of English grammatical structures, Brice (1992) recommended that the SLPs and teachers also focus on the grammatical aspects of language, including syntax, semantics, and morphology, in improving students' pragmatic skills.

In a follow-up study, Brice and Montgomery (1996) investigated the pragmatic performance of students from two adolescent groups: (1) non-language-learning-disabled, English-language-learning (ELL) students receiving English as a second language (ESL) classroom instruction versus (2) bilingual students receiving language therapy. All bilingual students spoke Spanish and English. The Adolescent Pragmatics Screening Scale (APSS) was used to measure their pragmatic performance. The findings of this study indicated that the bilingual language-learning-disabled students differed from the ELL students in expressing themselves, establishing greetings, initiating and maintaining conversations, listening to a speaker, and cueing the listener regarding topic changes. Both groups of students had difficulties regulating others through language. Thus, even bilingual students with no language learning disabilities may exhibit difficulty acquiring this U.S. school pragmatics feature. Academic failure and possible school dropout may be the result for bilingual students with communication disorders who experience these difficulties.

Bilingual students with language-learning disabilities may face alienation from their peers because of their inability to greet others appropriately, to begin and terminate personal discussions, to listen attentively to what others say, and to switch topics of conversation with ease. These problems place these bilingual students enrolled in language therapy at risk for academic failure and possible school dropout (Brice, 1992).

Narratives

Finally, in terms of their narratives, adolescents continue to refine their ability to tell and write stories in accordance with the standards of the cultural community or communities to which they are exposed. Stories become much longer in terms of the number of words used (Hughes, McGillivray, & Schmidek, 1997) and clause length. There is an increased reference to character emotions, mental states, thoughts, plans, and actions. The number of embedded episodes and number of complete episodes also increases (Nippold, 1998).

CONCLUDING REMARKS

The process that children from monolingual language backgrounds follow in acquiring their primary language is a very complex process that involves several different stages and phrases of development across a number of different areas of language development: phonology, morphology, syntax, semantics, and pragmatics. It is also a process that takes place over an extended period of time, from the first year of life into adulthood. As children are acquiring the various aspects of their native language, they are not only acquiring skills that are universal to all child language learners but also skills that are specific to the language or cultural community standards to which they have been exposed. Understanding the process of first language acquisition, the types of skills that are acquired, the sequence in which development proceeds, and the possible cross-linguistic and cultural variations that can occur is important to understanding related issues such as second language acquisition and communication disorder.

CASE STUDY PERSPECTIVES

Case Study One Background: Lela

Lela is a 4-year-old monolingual English-speaking child who, according to her parents, didn't say her first words until approximately 2 years of age. At present, she continues to have a very limited vocabulary of only 15 words. Her parents are concerned about her language development because they feel that she should be using more words to communicate her basic wants and needs. At present, she primarily uses vocalizations and gestures to communicate. Her parents also feel that she should be speaking in sentences by now. She has a medical diagnosis of cerebral palsy.

Observations of Lela's communication skills during play and conversational interactions with her parents revealed the following:

1. As reported by her parents, Lela primarily used gestures and vocalizations to express her basic needs and wants and to make requests. For example, she clapped her hands while looking at her parents to get them to clap their hands with her. She requested objects by reaching for them or pointing to them. She drew attention to objects of interest by pointing to them in books or in the playroom and then looking at her parents. She pointed to her pants to indicate that she needed to use the bathroom.

2. Most of her spoken words were imitated, although there were a few occasions where she was observed to spontaneously (independently) label objects or pictures on her own. All of her spoken communication involved single-word utterances. No multiword utterances were observed.

3. There were at least two occasions when Lela was observed to greet others. She said "hi" when picking up a toy phone. She waved "bye" when leaving her parents to go with the examiners.

4. During speech and language testing, which involved the labeling of pictured objects, Lela was able to imitate many of the words produced by the examiners. When the words were analyzed in terms of speech/sound productions, she displayed the ability to produce

the following sounds in at least one word position: /m, h, n, w, b, k, g, d, t, f, j, l, s/. An analysis of her imitative word productions also revealed use of the following syllable structures: CV, VC, CVC, CVCV, and V.

Case Study One Comments: Lela

Lela obviously displays speech and language delays in a number of areas. She appears to be displaying fairly normal speech/sound (phonological) development. However, she displays definite delays in the areas of semantics, morphology, syntax, and pragmatics. In the area of semantics, she displays limited vocabulary. By this age, Lela should have a spoken vocabulary of approximately 1,000 to 2,000 words. She should also be using single- as well as multiword utterances to convey all of the semantic content categories delineated by Bloom and Lahey (1978) and Lahey (1988).

According to the Brown's (1973) research, Lela should be using many, if not all, of the 14 morphemes identified by Brown as typical of English-speaking preschool language learners. She should also be producing, at minimum, simple sentences with some emerging complex sentence structures.

In the area of pragmatics, Lela should be using primarily words to code, at minimum, all of the primitive speech acts categories delineated by Dore (1978). She should also be starting to exhibit some of Dore's more advanced conversational speech act categories, and she should be starting to produce simple stories with additive and possibly temporal chain sequences.

Case Study Two Background: Jayden

Jayden is a 9-year-old monolingual Mainstream-American-English-speaking student who is currently in the fourth grade. According to his teacher's and parent's observations, Jayden has a number of language and learning difficulties that are affecting his progress in the classroom. At least some of his difficulties appear to be related to underlying attention issues. He has a previous diagnosis of attention deficit hyperactivity disorder (ADHD).

One of Jayden's academic weaknesses is in the area of narratives. According to Jayden's teacher, Jayden has difficulty retelling stories that are complete and easy to follow. He also has difficulties writing narratives that are clear and easy to understand during classroom assignments. Jayden's mother has noticed that when her son is attempting to retell a movie that he has just seen or something that happened during his day at school, his recounts or accounts are somewhat disorganized, and it is not always clear who did what to whom.

Administration of the "Short Narratives" subtest from the *Diagnostic Evaluation of Language Variation* (*DELV*) (Seymour, Roeper, & deVilliers, 2005), a standardized speech and language measure, revealed the following difficulties in Jayden's construction of narratives during testing. He rarely used grammatical forms such as antonyms, adjectives, prepositional phrases, and relative clauses to clearly contrast the actions and traits of characters in his story. He also failed to make explicit references to the thoughts and mental states of characters. Additional sampling of Jayden's narrative retelling skills using the book *Salt in His Shoes* (Jordan & Jordan, 2000), a story written by Michael Jordan's mother about her son's early basketball playing years, revealed difficulties with respect to the following: (1) clearly referencing and distinguishing characters by name; (2) being able to describe key character traits; and (3) including information about character mental states, internal responses, and reactions.

Case Study Two Comments: Jayden

Jayden's difficulties suggest weaknesses on a number of age-appropriate narrative skills and are likely to put him at risk for academic success on age-level state department of education content standards that need to be addressed in his curriculum. For example, if Jayden were a student in a California public school system, he would be at risk for the following fourth-grade-level content standard in the area of Reading (Literary Response and Analysis): "3.3 Use knowledge of the situation, setting, and of a character's traits and motivations to determine the causes for that character's actions" (California Department of Education, 2006).

The most appropriate type of intervention would be one that involves structured classroom narrative construction activities that would improve his ability to correctly identify or state key traits, thoughts, and beliefs expressed by characters within his narratives, as well as to make inferences about what characters might be thinking. Examples of recommended activities include:

1. Reading, writing, or listening to stories about key historical or fictional characters.
2. Prereading discussions that focus on making predictions about upcoming storyline and possible character background information, reactions, and thoughts.
3. Discussions about recently viewed movies, TV shows, or videos, with attention to key character names, background traits, thoughts, actions, and plans.
4. Role-playing situations where Jayden and other students have an opportunity to pretend to be a key character in a story they have read, written about, or seen via video, TV, movies, or a book and to respond to questions posed by others about what that character believes and feels.

INSTRUCTIONAL STRATEGIES

The following instructional and clinical strategies can be used in the general-education classroom or clinical settings, and/or the play setting (in the case of preschoolers).

Preschool-Age Children

1. Use a natural and child-centered approach to language modeling that is incorporated within activities that children are already doing or in which they are showing an interest. For example, if a child is playing with a toy, either label the toy ("truck") or describe something about the toy ("Oooh, a blue truck" or "The truck is moving").
2. Look for opportunities within child-centered routines to naturally improve vocabulary concepts and grammatical skills that children currently lack. For example, if you know that your child needs to work on size concepts, find opportunities to talk about the size of objects that he or she is using or playing with (e.g., "Oh, that's a big train, huh?").
3. Model language that is at an appropriate developmental and age level for the child. If your child is speaking in only one- to two-word utterances, model language using short one-, two-, or three-word utterances.
4. It is not always necessary to make a child repeat what you model for them. Simple exposure to enriched language can be equally powerful.

(continued)

5. Reinforce and encourage verbal productions from children by showing an active and positive interest in what they are talking about by using verbal acknowledgments like "Wow, that's great!" or "Really?"

6. One way to encourage verbal requests from children who do not use words to communicate is to withhold objects from them until they ask for what they want. Give them what they want once they have tried to imitate or say the name on their own at least once, even if it's not perfectly correct.

7. Use scaffolding and modeling to develop pragmatic and social communication skills by demonstrating to children what to say in certain situations. For example, if a child pushes another child who took away a toy, tell the first child something like "You need to tell her with your words that you had it first. Say, 'I had it first.'"

School-Age Children

8. Teach school-age children about inflectional prefixes and suffixes (e.g., *non-*, *dis-*) as well as derivational suffixes (e.g., *-er*, *-y*). Give them words and have them add prefixes or suffixes to form new words. Then have them use the new words in sentences.

9. Teach school-age students how to use sentence context to fast map the meaning of a new vocabulary word (McGregor et al., 2002). For example, have students listen to or read sentences containing new vocabulary words and have them try to figure out the meaning of the word. This exercise is most effective when the sentences used are related to classroom content.

10. When using stories in the classroom or therapy, emphasize characters' feelings and thoughts to develop cognitive perspective taking (Westby, 1998). Have school-age students infer what a character feels and thinks after important events in the story, and ask them why characters acted or reacted in the way they did. At the end of the story, ask students what lessons the characters may have learned from events and whether they believe the characters will continue to behave in the same way in the future. Ask students to explain the basis for their opinions.

11. Talk to school-age children about the importance of conversational etiquette such as staying on topic in conversation and not insulting others. Role-play situations in which conversational rules are violated and ones in which conversational rules are followed.

Adolescents

12. As with school-age students, it is important to make sure that language development goals, activities, and instructional approaches are tied to the curriculum and grade-level state department of education benchmark standards. Once you identify areas of language weakness through educational or speech testing, prioritize intervention and instructional goals to focus on those skills that are most likely to affect their progress toward one of the expected grade-level standards.

13. In the area of pragmatics, it is important for students to develop social communication skills that enable them to communicate effectively with peers, such as learning how to verbally negotiate and persuade.

14. Classroom activities built around understanding common group slang are not only useful for building social communication success with peers but also fun and interesting

for many students. One way to do this is to assign a class project where students have to write down, define, and create a dictionary of current slang vocabulary.

15. Develop language goals that are functional and related to future work needs for students transitioning into the workforce (e.g., emphasize the development of vocabulary and social language registers appropriate for that setting). For example, if you know that a student is going into a trade school that focuses on automotive skills, work on vocabulary associated with that trade. For students who are in the process of interviewing for jobs, discuss, practice, and role-play good communication strategies for partcipating in an interview.

REFLECTION QUESTIONS

1. Think of a child you know who is between the ages of 3 and 4 years. Reflect on some of the speech and language developments discussed in this chapter that are of typical of children who are in that age range. Then write down examples of communicative behaviors that you have observed being used by the child that reflect some of these communication developments.

2. Review some of the word learning strategies typically used by preschoolers to label new or unfamiliar objects or other referents (e.g., people, activities, events, actions). What are some strategies similar to those naturally used by children that you feel teachers can use in the regular classroom to enhance children's vocabulary development?

3. Review Lela's current level of language ability in the areas of semantics and pragmatics (see Case Study One). Identify some possible next-step intervention and/or instructional goals that you feel would be appropriate for Lela's teacher, parents, and school speech-language specialist in each of these areas that would be a logical next step for developing her language skills. The proposed goals should represent a natural developmental approach to intervention/ instruction (starting where she is and moving her to the next level of language development).

4. Six-year-old Tiffany confuses *I* and *me*, and *he*, *she*, *him*, and *her*. How would you prepare a lesson plan to teach her and other students the differences between these pronouns?

5. Justin, a first-grader, produces a mean of 4.01 words per communication unit. How would you prepare a lesson plan to increase the number of words he produces per communication unit?

6. Examine the proposed narrative intervention/instructional goals for Jayden as delineated in the comments section of Case Study Two. Outline an actual language instructional activity that a teacher or speech-language specialist could use in either the classroom or clinical setting to work on one of the proposed goals. Include a detailed discussion of the teaching strategies, activities, and materials that you would use for carrying out your proposed instructional activity.

7. Your 9-year-old students are having a great deal of difficulty understanding their science textbook, which is written in an expository style. They can sound out the words, but they have difficulty comprehending what they read. How would you prepare a lesson plan to teach them techniques for better understanding of expository texts?

REFERENCES

Amayreh, M. M., & Dyson, A. T. (1998). The acquisition of Arabic consonants. *Journal of Speech, Language, and Hearing Research, 41*, 642–653.

Anderson, R. T. (1995). Spanish morphological and syntactic development. In H. Kayser (Ed.), *Bilingual speech-language pathology: An Hispanic focus* (pp. 41–73). San Diego, CA: Singular Publishing Group.

Beck, I., & McKeown, M. (1991). Conditions of vocabulary acquisition. In R. Barr, M. Kamil, P. Mosenthal, & P. Pearson (Eds.), *Handbook of reading research* (Vol. 2, pp. 789–814). White Plains, NY: Longman.

Benelli, B., Arcuri, L., & Marchesini, G. (1988). Cognitive and linguistic factors in the development of word definitions. *Journal of Child Language, 15*, 619–635.

Bernthal, J. E., and Bankson, N. W. (1998). Analysis and interpretation of assessment data. In J. E. Bernthal & N. W. Bankson (Eds.), *Articulation and phonological disorders* (4th ed., pp. 270–298). Boston, MA: Allyn & Bacon.

Bishop, D. V. M., Chan, J., Adams, C., Hartley, J., & Weir, F. (2000). Conversational responsiveness in specific language impairment: Evidence of disproportionate pragmatic difficulties in a subset of children. *Development and Psychopathology, 12*, 177–199.

Blatchford, P., Baines, E., & Pellegrini, A. (2003). The social context of school playground games: Sex and ethnic differences, and changes over time after entry to junior school. *British Journal of Developmental Psychology, 21*, 481–505.

Bloom, L., & Lahey, M. (1978). *Language development and language disorders*. New York: John Wiley & Sons.

Botting, N., & Adams, C. (2005). Semantic and inferencing abilities in children with communication disorders. *International Journal of Language and Communication Disorders, 40*, 49–66.

Brice, A. (1992). The Adolescent Pragmatics Screening Scale: A comparison of language-impaired students, bilingual/Hispanic students, and regular education students. *Howard Journal of Communications, 4*, 143–156.

Brice, A., Miller, K., & Brice, R. G. (2006). Language in the English as a second language and the general education classroom: A tutorial. *Communication Disorders Quarterly, 27*, 240–247.

Brice, A., & Montgomery, J. (1996). Adolescent pragmatic skills: A comparison of Latino students in ESL and speech and language programs. *Language, Speech, and Hearing Services in Schools, 27*, 68–81.

Brinton, B., Fujiki, M., Loeb, D. F., & Winkler, E. (1986). Development of conversational repair strategies in response to requests for clarification. *Journal of Speech and Hearing Research, 29*, 75–81.

Brown, R. (1973). *A first language: The early stages*. Cambridge, MA: Harvard University Press.

Cain, K., Oakhill, J. V., & Elbro, C. (2003). The ability to learn new word meanings from context by school-age children with and without language comprehension difficulties. *Journal of Child Language, 30*, 681–694.

California Department of Education. (2006). *Teaching reading: A balanced, comprehensive approach to teaching reading in pre-kindergarten through grade three*. Sacramento, CA: Author.

Carey, S. (1978). The child as word learner. In M. Halle, J. Bresnan, & G. Miller (Eds.), *Linguistic theory and psychological reality* (pp. 264–297). Cambridge, MA: MIT Press.

Champion, T. B. (2003). *Understanding storytelling among African American children: A journey from Africa to America*. Mahwah, NJ: Lawrence Erlbaum Associates.

Craig, H. K., Washington, J. A., & Thompson, C. A. (2005). Oral language expectations for African American children in grades 1 through 5. *American Journal of Speech-Language Pathology, 14*, 119–130.

Cronin, V. S. (2002). The syntagmatic-paradigmatic shift and reading development. *Journal of Child Language, 29*, 189–204.

deVilliers, J., & deVilliers, P. (1973). A cross-sectional study of the acquisition of grammatical morphemes in child speech. *Journal of Psycholinguistic Research, 2,* 267–278.

Dews, S., & Winner, E. (1997). Attributing meaning to deliberately false utterances: The case of irony. In C. Mandell & A. McCabe (Eds.), *The problem of meaning: Behavioral and cognitive perspectives* (pp. 377–414). Amsterdam, The Netherlands: Elsevier Science.

Dore, J. (1978). Requestive systems in nursery school conversations: Analysis of talk in its social context. In R. Campbell and P. Smith (Eds.)., *Recent advances in the psychology of language: Language development and mother-child interaction* (pp. 343–350). New York: Plenum Press.

Dorval, B., & Eckerman, C. O. (1984). Developmental trends in the quality of conversation achieved by small groups of acquainted peers. *Monographs of the Society for Research in Child Development, 49* (1, Serial No. 206).

Francis, B. (1997). Power plays: Children's constructions of gender and power in role plays. *Gender and Education, 9,* 179–192.

Garner, P. W. (1996). The relations of emotional role taking, affective/moral attributions, and emotional display rule knowledge to low-income school-age children's social competence. *Journal of Applied Developmental Psychology, 17,* 19–36.

Goodwin, M. H. (2002). Building power asymmetries in girls' interaction. *Discourse & Society, 13,* 715–730.

Goodwin, M. H., Goodwin, C., & Yaeger-Dror, M. (2002). Multimodality in girls' game disputes. *Journal of Pragmatics, 34,* 1621–1649.

Green, L. J. (2002). *African American English: A linguistic introduction.* Cambridge, UK: Cambridge University Press.

Guasti, M. T. (2002). *Language acquisition. The growth of grammar.* Cambridge, MA: MIT Press.

Gutierrez-Clellen, V. F., & Quinn, R. (1993). Assessing narratives of children from diverse cultural/linguistic groups. *Language, Speech, and Hearing Services in Schools, 24,* 2–9.

Haynes, W., & Moran, M. (1989). A cross-sectional developmental study of final consonant production in southern black children from preschool through third grade. *Language, Speech, and Hearing Services in Schools, 20,* 400–406.

Hughes, D., McGillivray, L., and Schmidek, M. (1997). *Guide to narrative language: Procedures for assessment.* Eau Claire, WI: Thinking Publications.

Hunt, K. (1970). Syntactic maturity in school children and adults. *Monographs of the Society for Research in Child Development, 35* (1, Serial No. 134).

Hyter, Y. D., & Westby, C. E. (1996). Using oral narratives to assess communicative competence. In A. G. Kamhi, K. E. Pollock, & J. L. Harris (Eds.), *Communication development and disorders in African American children* (pp. 247–284). Baltimore, MD: Paul H. Brookes.

Iglesias, A., & Goldstein, B. (1998). Language and dialectal variations. In J. E. Bernthal and N. W. Bankson (Eds.), *Articulation and phonological disorders,* (4th ed., pp. 148–171). Boston: Allyn & Bacon.

Johnson, C., & Anglin, J. (1995). Qualitative developments in the content and form of children's definitions. *Journal of Speech and Hearing Research, 38,* 612–629.

Jordan, D., & Jordan, R. (2000). *Salt in his shoes: Michael Jordan in pursuit of a dream.* New York: Simon & Schuster Books for Young Readers.

Kuczaj, S. (1979). Influence of contractibility on the acquisition of be: Substantial, meager or unknown? *Journal of Psycholinguistic Research, 8,* 1–11.

Lahey, M. (1988). *Language disorders and language development.* New York: Macmillan.

Lane, V. W., & Molyneaux, D. (1992). *The dynamics of communicative development.* Englewood Cliffs, NJ: Prentice Hall.

Langdon, H. W., & Merino, B. J. (1992). Acquisition and development of a second language in the Spanish speaker. In H. W. Langdon & L. L. Cheng (Eds.), *Hispanic children and adults with communication disorders: Assessment and intervention* (pp. 132–167). Gaithersburg, MD: Aspen.

Larson, V. L., & McKinley, N. L. (2003). *Communication solutions for older students: Assessment and intervention strategies.* Eau Claire, WI: Thinking Publications.

Leaper, C., & Smith, T. E. (2004). A meta-analytic review of gender variations in children's language use: Talkativeness, affiliative speech, and assertive speech. *Developmental Psychology, 40,* 993–1027.

Leman, P. J., Ahmed, S., & Ozarow, L. (2005). Gender, gender relations, and the social dynamics of children's conversations. *Developmental Psychology, 41,* 64–74.

Lewis, D. J., & Windsor, J. (1996). Children's analysis of derivational suffix meanings. *Journal of Speech and Hearing Research, 39,* 209–216.

Lloyd, P., Camaironi, L., & Ercolani, P. (1995). Assessing referential communication skills in the primary school years: A comparative study. *British Journal of Developmental Psychology, 13*, 13–29.

Loban, W. (1976). *Language development: Kindergarten through grade twelve*. Research Report No. 18. Urbana, IL: National Council of Teachers of English.

Marinellie, S. A. (2004). Complex syntax used by school-age children with specific language impairment (SLI) in child-adult conversation. *Journal of Communication Disorders, 37*, 517–533.

Marinellie, S. A., & Johnson, C. (2003). Adjective definitions and the influence of word frequency. *Journal of Speech, Language, and Hearing Research, 46*, 1061–1076.

McCabe, A., & Rollins, P. R. (1994). Assessment of preschool narrative skills. *American Journal of Speech-Language Pathology, 3*, 45–56.

McGregor, K., Friedman, R., Reilly, R., & Newman, R. (2002). Semantic representation and naming in young children. *Journal of Speech, Language, and Hearing Research, 45*, 998–1014.

McLaughlin, S. (1998). *Introduction to language development*. San Diego, CA: Singular.

McLaughlin, S. (2006). *Introduction to language development* (2nd ed.). Clifton Park, NY: Thomson Delmar Learning.

Miller, J. F. (1991). *Assessing language production in children: Experimental procedures*. Boston, MA: Allyn and Bacon.

Munro, P. (2002, April). *What slang can teach us about language*. Paper presented at the annual California State University, Fullerton Linguistics Symposium, Fullerton, CA.

Nippold, M. A. (1995). School-age children and adolescents: Norms for word definition. *Language, Speech, and Hearing Services in Schools, 26*, 320–325.

Nippold, M. A. (1998). *Later language development: The school-age and adolescent years* (2nd ed.). Austin, TX: Pro-Ed.

Nippold, M. A., Hegel, S., Sohlberg, M., & Schwarz, I. E. (1999). Defining abstract entities: Development in preadolescents, adolescents, and young adults. *Journal of Speech, Language, and Hearing Research, 42*, 473–481.

Nippold, M. A., Hesketh, L., Duthie, J., & Mansfield, T. (2005). Conversational versus expository discourse: A study of syntactic development in children, adolescents, and adults. *Journal of Speech, Language, and Hearing Research, 48*, 1048–1064.

Nippold, M. A., Moran, C., & Schwarz, L. (2001). Idiom understanding in preadolescents: Synergy in action. *American Journal of Speech-Language Pathology, 10*, 169–179.

Nippold, M. A., & Rudzinski, M. (1993). Familiarity and transparency in idiom explanation: A developmental study of children and adolescents. *Journal of Speech and Hearing Research, 36*, 728–737.

Nippold, M. A., & Sullivan, M. (1987). Verbal and perceptual analogical reasoning and proportional metaphor comprehension in young children. *Journal of Speech and Hearing Research, 30*, 367–376.

Owen, A. J., & Leonard, L. B. (2006). The production of finite and nonfinite complement clauses by children with specific language impairment and their typically developing peers. *Journal of Speech, Language, and Hearing Research, 49*, 548–571.

Owens, R. E. (2005). *Language development: An introduction* (6th ed.). Boston, MA: Pearson Education.

Pan, B. A., & Snow, C. E. (1999). The development of conversational and discourse skills. In M. Barrett (Ed.), *The development of language* (pp. 229–249). East Sussex, UK: Psychology Press.

Peña-Brooks, A., & Hedge, M. N. (2000). Assessment and treatment of articulation and phonological disorders in children. Austin, TX: Pro-Ed.

Peterson, C., & McCabe, A. (1983). *Developmental psycholinguistics: Three ways of looking at a child's narrative*. New York: Plenum.

Prather, E. M., & Hedrick, D. L. (1975). Articulation development in children aged two to four years. *Journal of Speech and Hearing Disorders, 40*, 179–191.

Redmond, S. M. (2003). Children's productions of the affix *-ed* in past tense and past participle contexts. *Journal of Speech, Language, and Hearing Research, 46*, 1095–1109.

Sander, E. K. (1972). When are speech sounds learned? *Journal of Speech and Hearing Disorders, 37*, 55–63.

Schelletter, C., & Leinonen, E. (2003). Normal and language-impaired children's use of reference: Syntactic versus pragmatic processing. *Clinical Linguistics and Phonetics, 17*, 335–343.

Scott, C. M. (1988a). Producing complex sentences. *Topics in Language Disorders, 8*, 44–62.

Scott, C. M. (1988b). Spoken and written syntax. In M. Nippold (Ed.), *Later language development: Ages nine through nineteen* (pp. 49–95). Austin, TX: Pro-Ed.

Scott, C. M., & Stokes, S. (1995). Measures of syntax in school-age children and adolescents. *Language,*

Speech, and Hearing Services in Schools, 26, 301–319.

Seymour, H. N., Roeper, T. W., & deVilliers, J. (2005). *Diagnostic Evaluation of Language Variation—Norm Referenced.* San Antonio, TX: Harcourt Assessment.

Smith, T. T., Lee, E., & McDade, H. L. (2001). An investigation of T-units in African American English-speaking and Standard American English-speaking fourth-grade children. *Communication Disorders Quarterly, 22,* 148–157.

Spackman, M. P., Fujiki, M., & Brinton, B. (2006). Understanding emotions in context: The effects of language impairment on children's ability to infer emotional reactions. *International Journal of Language and Communication Disorders, 41,* 173–188.

Stein, N., & Glenn, C. (1979). An analysis of story comprehension in elementary school children. In R. Freedle (Ed.), *New directions in discourse processing* (Vol. 2, pp. 53–120). Norwood, NJ: Ablex.

Sutter, J., & Johnson, C. (1990). School-age children's metalinguistic awareness of grammaticality in verb form. *Journal of Speech and Hearing Research, 33,* 84–95.

van Kleeck, A. (1994). Metalinguistic development. In G. Wallach & K. Butler (Eds.), *Language learning disabilities in school-age children and adolescents: Some principles and applications* (pp. 53–98). Boston, MA: Allyn & Bacon.

Verhoeven, L., Aparici, M., Cahana-Amitay, D., van Hell, J., Kriz, S., & Viguié-Simon, A. (2002). Clause packaging in writing and speech: A cross-linguistic developmental analysis. *Written Language & Literacy, 5,* 135–162.

Vogel, I., & Raimy, E. (2002). The acquisition of compound vs. phrasal stress: The role of prosodic constituents. *Journal of Child Language, 29,* 225–250.

Wallach, G. (1984). Later language learning: Syntactic structures and strategies. In G. Wallach & K. Butler (Eds.),

Language learning disabilities in school-age children (pp. 82–102). Baltimore, MD: Williams & Wilkins.

Westby, C. E. (1994). The effects of culture on genre, structure, and style of oral and written texts. In G. P. Wallach & K. G. Butler (Eds.), *Language learning disabilities in school-age children and adolescents* (pp. 180–218). New York: Macmillan.

Westby, C. E. (1998). Communication refinement in school age and adolescence. In W. O. Haynes & B. B. Shulman (Eds.), *Communication development: Foundations, processes, and clinical applications* (pp. 311–360). Englewood Cliffs, NJ: Prentice-Hall.

Wyatt, T. A. (1991). Linguistic constraints on copula production in Black English child speech (Doctoral dissertation, University of Massachusetts, Amherst, 1991). *Dissertation Abstracts International, 52*(2), 781B.

Wyatt, T. A. (1999). An Afro-centered view of communicative competence. In D. Kovarsky, J. Duchan, & M. Maxwell (Eds.). *Constructing (in)competence: Disabling evaluations in clinical and social interaction* (pp. 197–221). Mahwah, NJ: Lawrence Erlbaum.

Wyatt, T. A. (2001). The role of the family, community, and school in children's acquisition and maintenance of African American English. *Sociocultural and historical contexts of African American English.* Amsterdam/Philadelphia: John Benjamins.

Wyatt, T. A., & Seymour, H. N. (1990). The implications of code-switching in Black English speakers. *Equity and Excellence, 24,* 17–18.

Zimmerman, I. L., Steiner, V. G., & Pond, R. E. (2002a). *Preschool Language Scale—Fourth Edition (English).* San Antonio, TX: Psychological Corporation.

Zimmerman, I. L., Steiner, V. G., & Pond, R. E. (2002b). *Preschool Language Scale—Fourth Edition (Spanish).* San Antonio, TX: Psychological Corporation.

Chapter 4

Second-Language Acquisition

Alejandro Brice and Roanne G. Brice

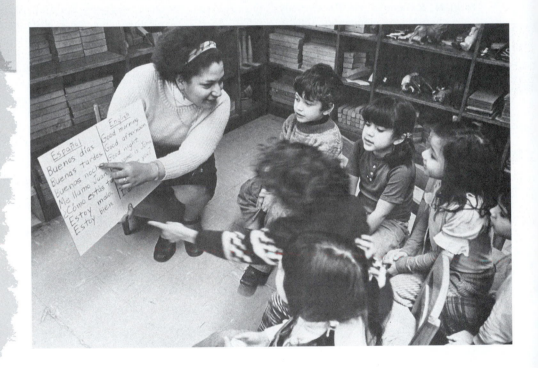

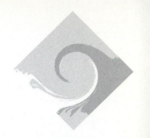

CHAPTER OUTLINE

Introduction

Definitions

Spanish Phonology and Phonological Transfer

Morphological and Semantic Transference

Syntactic and Pragmatic Transference

Case Study Perspectives

Concluding Remarks

INTRODUCTION

One of the largest waves of immigration in United States history took place during the 1990s, filling the nation's schools with the largest-ever influx of students who did not speak English as their first language. A recent U.S. Census Bureau (2000) report indicated that culturally and linguistically diverse (CLD) individuals accounted for up to 80% of the nation's population growth from 1990 to 2000. Of particular interest is the Hispanic population, which has now increased to become the largest minority group in the United States. The U.S. Census Bureau

(2003) reported that from April 1, 2000, to July 1, 2002, the Hispanic population increased by a total of 35.3 million. The U.S. Census Bureau (2001) also stated that 35.7% of Hispanics were less than 18 years of age (i.e., of preschool or school-age populations), compared with 23.5% of non-Hispanic Whites. A large percentage of these young Hispanic children are students who do not have a strong command of English. According to data from the U.S. Department of Education, the number of all English language learning (ELL) students (including Spanish speakers and speakers of other languages) in U.S. schools has almost doubled over the past decade (Padolsky, 2002). In addition, within the past decade, the ELL enrollment has increased at nearly eight times the rate of all student enrollment.

The U.S. Department of Education (2000) reported that in 2000 there were approximately 4 million students learning English, or classified as English language learning (ELL), in the nation's schools. Most of these students were acquiring Spanish as their first language (L1) and English as their second language (L2). The majority (86%) of these Hispanic, Spanish-English-speaking students attended elementary schools, while 14% of these students were in grades 10 through 12 (Zygouris-Coe, 2001). Some reasons for the larger numbers of Hispanic students in elementary school may be higher birth rates, increased immigration, and higher retention rates among Hispanics. Snow, Burns and Griffin (1998), in the National Research Council (1998) report, stated that the fact that ELL students have limited English skills is most likely a factor in the high percentage of Hispanic students who do not succeed in school. A large number of Hispanic children seen in the U.S schools come to school and do not speak English as their first language; thus, they are also at risk for school failure. Consequently, knowledge of Spanish, that is, developmental factors affecting English learning, is important for all professionals who teach, assess, and treat these Hispanic students.

DEFINITIONS

Before a discussion of language factors proceeds, it is necessary to define some key components affecting bilingual language acquisition and development. These components include (1) English-language learner and limited English proficiency; (2) bilingualism; (3) language proficiency; (4) interlanguages, common versus separate underlying proficiencies, BICS, and CALPS; (5) interaction of two languages; (6) fossilization, (7) language transference and interference, and (8) language alternation (including code switching and code mixing).

English-Language Learner and Limited English Proficiency

An **English-language learner (ELL)** is a language minority student whose English-language skills are limited, so that he or she cannot fully profit from instruction delivered entirely in English. The student's curriculum requires some type of program modification (Baca & Cervantes, 1998). ELL is a term that is often used in place of the term *limited english proficient (LEP)*.

Limited english proficient (LEP) is a lack of facility, fluency, or linguistic competence in English relative to a fluent native English speaker (Hamayan & Damico, 1991).

Note that this term is commonly used by federal, state, and local education agencies to identify students who are English-language learners. Throughout this chapter, the term *English-language learners* will be used to designate those students who are not fully competent in the English language.

The terms *first language* and *second language* are sometimes referred to as either L1 or L2. **L1** designates the first or native language, while **L2** designates the second language acquired.

Bilingualism

Students who possess fluency in more than one language may show proficiency levels from minimum ability in one language to complete fluency in both languages (Gutierrez-Clellen, 1999). Language is more than its oral component, that is, speaking. Professionals in schools tend to view language according to the different domains of speaking, listening, reading, and writing (Brice & Rivero, 1996; Brice, 2004b). **Bilingualism** is defined here as the ability to speak, listen, read, and/or write in more than one language with varying degrees of proficiency.

Language Proficiency

Language proficiency refers to a person's level or ability to listen, speak, read, and write in a language. Language proficiency can be categorized along multiple levels (Skutnabb-Kangas, 1981). Measurement of language dominance seems to be universally questioned by experts in the field and has lost favor to measurements of language proficiency (Döpke, 1992; Miller, 1988). One needs to ask if one language is really dominant for all aspects of communication (i.e., speaking, listening, reading, writing). Therefore, measuring proficiency in each of the child's languages (e.g., Spanish and English) seems to be a better indicator of overall ability than dominance.

A bilingual student may exhibit one of five degrees or levels of proficiency. (We are not limited to five; however, these seem to be the most basic levels.) An **L1 advantaged** speaker shows proficiency in Spanish, yet very little proficiency in English. This corresponds to someone performing at a low level in English (0–2 on the International Second Language Proficiency Rating [ISLPR] system; Wylie & Ingram, 1999). An **L2 advantaged** speaker shows the opposite, with proficiency in English but not in Spanish. A **balanced advantaged** speaker shows a high degree of proficiency in both English and Spanish. The level of proficiency is at a level of 3 or higher on the ISLPR (Wylie & Ingram, 1999). A **mixed advantaged** speaker shows limited proficiency in both languages (e.g., 2 on the ISLPR), whereas a **bilingually disadvantaged** speaker shows minimal proficiency, less than 2 on the ISLPR, in both Spanish and English. This speaker may demonstrate 0 to 0+ abilities on the ISLPR (Wylie & Ingram, 1999), and may appear to be language disordered or language-learning impaired (LLI) to the speech-language pathologist, special education teacher, or the classroom teacher. The student's low ability may or may not be the result of a language disorder/impairment in both languages. Consequently, this determination must be made through extensive language testing in both languages.

Interlanguages, Common Versus Separate Underlying Proficiencies, BICS, and CALPS

Interlanguages (ILs) are approximations of the target language (L2) (e.g. English in the United States, Canada, Australia, and the United Kingdom) when it is still being learned. In this case, the interlanguage would be an approximation of English. The IL would show errors because the learner is still in the process of acquiring English. Children who have not quite developed a proficiency in the second language may be still be using an interlanguage system or approximation of English (Selinker, 1991). Selinker stated the strong interlanguage transference hypothesis (to be defined later in this chapter) to be where "non-native (NN) speaking students do not learn to produce second languages; what they do in fact is to create and develop ILs in particular contexts" (p. 23). Several different interlanguages may co-exist, and each interlanguage may be used for specific purposes.

According to Cummins (1984), "a 'common underlying proficiency' is hypothesized to underlie the surface manifestations of both L1 and L2 and make possible transfer of cognitive and academic skills across languages" (p. 6). In essence, **common underlying proficiencies (CUPs)** allow for knowledge attained in one language to be transferred to the other (i.e., language transference). **Separate underlying proficiencies (SUPs)** refer to the inability of the two languages to interact and transfer information (i.e., language interference). Refer to the section later in this chapter on language transference and interference. See Figure 4–1 for an illustration of Cummins's CUP and SUP models.

FIGURE 4–1
Common Underlying Proficiencies Versus Separate Underlying Proficiencies

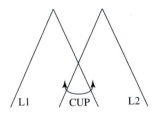

Common Underlying Proficiencies

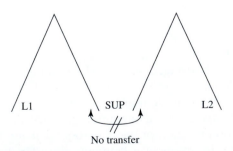

Separate Underlying Proficiencies

Source: Cummins, (1984)

An extension of the common underlying proficiencies (CUPs) model is useful to the following discussions. Refer to Figure 4–2. Cummins's original model is seen in **Stage D** of the new extended model. It should be noted that his model illustrates the terminal stage of dual language development. Children begin language learning with **Stage A**. Here, children show an underdeveloped first language, that is, a language system still in acquisition. As can be seen in the new model, second language acquisition or development is not immediate and appears to move through various stages of development. As also can be seen in this model, **Stages B and C** illustrate the evolution of the interlanguages until a fully developed L2 has emerged in **Stage D**.

Culturally and linguistically different children and students initially learning a second language are typically able to function only in quadrant A (context embedded and cognitively undemanding). Language of this type is what Cummins (1984) refers to as **basic interpersonal communication skills (BICS)**. BICS is oral language or language that one uses in conversation with others.

Language in quadrant D (context reduced and cognitively demanding) is language that is typically used in classrooms. It has an academic language orientation: it is language used in a typical learning environment. Cummins refers to students using language in this realm as having **cognitive academic language proficiency (CALP)** abilities. Students who learn English as a second language typically acquire oral language proficiency (BICS) in two or three years' time (quadrants A and B), while academic language (CALP) may require between five and seven years or up to ten years to acquire (quadrant D) (Collier, 1987; Cummins, 1984; Cummins, 1999; Thomas & Collier, 2002). The ability to use language may vary according to the length of time a student has been in the country and the degree of environmental cues presented.

It should be noted that, generally, second-language learners acquire oral conversational skills in English prior to acquiring academic English-language skills. However, high levels of academic language occasionally can precede attainment of fluent oral language. An example of this would be a student who can read in English before he or she can speak fluently. Yet phonological skills in the second language seem to reach a plateau in a child's first ten years of speaking a second language (e.g., English)

FIGURE 4–2

Stages of Second-Language Growth: Interlanguages and Common Underlying Proficiencies

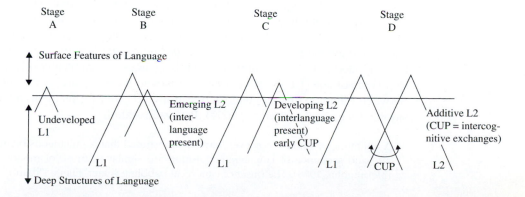

(Cummins, 1999). However, vocabulary knowledge (i.e., semantics), morphology, syntax, pragmatics, literacy, and other cognitively demanding aspects of language continue to develop. An instructional program for bilingual students where language growth is viewed as vital would emphasize growth in cognitive skills, academic topics, and critical language skills.

Interaction of Two Languages

The issue of how and when the second language should be learned has long been debated. Should children learn two languages simultaneously, or should they learn them in sequential fashion? Should the two languages be kept separate or allowed to be used in conjunction with each other? Patterson (1999) concludes that "families should be supported in their choice of either language input strategy" (p. 37). However, Wong-Fillmore (1992) stated that for English to be added to the native language and not replace it, a well-developed native language has to be in place. She also indicated that societal pressures to learn English and societal pressures to assimilate are prevalent. Hence, the notion of bilingual education may be questioned by some educators. However, maintenance of the home language and native culture is important to children's self-esteem and building a strong language foundation (Brice, 2002; Wong-Fillmore, 1992).

Parents of English-language-learning children may not be aware of proper educational decisions affecting their children. Parents may ask school personnel for guidance in this area. They may want their children to succeed and therefore may allow English to be used in the home as the language of communication (Wong-Fillmore, 1992). Parents of English-language-learning children may need to be encouraged to be educated consumers of education and also to seek to maintain the use of their native language in the home. The issue of how two languages are acquired is discussed next.

Second-language acquisition may occur in two ways: that is, simultaneously (referred to as simultaneous acquisition) or sequentially (i.e., sequential acquisition) (Brice, 2002). **Simultaneous acquisition** occurs when the first or home language (L1) is acquired about the same time as the L2. The child may learn Spanish and English in the home at the same time. An example is where the father may speak English to the child and the mother may speak Spanish to him or her. This has been referred to as the one-parent-one-language rule (Patterson, 1999). Also, under simultaneous acquisition, both languages are usually acquired prior to 3 years of age (McLaughlin, 1995). McLaughlin also stated that children exposed to two languages before 3 years of age were to be considered simultaneous language learners and older children as successive language learners. The term *bilingual first-language acquisition* has also been applied to the situation when both languages are simultaneously acquired prior to 3 years of age (De Houwer, 1990). However, most researchers do not distinguish between bilingual first-language acquisition and other forms of simultaneous acquisition (Brice, 2002; Patterson, 1999). Patterson stated:

> A multitude of studies, however, have demonstrated that simultaneous bilingual children's rate and sequence of language acquisition are similar to those of monolingual children (McLaughlin, 1988). The onset of canonical babbling (Oller, Eilers, Urbano, & Cabo-Lewis,

1997), use of first words (Doyle, Champagne, & Segalowitz, 1978), expressive vocabulary spurts (Pearson & Fernandez, 1994), onset of word combinations (Patterson, 1998), and the acquisition of a wide range of syntactic structures and grammatical morphemes (De Houwer, 1995) occur at the same age, and in the same sequence in bilingual as in monolingual children (p. 33).

Therefore, it appears that simultaneous acquisition of two languages is not detrimental to a child's language growth in either of the two languages.

Sequential acquisition occurs when the native language is acquired first, followed by learning of the second language. The second language is typically acquired after 3 years of age (McLaughlin, 1995). It would also appear that children acquiring language sequentially are not at risk for language delays. It has been frequently noted that there are changes in the ease of language acquisition with age. According to Lenneberg (1967), the difficulty in acquiring language after the early teens suggests that there is a critical period for language learning. To test this hypothesis, many researchers have undertaken studies to examine the relationship between age and the second-language acquisition process (Johnson & Newport, 1989). For second-language learners, early versus late learning depends on two main variables, that is, age upon arrival (AOA) (i.e., at what age did the child come to the new country?) and length of residence (LOR) in the new country (i.e., how long has the child been living in the new country?).

Most of these studies have focused on the early stages of learning and tend to show an initial adult advantage in both phonology (Asher & Price, 1967; Olson & Samuels, 1973; Snow & Hoefnagel-Hohle, 1977) and syntax (Snow & Hoefnagel-Hohle, 1977). This suggests that adults move toward second-language proficiency more quickly (Johnson & Newport, 1989) than do children. However, when studies focused on eventual proficiency or ultimate language attainment in the second language, an advantage was seen in both phonology (Asher & Garcia, 1969; Seliger, Krashen, & Ladefoged, 1975; Oyama, 1976) and syntax (Oyama, 1976; Patkowski, 1980) for subjects who began learning in childhood (Johnson & Newport, 1989).

Some studies have specifically investigated child–adult differences in the ultimate or final attainment of grammar (Patkowski, 1980; Oyama, 1976; Johnson & Newport, 1989). Patkowski (1980) assessed participants' syntactic ability by assigning syntactic ratings to written transcripts of the participants' speech from tape-recorded interviews. Results from the analysis of variance showed that age of arrival (AOA) (age at which participants came to the United States and were exposed to English) was the only significant predictor of syntactic proficiency. Oyama (1976) measured participants' ability to repeat spoken English sentences that had been masked with white noise. Results from this study matched those of Patkowski's study; age of arrival was the only significant predictor of test performance. The other variables investigated in these studies included exposure to English in natural versus classroom settings, motivation, self-consciousness, and cultural identification. Johnson and Newport (1989) used a grammaticality judgment task to test whether young children are better second-language learners than adults and consequently achievers of higher levels of final proficiency in the second language. Results of the study demonstrated a strong advantage for earlier arrivals over the later arrivals (Johnson & Newport, 1989). Although these studies used very different measures of English proficiency, they complement each other well because each emphasized a different aspect of language use (processing in comprehension, free production, and underlying grammatical competence via sentence judgments). Results from these studies provide strong evidence for the conclusion that children are more successful in their ultimate attainment of a second language; however, adults are also capable of acquiring second languages with high levels of proficiency. One point, however, is typically conceded in the early-versus-late language-learning debate. Krashen, Long, and Scarcella (1992) stated, "Pronunciation is one aspect of language learning where the younger is better hypothesis may have validity." This would explain why some individuals have accents in English even after many years of speaking English.

In conclusion, there does not appear to be a critical period for second-language learning, although there may be sensitive periods for optimal learning or windows of opportunity for best learning. Nonetheless, learners can typically acquire most features of a second language, given appropriate input, motivation, and opportunities to practice their second language. Acceptance of the Lenneberg (1967) hypothesis is highly questioned.

General characteristics that involve both types of language acquisition (i.e., simultaneous or sequential) include (1) the influence of one language on the other, especially when one is favored outside the home (e.g., English); (2) avoidance of difficult words and constructions in the weaker language; and (3) rapid shifts in dominance of either language with environmental shifts (e.g., returning to Puerto Rico) (Wong-Fillmore, 1992). The key to dual-language development is the continuous use of the two languages by parents and caregivers within their home environments (Patterson, 1999).

Lambert (1977) defined two basic types of bilingual learning effects resulting from bilingual language development, that is, subtractive and additive bilingualism. **Subtractive bilingualism** occurs when, at some stage, the development of the native language (L1) is displaced by the more prestigious dominant language (L2). The first language is subtracted from language abilities. **Additive bilingualism** is when another language (L2) is added to the native language (L1), with neither in jeopardy of being lost. The second language is added to the first.

When children are exposed to two languages, what happens to the language of the home? What happens when English becomes the language of the home? Should children have intensive English teaching when they are English-language learning (ELL)? These are complex questions. The answers may not always be definitive.

Wong-Fillmore (1991) stated that English can often replace the language of the home "especially when the second language is promoted in a way that suggests that it is more socially desirable and valued than their primary language" (p. 14). Children are encouraged to speak only English and not speak their native language when instruction in school is entirely in English and when the child is told not to speak Spanish at school. As a consequence, children may not actively maintain their native language.

Certain problems are most likely to occur when English becomes the language of the home and the parents are not proficient in English. This occurs often when parents are told that switching to English at home may help their children become more proficient in English. The parents may lose the best avenue of communication with their child, especially if the parents are not English-proficient. Wong-Fillmore (1991) also stated that if **L1 attrition** (language loss) occurs when it is the only language the parents speak, then the "children stand to lose much of what the parents can teach them" (p. 14). This point was also addressed by Ortiz (1991) when she noted that, if parents who are not proficient in English speak only English to their children, then they may be limiting their children's cognitive development. In addition, the parents may teach a model of English that will need to be corrected and may cause the child to appear as language-learning disabled (LLD).

Fossilization

Roseberry-McKibbin (1995) stated, "Fossilization occurs when specific second language 'errors' remain firmly entrenched despite good proficiency in the second language (Pica, 1994)" (p. 132). **Fossilization** of sounds, words, phrases, or sentences can be idiosyncratic to a child or it can be a common language practice within a child's or adult's language community. An example in Spanish would be *El gobierno reducio el impuesto* ("the government reduced the taxes"). The correct grammatical form would be *El gobierno redujo el impuesto*. An example in English would be "I *seen* you playing at the ball game last night." Although individuals may be exposed to more grammatically correct language, they may persist in using the incorrect form. Thus, fossilized forms are defined as being resistant to change despite modeling and instruction.

Language Transference and Interference

Language transference is the cross-linguistic effect or influence that two or more languages have on each other. Transfer may occur in either direction, that is, between the first (native, L1) and second language (L2), or between the second and first language. Transfer may be positive or negative. **Positive transfer** occurs when one of the languages has a facilitating effect on abilities in the other language, while **negative transfer** (sometimes referred to as **interference**) occurs when one language does not help or facilitate exchange of information to the other language. An example of positive transference is a child learning to read in English after he or she has already become capable of reading in Spanish. The Spanish-speaking student already had skills of print awareness (e.g., how to hold a book, left-to-right orientation of words on the page, the symbolism of words, etc.), phonological awareness, phonemic awareness, phonics skills, oral and written vocabulary associated with reading, fluency in reading, and comprehension of what was read. Hence, the English-language-learning student would simply have to transfer many of these skills to learning the new language. An example of interference is when the student says, "This house no is my" when he or she wished to say, "This is not my house."

Cummins (1979) popularized the notion of a strong **positive transference hypothesis** or **interdependence hypothesis** (i.e., the two languages are interdependent with each other) when he stated:

> When the usage of certain functions of language and the development of L1 [native language] vocabulary and concepts are strong, as in the case in most middle-class children in immersion programs, then the intensive exposure to L2 is likely to result in high levels of L2 [second language] competence at no cost to L1 competence (p. 233).

Cummins's notion of a strong positive transference hypothesis is reflected in his terminology of common underlying proficiencies (CUPs) versus separate underlying proficiencies (SUPs). Cummins (1984) strongly supports the common underlying proficiency model, as reflected in his comments that "a theoretical model of bilingual proficiency is proposed in which a 'common underlying' proficiency is hypothesized to underlie the surface manifestations of both L1 and L2 and make possible transfer of cognitive/academic skills across languages" (p. 6).

Cummins (1979) cited the example of middle-class majority-language children (Canadian-English-speaking students learning French) who demonstrated an ability to extract meaning from printed text. He proposed that this ability can be transferred from one language (English) to another (French). For the English-language-learning student, the primary academic task is learning how to extract information efficiently from printed text. As Cummins stated, subsequent school progress depends on how well this task is accomplished.

Cummins's positive transference hypothesis (1984) predicts that older learners, who are more cognitively mature, are better at acquiring a second language (L2) proficiently. His theory seems to suggest that older children's underlying proficiency in their first language assists with the process of second-language acquisition. Thus, Cummins states that, for older students, skills and concepts acquired in the native language transfer to English in an accelerated process (McLaughlin, 1988; Skutnabb-Kangas, 1981). Note that this idea is not widely accepted, and the concept of sensitive language periods for young or older language learners is still being researched.

Current investigations do not refute language transference; however, they support a model where skills and information do not readily and easily transfer. Hence, a **weaker transference model** is proposed (Brice & Rivero, 1996; Carson, Carrell, Silberstein, Kroll, & Kuehn, 1990; Hakuta, 1986; Major, 1992; Pica, 1994). Hakuta (1986) questioned the value of the dichotomy of interdependent (strong transference) versus independent (little or no transference) language use. He stated, "The real question is the identification of the conditions under which the two languages maintain separation and those under which they are apparently merged" (pp. 94–95). Carson et al. (1990) stated that the pattern and strength of language transference varies according to the person's first language background, educational level, and personal background. Thus, it appears that several nonlinguistic factors may affect transference skills.

Language Alternation

Communication in English can be a barrier for English-language-learning students because English serves as a content subject and also as the means of instruction. One manner of overcoming this communication (language) barrier is for bilingual students to alternate use of their two languages (referred to as **language alternation**) as a bridge between their two languages (Brice, 2002; Faltis, 1989). Language alternation can consist of code switching or code mixing (Brice, 2002).

According to Aguirre (1988), code switching in the classroom is obvious and unavoidable with bilingual children, and school professionals should regard code switching as examples of communication strategies employed by students. Unfortunately, true understanding of language alternation behaviors is possessed by few speech-language pathologists, special educators, and general education teachers. Cheng and Butler (1989) stated, "Professionals in speech-language pathology have viewed the use(s) of . . . code-switching as indicators for relative proficiency or, on occasion, as the lack thereof. Some practitioners view code-switching as a symptom of language deficiency" (p. 293). Clearly, speech-language pathologists (SLPs) and teachers need to continually increase their understanding of second-language acquisition issues such as the interrelationship between two languages used by culturally and linguistically diverse (CLD) bilingual students.

Language alternation can be divided into the two linguistic categories of **code switching** (CS) and **code mixing** (CM) (Brice, Mastin, & Perkins, 1997; Kamwangamalu, 1992). Language alternation across sentence boundaries is known as intersentential code switching (CS), while language alternation within a sentence is known as intrasentential code mixing (CM) and has been referred to as intrasentential alternation (Brice, Mastin, & Perkins, 1997; Grosjean, 1982; Torres, 1989). In code switching, the student may say, "I know a lot of people that are smart. Como ellos dicen siempre [Like they always say]." Thus, the transition from the English sentence of people being smart to the Spanish sentence of "Like they always say" constitutes an intersentential (i.e., across sentences), code-switched language alternation. Embedded words, phrases, and sentences from two languages can also be found within sentences, forming an intrasentential (i.e., within a sentence), code-mixed language alternation. For example, the student or teacher may incorporate words or phrases into her or his English from another language. She or he may say, "They will be speaking Spanish and my dad will say que el es Cubano y esposa es Portorriquena [that he is Cuban and his wife is Puerto Rican]." Another example of code mixing is when the teacher says, "Do you know what *traer* [to bring] means?"

In sum, use of language alternation by itself is not indicative of a language disorder (Brice, 2002; Cheng & Butler, 1989; Reyes, 1995). On the contrary, language alternation in the proficient bilingual speaker's discourse indicates his or her knowledge of the two languages, including the semantic, morphological, syntactic, and pragmatic dimensions of both languages. Most important, it can be argued that the code-mixed combination of English and Spanish constitutes a unique third language form. Language alternation (e.g., code switching, or code mixing) in some individuals may indicate a sophisticated exhibition of sound cognitive and linguistic functioning.

This review has examined various phenomena common to bilingual speakers acquiring a second language. What should have become evident is the complex nature of how the two languages interact and influence each other. The rest of this chapter is devoted to an understanding of phonological, morphological, semantic, syntactic, and pragmatics development between Spanish and English. Two case studies, along with strategies for eliciting language, will be presented.

Phonological transference is the beginning point to illustrate the influence of Spanish on learning English. In addition, phonological transference between Spanish and English has not been extensively investigated. Therefore, a discussion of Spanish phonology and phonological transfer follows.

SPANISH PHONOLOGY AND PHONOLOGICAL TRANSFER

"**Phonology** [emphasis added] is the study of the speech-sound system, including the rules and patterns by which the phonemes (speech sounds) are combined into words and phrases (Moats, 2000)" (Brice, 2004a, p. 39). Hence, phonology refers to rules governing how sounds can be combined in making words (Bernthal & Bankson, 1998). Speech-language pathologists, special educators, and other language professionals require current information about Spanish phonology to provide appropriate assessment and therapeutic intervention for English-language-learning children (Brice & de la Paz, 1997; Goldstein, 1995; Goldstein & Iglesias, 1996). Goldstein (1995) stated:

> Due to a lack of information on phonological acquisition in the Latino population in general and across the various Spanish dialects in particular, speech-language pathologists face a difficult task in providing appropriate diagnostic and intervention services to Spanish speaking children (p. 18).

Fantini (1985) conducted a longitudinal investigation of his own son's bilingual language (Spanish and English) development from birth to 5 years of age. His son, Mario, was a sequential bilingual learner; that is, he was not exposed to English until he was approximately 2 and a half years of age (Fantini, 1985). What is of interest here is Mario's early Spanish phonetic and phonological acquisition. Fantini reported that Mario was able to acquire all the basic vowels and consonants for Spanish by 2 years 7 months. However, he did not have the sounds of /r/ and /R/ (tap and trill r's in the words "da*r*" and "ca*rr*o"). Tap sounds are similar to stop sounds but consist of shorter duration. Trills have been described as vibrants and are what the layperson thinks of when the Spanish *r* is mentioned. Fantini reported that these two sounds are (not surprisingly) acquired late "for it is well known to be the last sound acquired by monolingual Spanish-speaking children" (p. 131). Unfortunately, a paucity of studies dealing with normal and disordered Spanish phonology exists. However, several existing studies will be discussed next.

Normal Spanish Phonology

Only a few studies have examined normal Spanish phonological development (Diamond, 1983; Martinez, 1986; Rivera-Umpierre, 1988; Paulson, 1991). Three of these four studies (Diamond, 1983; Martinez, 1986; and Paulson, 1991) used Mexican Spanish speakers for their sample, while Rivera-Umpierre used Puerto Rican Spanish speakers in her study. A brief description of each study will be presented.

Diamond (1983) studied normally developing 4-year-old bilingual Mexican-American children in San Diego, California. She used the *Assessment of Phonological Processes—Spanish (APP—S)* developed by Hodson (1985). Diamond found that consonant sequence reduction (e.g., "br" to "b_") was the most prevalent omission process, with tap/trill /r, R/ deviation also a frequent omission process. She concluded that the phonological performance of the bilingual children "appeared to approximate closely the speech of adult models in their community" (p. 93).

Martinez (1986) also studied normal Mexican-American Spanish phonological development in San Diego, California. However, her study employed younger 3-year-old children. Ten children served as the participants, with ages ranging from 3:6 to 3:11. She also used the *APP—S* for data collection. Percentage-of-occurrence scores were as follows: (1) tap/trill /r, R/, 37%; (2) consonant sequence reduction, 16%; (3) postvocalic singletons (i.e., consonants following a vowel), 8%; (4) lateral

(l) and stridents (e.g., /s, z, ʃ/), 7%; (5) syllable reduction, 6%. Velars, glides, nasals, and prevocalic singletons (consonants preceding the vowel) were all at or below 4%. The high percentage-of-occurrences errors for the tap/trill /r, R/ and postvocalic singletons appeared to be due to the Mexican Spanish dialect and were not considered to be phonological errors. These errors were thought to be negative transference (interference) errors. Canfield (1981) noted the occurrence of vowel reduction in unstressed syllables in highland Mexico, and hence most of Mexico. This feature appears to occur quite frequently in Mexican Spanish and may yield some deletions affecting postvocalic deletions. The fact that the tap/trill /r, R/ had high percentage-of-occurrence scores also indicates that it is an aspect of Mexican Spanish phonology.

Rivera-Umpierre (1988) studied ten 3-year-old and ten 4-year-old Puerto Rican Spanish-speaking children. She also utilized the *APP—S* protocol. The results from her study indicated that substitutions of /l/ for /r/ and substitutions of posterior fricatives for the Puerto Rican /r/ occurred. According to Canfield (1981), these are normal Puerto Rican Spanish occurrences. Stridency deletion of word final /s/ also affected phonological process scores. Canfield (1981) stated, "/s/ syllable final tends to be aspirated or dropped entirely" in Caribbean dialects of Spanish (p. 79).

Paulson (1991) studied three groups of Mexican Spanish-speaking children ($n = 30$) in Dallas–Fort Worth, Texas. The group ages were 2:4 to 2:8, 3:1 to 3:5, and 3:10 to 4:2. She also used the *APP—S* test. Her immediate findings were that the phonological processes most affected were consonant sequence reduction, tap/trill /r, R/ sounds, and strident sounds. As noted above, processes with the tap/trill /r, R/ and stridents are highly affected by the Mexican Spanish dialect and are not necessarily disordered phonological processes. In sum, several phonological processes are influenced by Mexican and Puerto Rican dialects of Spanish, including tap/trill sounds; postvocalic singleton omissions, particularly /s/ finals; and strident omissions. The phonological process of consonant sequence reduction appears to be a phonological deficiency that is common to both the Mexican and Puerto Rican Spanish dialects. Refer to Table 4–1 for a summary of these features.

Phonetic and Phonological Transference

Phonological transfer refers to the ability of phonological processes to migrate from one language to another. Features that are easily capable of transferring from Spanish to English include some consonants that are shared between both languages, including:

1. The English consonants of /t ʃ, f, s, m, n, p, and k/ can transfer to Spanish in unaspirated productions (unaspirated sounds do not release a puff of air associated with its production) (Lafford & Salaberry, 2003; Stockwell & Bowen, 1965; Whitely, 2002).
2. The English and Spanish /b, d, g/ can be transferred; however, Spanish has allophonic variations of both /b/ and /g/ (allophones are variations of a sound that do result in a change in meaning) . The allophonic variations of /b/ include /β/, a bilabial voiced fricative, while the variation of /g/ includes a voiced glottal /ɡ/.

TABLE 4–1
Comparison and Contrast of Spanish Versus English Phonology

Spanish Phonology	English Phonology
1. Dialect is primarily affected by consonantal changes seen in fricatives, liquids, and nasals.	1. English dialects are primarily affected by vowel differences.
2. Spanish has few single-syllable words.	2. English has many single-syllable words.
3. Spanish is more syllable timed. Stress is present or absent.	3. English is more stressed timed. English is more complicated in stress.
4. Spanish syllables and words tend to end with vowels. In Spanish /s, z/ are the only fricatives allowed in the final position of words. Other sounds that end in Spanish words include /r/ and nasals.	4. Most English words and syllables end with consonants. English has 20 or more consonants that end in the syllable final position.
5. Spanish /s/ is a high-frequency-occurring sound found in single syllables *(los, las, ellos, ellas, estos, estas)*.	5. The English voiced "th" /ð/ tends to occur with high frequency, as seen in function words and articles *(the, this, that, those, there)*.
6. Spanish does not have many true consonant clusters. The consonants are contiguous and typically occur at intersyllable boundaries.	6. English has many true consonant clusters.
7. Syllable initial positions are more tense, while syllable final positions tend to be more lax and prone to aspiration, deletion, or reduction (Madrid → Madri_; mas → ma_). Morphological marking occurs in articles, nouns, pronouns, verb tenses, and adjectives. Final syllable production is not as critical as in English.	7. Word final positions tend to mark morphological marking and are important to meaning.
8. Consonantal productions are generally more tense (precise) than English.	8. Consonantal productions are generally more lax than in Spanish.

Source: Developed by A. Brice & R. Brice.

Spanish and English vary on some consonantal and vocalic elements. Specifically, Spanish has fewer vowels and consonants than does English. Spanish has 21 consonants, while English has 24 consonants (Garn-Nunn & Lynn, 2004; Stockwell & Bowen, 1965; Whitley, 2002). In addition, Spanish does not contain the following consonant sounds in the final position of words: /p, b, f, v, tʃ, and m/. Most Spanish words tend to end with /r, s, d, n, l/, or vowels. In addition, Spanish sounds tend to be more frontally produced in the oral cavity, as evidenced in the sibilant sound /s/, stop or stop/obstruent sounds /t, d/, and other sounds /n, l, r/ (Canfield, 1981; Whitely, 2002). Spanish has additional sounds of the tap /r/, trill or vibrant /R/, and the nasal /ñ/. Spanish does not possess the English sound of /ʃ/, with the most common substitution by English-language learners consisting of /tʃ/ for the /ʃ/ sound (Goldstien & Iglesias, 1996). All Spanish dipthongs (where two vowels are pronounced as one) involve a glide where the tongue moves farther than it does for English dipthongs (Stockwell & Bowen, 1965; Whitely, 2002). Spanish consonants in the syllable final position tend to be lax and subsequently aspirated (i.e., a puff of slightly audible air is released in place of the phoneme) or deleted (Brice & de la Paz, 1997). As a result, differences between Spanish and English may cause difficulties for young children in the perception, discrimination, and production of phonemes necessary for speaking. Consequently, some separate underlying proficiencies or interference features between Spanish and English phonology or phonetics occur, including:

1. Spanish has something that resembles the English /ð/ as an allophone of /d/ (Stockwell & Bowen, 1965). The "th" sounds /ð, θ/ may become /d/ or /f/.

2. Spanish has allophones of /b/ and /ß/ and /g/ and /g̱/ (glottal) (Stockwell & Bowen, 1965).

3. Spanish sounds tend to be more frontally (forward) produced, as evidenced in the sibilant sound /s/; stop or obstruent sounds /t, d/; and other sounds /n, l, r/.

4. Spanish syllables end with fricatives of /s/; nonfricative endings, including nasals; and /r/ (Eblen, 1982).

5. Consonant clusters (e.g., /pl/) are few in Spanish (Stockwell & Bowen, 1965). Spanish has different phonemes from English, for example, the tap /r/ and trill /R/.

6. Spanish has additional sounds of the tap /r/, trill or vibrant /R/, and the nasal /ñ/.

7. Spanish does not possess the English sound of /ʃ/, with the most common substitutions consisting of /ʃ/ to /tʃ/.

8. All Spanish dipthongs involve a glide in which the tongue moves farther than it does for English dipthongs (Stockwell & Bowen, 1965; Whitely, 2002).

9. Spanish consonants in the syllable final position tend to be lax and hence are either aspirated or deleted. Spanish vowels consist of: /a/ (año, father), /e/ (eco, bet), /i/ (hija, heat), /o/ (ojo, boat), and /u/ (humo, food).

10. Spanish consonant blends cannot begin words with /s/, resulting in a vowel-consonant combination of /es/. Therefore, the word *stop* becomes *estop.*

Some general, universal phonological truths seem to exist across languages (Carey, 2002; Greenburg, 1966; Jakobson, Fant, & Halle, 1952): fricatives are harder to produce than nasals or stops, and consonants are easier in syllable onsets than in syllable final positions. The form of these processes may differ from language to language; however, the differences in phonological processes are determined by each language.

In sum, phonological rule variations of Caribbean Spanish (which may apply to other dialects of Spanish) as noted by Hammond (1989) include: (1) syllable final, word final aspiration of /s/; (2) general word final deletion; (3) /r/ and /l/ confusion; (4) vocalization of word final liquids; (5) word final /n/ velarization; and (6) alteration of /tʃ/ and /ʃ/. Hence, the following noted processes seem to be most affected by Spanish dialect and interlanguage phonological interference: (1) consonant sequence reduction (CSR)—dialect and interference, (2) postvocalic omission—dialect, (3) stridents—interference, and (4) /l, r/—dialect and interference.

MORPHOLOGICAL AND SEMANTIC TRANSFERENCE

Morphology

"**Morphology** [emphasis added] is the study of word structure and describes how words are formed from morphemes. Morphemes . . . can be manipulated to modify word structures in order to change the meaning of the word" (Brice, 2004a, p. 40). Spanish morphology differs from English morphology in a number of ways. In Spanish, subjects or noun phrases are optional (i.e., sentences do not always require a stated subject). English almost always requires the subject noun or pronoun. Spanish verb inflections are used to encode information about person (e.g., *I* versus *you*, versus *he/she* versus *we*), number (i.e., singular versus plural), or other tense information. English verb inflection encodes numbers in a more reduced fashion (e.g., first person singular versus third person singular; I wal*k*, he/she wal*ks*). Spanish requires gender and number agreement for determiners (e.g., *el* [the], *la* [the], *un* [a], *una* [a], *los* [the], *las* [the], *unos* [a few], *unas* [a few]), articles, adjectives, and past participles. English does not require gender agreement and uses a much more limited number agreement (e.g., *a, the, a few, some*). Past participles that form the passive tense or perfect tense are present in both Spanish and English (e.g., "Yo he caminado"/"I have walked"). However, past participles in English are not as obvious as in Spanish because they often take the same form as the regular past tense verb ending in *-ed*. In English, the past participle combines with some form of the verb "to have." For example, *worked* is a past tense verb in the sentence "I worked at home," but the English past participle would be "I have worked." Spanish past participles typically end in *-ado* or *-ido*. Despite the complexity of Spanish, most children acquire these morphological features without any difficulties and typically acquire gender agreement for articles and verbal conjugations by 3 years of age and most complex morphological operations by 4 years of age (Jacobson & Schwartz, 2002).

Studies describing general Spanish morphology or English morphological acquisition by Spanish-speaking children have been limited. However, studies have investigated the acquisition of common Spanish morphemes (Kvaal, Shipstead-Cox, Nevitt, Hodson, & Launer, 1988), Spanish morphology acquisition in a young child via a descriptive case study investigation (Restrepo & Kruth, 2000), and use of Brown's 14 grammatical English morphemes (Bland-Stewart & Fitzgerald, 2001).

Kvaal, Shipstead-Cox, Nevitt, Hodson, and Launer (1988) investigated the acquisition of common Spanish morphemes in 15 Mexican-American monolingual Spanish-speaking children between the ages of 2:0 and 4:8. Due to the limited number of participants in this study ($n=15$), these results should be viewed with caution and should be seen as preliminary. Spontaneous language samples were gathered in informal play settings. The children were divided into three groups based on their MLU level, 2.6 to 3.5, 3.6 to 4.5, and 4.5 to 7.9. The authors did not state how MLU was calculated in Spanish (i.e., in words or morphemes). The order of acquisition for the most common Spanish morphemes follows:

1. Demonstratives were acquired by all participants in this study. The most commonly used form consisted of the masculine singular forms *ese* (that), *este* (this), and the neutral form *eso* (that one). Feminine plurals were rarely used.

2. Articles were used in 95.6% of obligatory contexts (when the article should have been used). Most of the participants had acquired the Spanish definite article *el*.

3. Copulas *estar* (to be) and *ser* (to be) were acquired by most participants.

4. *De* (of) was acquired at an approximate age 2.3.

5. *En* (in, on) was consistently used when the participants had an MLU of 4.0. The children used *en* as "in" more often than they used *en* for "on."

6. Regular present indicative was acquired by an MLU of 2.6. The present indicative tense consists of *yo hablo* (I speak), *tu hablas* (informal-you speak), *el/ella habla* (he/she speaks), *nosotros hablamos* (we speak), *usted habla* (formal-you speak), *ellos/ellas hablan* (they speak).

7. Irregular present indicative becomes productive at an early MLU of 2.6 and is acquired after the regular past tense. This morphological feature is developed at an MLU of 2.8. The verb *ir* (to go) was the most frequently used present indicative.

8. Regular and irregular preterite was acquired when children reached an MLU between 2.8 and 3.2. The preterite tense in Spanish is the past tense that indicates that actions were completed, e.g., *yo compré* (I bought).

9. Plurals were found to be productive at an early age of approximately 2.4 to 2.6. The short form plural *-s* was found to be the most frequently used.

Bland-Stewart and Fitzgerald (2001) investigated the development of Brown's grammatical morpheme acquisition in a group of 15 bilingual Hispanic preschoolers. Spontaneous language samples were gathered and analyzed. The children were between the ages of 2.6 years and 5.0 years old. These children were of Central or South American Spanish origin. It should be noted that a child's dialect of Spanish from their birth country may affect the rate and ease of acquiring English morphology. Because this study did not include a diverse sample of Spanish speakers from different countries and the sample size was small ($n=15$), the results should be viewed as tentative. The response for the grammatical morphemes in English follow:

1. Present progressive *-ing* acquisition by the Spanish-speaking children met American English age and MLU benchmarks.

2. Plurals did not meet the American English normative standards; however, plurals were found to be an emergent skill.

3. Use of the preposition *in* did not meet the American English standards.

4. The use of the preposition *on* did not meet the American English normative standards. The Spanish *en* (on) was cited by Kvaal et al. (1988) to be a later emerging morpheme in Spanish, perhaps due to extended use of contextual cues in Spanish. Prepositions are not as clearly marked in Spanish as they are in English.

5. Possessive *s* did not meet the American English normative standards. Spanish speakers denote possession with *de*; hence, possible Spanish interference may have delayed acquisition of the English possessive.

6. Regular past tense *-ed* did not meet the American English normative standards. Spanish phonology may have had an interfering influence because final stops may be aspirated or deleted (Brice, 2002). However, the regular past tense was found to be an emergent skill.

7. Irregular past tense did not meet the American English normative standards. It was also found to be an emergent skill. The irregular Spanish past tense is typically acquired at a later age (Kvaal et al., 1988).

8. The regular third person singular did not meet the American normative English standards. However, this morphological feature is not singled out in Spanish as much as it is in English (i.e., a different ending for first versus third person). For example, Spanish marks changes in person and number in the verb form (yo habl<u>o</u>, tu habl<u>as</u>, el/ella habl<u>a</u>, nosotros habl<u>amos</u>, usted habl<u>a</u>, ellos/ellas habl<u>an</u>).

9. Articles <u>a</u> and <u>the</u> did not meet the American normative standard; however, this morpheme was noted to be emerging. Note that Spanish articles <u>el</u>, <u>la</u>, <u>los</u>, and *las* denote number and gender. In addition, the masculine pronoun *el*, the feminine article <u>la</u>, and the direct object <u>la</u> make article acquisition in Spanish more complex. Despite the complexities, Spanish articles are typically acquired earlier than are English pronouns, perhaps due to their high frequency of use in spoken Spanish.

10. The contractible and auxiliary <u>to be</u> did not meet the American English normative standards. The Spanish copula and auxiliary morphemes are <u>ser</u> and <u>estar</u>. Spanish speakers also use <u>tener</u> (to have) to denote state of being (e.g., <u>yo tengo sed</u>—literally, "I have thirst"). The difference and complexity of the Spanish and English copula/auxiliary verbs may have caused some language interference difficulties.

11. Irregular third person singular did not meet the American English normative standards. Irregular Spanish verbs tend to maintain their irregularity throughout all persons and number. Hence, some language interference difficulties also may have occurred.

12. The uncontractible copula and auxiliary <u>to be</u> did not meet the American English normative standards. Spanish does not contain uncontractible forms. Contractions do exist in Spanish (e.g., <u>de</u> + <u>el</u> = <u>del</u>). However, some language interference difficulties again may have occurred.

Use of American English norms for English-language-learning children may be inappropriate due to the unique influences that Spanish may have on English morpheme acquisition. Speech-language pathologists and special educators should take into account second-language learning patterns when evaluating the language skills of bilingual children.

Restrepo and Kruth (2000) investigated the developing morphological skills of two bilingual, Spanish-English-speaking children with and without language impairments. Of particular interest is their investigation of a 7-year-old participant (Hilda) who did not present any language impairments. Spontaneous language samples were gathered and analyzed. Hilda used the following English morphemes in her language with 100% accuracy: *-ing*, plural *-s*, definite article (*the*), indefinite article (*a, an*), regular third person, uncontractible copula, and contractible copula. Other morphological features were as follows: contractible auxiliary, 92%; uncontractible auxiliary, 88%; irregular third person, 83%; irregular past, 77%; and regular past, 65%.

Some other studies have reported the acquisition of Spanish morphology. However, several studies have investigated singular morphological features. Therefore, those results are deemed to be too item-specific and are not reported here (Anderson, 1996; Restrepo, 1998; Restrepo & Gutierrez-Clellen, 2001). However, more general information regarding Spanish-language development from Gonzalez (1981); Kvaal, Shipstead-Cox, Nevitt, Hodson, and Launer (1988); and Radford and Ploenig-Pacheco (cited in Bedore, 1999) is compiled and presented in Tables 4–2 and 4–3.

Semantics: Language Differentiation and Transference

"**Semantics** [emphasis added] encompasses vocabulary, the ability to distinguish between word meanings (including multiple meanings and subtle nuances), and the

TABLE 4–2
Spanish Morphological Development

Morpheme	MLU Achievement (Correct Use of Form in 80% of Obligatory Contexts)	Approximate Age (Emerging/Acquired)
Demonstrative *esa*, *ese* (that) *esas*, *esos* (those) *esta*, *este* (this) *estas*, *estos* (these)	2.6	
Nongendered *eso* (that one) *esos* (those) *esto* (this one) *estos* (those)		
Articles Definite Article *la, las, el, los*	2.6	
Indefinite Article *una, uno, unas, unos*		
Copulas (*ser, estar*)	2.6	
Regular Present Indicative *Son pollos* They are chickens	2.7	2.6 years /4.6
Irregular Present Indicative Pido **I ask**	2.8	
Regular past Preterit Indicative *Agarró* He grabb**ed**	2.8–3.2	2.6 years /4.6

(continued)

TABLE 4–2 (*continued*)

Morpheme	MLU Achievement (Correct Use of Form in 80% of Obligatory Contexts)	Approximate Age (Emerging/Acquired)
Present Progressive *Estoy pint**ando*** I *am* paint*ing*		2.6 years /4.6
Periphrastic future ***Van** a tomar* They *are go**ing to drink***		2.6 years /4.6
Plurals	3.2	
Imperfect Camin**aba** I ***used to walk***		3.0 years /4.6
Present Subjunctive Acab**emos** That we finish		3.0 years /4.6
Possessive /de/	3.2	
Periphratic Past ***iba a** peg**ar*** *was going to spank*		3.0 years /4.6
Periphratic Future Progressive ***Voy** a esta**r vie**ndo* *I am going to see*		3.0 years /4.6
Preposition /en/ /in/	4.2–4.5	
Irregular preterite	4.6	
Past Subjunctive Hic**ieras** That I do		?/4.6 years

Source: Brice, A. (2002). *The Hispanic child: Speech, language, culture and education.* Boston, MA: Allyn & Bacon.

TABLE 4–3
Spanish Syntactic Development

Syntactic Structure	Approximate Age That Feature Is Acquired
Simple Imperative Command Tom**alo** *Take it*	2.0 years
Third Person Singular *No vien**e*** *He do**es** not come*	2.0 years
Indirect object *Me está pintando **los zapatos*** *He is shining **my shoes** (for me)*	2.6 years

TABLE 4–3 (*continued*)

Syntactic Structure	Approximate Age That Feature Is Acquired
Direct object **La** agarró esta muchacha This girl took **it**	2.6 years
Yes/no questions	2.6 years
Information Questions *Qué* (What) *Dónde* (Where) *Cuándo* (When) *Quién* (Who) *Por qué* (Why)	2.6 years
Gerund	2.6–3.0 years
Full Sentence Negation	2.6 years

Subject-verb-object Position Changes
S-V-DO
Yo tengo zapatitos
    I have little shoes
    V-S-DO
Omí yo huevos
    I ate eggs
    V-DO-S
        Perdío las gomas el autobus
        The bus lost its tires
	2.9 years

Imperatives
Verb + indirect object pronoun + direct object pronoun
    Dámela
    Give it to me
Verb = reflexive pronoun + direct object pronoun
    Tómatelo tu
    You drink it
	3.0 years

Compound sentences with use of y	3.0 years

Locative verb clauses
    Allá dondé esta la casa ver
    There where the house is
	3.0 years

Conditional clause with use of si ("if") *Si no el me pretas atencíon, le voy a castegar* *If he does not pay attention to me,* I am going to punish him	3.0 years

Tag questions with use of verdad right/correct
    Este niño se porta bien, verdad?
    This boy behaves well, right?
	3.3 years

Comparative "mas more" or "-er" comparative	3.3 years
Compound sentences with use of pero (but)	4.6 years
Comparison of equalities with use of como (like)	4.6 years

Source: Brice, A. (2002). *The Hispanic child: Speech, language, culture and education.* Boston, MA: Allyn & Bacon.

relationships between different words (Palloway & Smith, 1992)" (Brice 2004a, p. 42). Research in early bilingual semantic acquisition has been studied in order to address the early language needs of young bilingual children. This research information benefits bilingual children, speech-language pathologists, and other professionals, and contributes to the general understanding of language development among bilingual children (Lanza, 1997; Miesel, 1989).

Language differentiation (i.e., the question of whether young bilingual children initially use one or two language systems) has been investigated in order to examine normal language acquisition in bilingual children, particularly at the semantic level. Researchers have disputed whether the ability to communicate with two languages as separate entities is an inherent ability or acquired later with growth and maturity. A child's ability to process and use his or her two languages separately has been studied by numerous child language researchers (Döpke, 1992; Genesee, Nicoladis, & Paradis, 1995; Jackson-Maldonado, Thal, Marchman, Bates, & Gutierrez-Clellen, 1993; Lanza, 1992; Lindholm & Padilla, 1978; Meisel, 1989; Pearson, Fernandez, & Oller, 1993 & 1995; Quay, 1995; Redlinger & Park, 1980; Vihman, 1985; Volterra & Taeschner, 1978). Consensus on whether bilingual children acquire their two languages initially as one system or are capable of immediately differentiating between the two has not been achieved.

The data obtained on early language development have included the following procedures: (1) diary entries (Quay, 1995; Vihman, 1985; Volterra & Taeschner, 1978); (2) parent questionnaire forms (Jackson-Maldonado, Thal, Marchman, Bates, & Gutierrez-Clellen, 1993; Pearson, Fernandez, Lewedeg, & Oller, 1997; Pearson, Fernandez, & Oller, 1993, 1995); and (3) language samples (Döpke, 1992; Genesee, Nicoladis, & Paradis, 1995; Lanza, 1992).

Research in the area of bilingual language differentiation has been divided into two main schools of thought, that is, the initial one system school and the immediate differentiation school. The **initial one system hypothesis** postulates that the bilingual child has one language system (i.e., his or her two languages are initially molded together as one). Differentiation between the two systems occurs later during the child's language development and cognitive maturation (e.g. around 3 years of age). According to this theory, differentiation occurs at the word level and then at the syntactic level. This hypothesis has also been called the unitary language system (Genesee, 1989).

The **immediate differentiation hypothesis** states that young bilingual children are capable of immediately differentiating between their two languages. In addition, they do not initially seem to use a single unitary system (Döpke, 1992). This approach maintains that children's use of translation equivalent words (words that are common to both languages) serves as evidence of their understanding and use of two language systems (Genesee, 1989).

Initial One System Hypothesis

Volterra and Taeschner's (1978) study analyzed how young bilingual children differentiated the use of their two languages. The authors believed that children between 1 and 4 years of age progressed through specific language stages before their two languages were notably distinct. Volterra and Tasechner collected data from three children using language samples and/or notes from comprehensive parent diaries. Audio recordings were gathered in both languages during daily activities in the home. The language samples were then transcribed. Their results indicated that the young bilingual children used a limited number of doublets or translation equivalents (i.e., a pair of words, one from each language, that shares the same meaning). Volterra and Taeschner (1978) stated that the children in their study had only one unitary and combined vocabulary in their communication. They concluded that the children's limited number of translation equivalents was evidence that these children were not cognizant of their two languages.

Redlinger and Park's (1980) study indicated that initially the children they studied had a large number of mixed utterances, which suggested a lack of language differentiation in their children. Vihman (1985) also noted a limited number of translation equivalents in her study participant's language and concluded this to be evidence of the unitary or initial one system hypothesis. Results from her study indicated that by the time the child was able to differentiate between the two lexicons, she was also beginning to use syntax for each language appropriately. Redlinger and Park also observed a decrease in the use of code-mixed utterances as the child's pragmatic knowledge improved. The authors concluded that the child could distinguish both languages at an early age and that the process seemed to be sequential. It can be stated that the above-mentioned studies (Redlinger & Park, 1980; Vihman, 1985; Volterra & Taeschner, 1978) are limited because they did not incorporate many participants; thus, external validity and generalizability were affected.

Immediate Differentiation Hypothesis

Lindholm and Padilla (1978) wished to establish that language alternations did not prohibit a child from becoming bilingual. They observed five Spanish-English-speaking, children 2:10 to 6:2 years of age. They collected a spontaneous language sample as each child interacted with two speakers, one speaking, Spanish and one speaking English. The children exchanged and translated information between the two adult speakers, whom they thought to be monolingual. The authors concluded that the children used translation equivalents as compensation for a lack of vocabulary in one of their languages (Lindholm & Padilla, 1978). Unfortunately, this study also observed few children. In addition, the participants' age range was too wide to permit generalization.

Regarding language differentiation, Genesee (1989) contends that a gradual acquisition process or progression through stages is not established in the studies that he reviewed because they lacked contextual analysis. To declare that language differentiation occurred, the following should be considered: (1) pragmatics rules of both languages, (2) the role of context on language use, and (3) the effect of maturity on lexical-vocabulary systems. He also stated that "in order to uphold the unitary-system hypothesis [initial one hypothesis] one would need to establish that, all things being equal, bilingual children use items from both languages indiscriminately in all contexts of communication" (Genesee, 1989, p.165).

Quay (1995) challenged the belief that children under 2 years of age could not distinguish their two languages. She stated that children early in their development are able to keep their two languages apart, as demonstrated by a high number of translation equivalents in their communication. Quay stipulated that some bilingual children may not speak in their second language, even if they know of an appropriate translation equivalent. This may happen when the parents use the one-parent-one-language system or when the child knows that the parent is bilingual.

Quay's (1995) research supports the immediate differentiation hypothesis because a significant number of translation equivalents were observed in her participant's language. The large occurrence of translation equivalents in this child's language contradicts the conclusions made by Volterra and Taeschner (1978).

Pearson, Fernandez, and Oller (1995) examined expressive vocabularies of 27 bilingual children (ages 0:8–2:6) using the *MacArthur Communicative Developmental Inventory (CDI)* (1989) and its Spanish version, *Inventario del Desarrollo de las Habilidades Communicativas*. The Spanish version, developed by Jackson-Maldonado and Bates (1988), was given to the bilingual parents to complete. Each parent completed a form in one language indicating the child's lexical abilities in both Spanish and English. The vocabularies in the two languages were then compared. Only 2 of the 27 children exhibited the developmental pattern proposed by Volterra and Taeschner, that is, demonstrated few translation equivalents in the first stage of development and more in the second stage. The results from this study indicated that a high percentage of translation equivalents were found in the language of the other 25 participants. The translation equivalents did not change over time, as Vihman (1985) had indicated.

Döpke (1992) also contributed to the immediate differentiation hypothesis in her case study of a young child. The child was observed from the age of 2;0 to 2;5. The child used a higher amount of translation equivalents (TEs) in German with a lower incidence of TEs in English. Döpke stated that this was the result of the child's personal preference and not necessarily a deficit in linguistic knowledge. This was supported by the child's attempt to adhere to the one-person-one-language rule. For example, the child predominantly selected German words with the mother and English words with the father. Another instance was when the child corrected his mother when she mistakenly used English words for German words.

Döpke (1992) mentioned that the child in her study displayed limited linguistic abilities (in the less dominant language of English) when he mixed utterances. According to Döpke, this was not due to his lack of understanding. Nicoladis and Genesee's (1996) study provided support for Döpke's (1992) claim that young bilingual children can also demonstrate pragmatic language differentiation. Their results indicated that the four children partially differentiated their languages with their parents. Emergence of differentiation was observed between the ages of 1:9 and 2:4.

Genesee, Nicoladis, and Paradis (1995) and Genesee, Boivin, and Nicoladis (1996) provided evidence for the notion that bilingual children (1:10 to 2:2 years of age) are able to differentiate their languages with familiar speakers. In addition, these speakers were able to identify a monolingual speaker's inability to understand the child's second language. These studies stated that if children were capable of adjustments in their language (with other speakers beside the parents), then this would indicate the child's conscious language choice. Genesee, Nicoladis, and Paradis (1995); Döpke (1992); and Lanza (1992) also claimed that language dominance might be an important factor in the child's use of code mixing and translation equivalents.

Brice and Wertheim (2004/2005) investigated whether young bilingual children were able to differentiate between their two languages. Specific questions from their study included whether young children were able to differentiate between their two languages based on analyses of total vocabulary and translation equivalents (TEs, or pairs of words with the same meaning; e.g., gato/cat), as measured by the English and Spanish versions of the short forms of the *MacArthur Communication Development Inventory (CDI)*.

Sixteen Spanish-English-speaking bilingual children were selected for this study. The parents completed a case history questionnaire for their child's speech and language development. None of the participants selected showed a history for speech and/or language problems. Data was collected with parental questionnaires and administration of the Spanish and English versions of the *MacArthur CDI*. It was found that the children displayed a high number of translation equivalents, supporting the hypothesis that young children could differentiate between their two languages. Results also suggested that the young bilingual children seemed to use the translation equivalents (TEs) as a bridge between their two languages. This study found that TEs acted as a bridge between the preferred and less preferred languages spoken by the children. In addition, TEs appeared to be normal occurrences in the children's vocabulary. The children with strong preference for one language tended to show fewer occurrences of TEs. The children who did not show such an extreme preference showed a higher occurrence of TEs. Thus it appeared that as children gained higher proficiency in the second language, they were more apt to use translation equivalents.

If the TEs act as a bridge between the languages, then they are examples of transference at the word level. The concept and actualization of transference via the TEs supports Cummins's interdependence hypothesis or common underlying proficiency model whereupon lexical items transfer (Cummins, 1984; Cummins, 1979; Thomas & Collier, 2002). Hence, improvements in one language at the vocabulary level may transfer to the next (Collier, 1987; Cummins, 1979; Thomas & Collier, 2002). In summary, the study by Brice and Wertheim supported the notion that translation equivalents occur in young children's bilingual language use, in turn supporting the immediate differentiation hypothesis.

SYNTACTIC AND PRAGMATIC TRANSFERENCE

Syntax

"**Syntax** [emphasis added] is the rule system that governs how words are combined into larger meaningful units of phrases, clauses, and sentences" (Brice, 2004a, p. 42). Collentine (2003) stated that the second-language acquisition literature documents that "syntactic abilities tend to outpace morphological abilities" during the initial stages of learning, especially when both languages are Indo-European in origin (as in Spanish and English) (p. 88). Ellis (1987) postulated that learners of Spanish generally progressed through four sequential stages of syntactic acquisition: (1) development of basic syntactic knowledge such as subject-verb-object order, (2) acquisition of variant word order, (3) development of morphological knowledge, and (4) acquisition of knowledge and information governing complex sentence structure.

Anderson (1995) reported the specific sentence types that emerged developmentally in Spanish. For example, by 2:6, a Spanish-speaking child demonstrates negatives, questions, imperatives, and embedded sentences (Anderson, 1995). Children as early as 2 years of age use rising intonation to indicate yes/no questions. Spanish wh- question forms are also seen at this age (*qué* [what]; *quién* [who]; *donde* [where]). At 2 and half years of age, Spanish-speaking children also exhibited instances of other question forms (*para qué* [for what]; *cuando* [when]; *por qué* [why]; *como* [how]) (Anderson, 1995).

Pragmatics Development in Bilingual Students

It is important for school personnel to be aware of student pragmatics in order to assist students in their education, particularly students at risk for academic failure or social adjustment problems. Brice and Montgomery (1996) define **pragmatics** "as the ability to use language in specific contexts and for specific purposes" (p. 68). Pragmatics refers to the use of language that encompasses cognitive thoughts, social-environmental influences, and language choice. Pragmatics is also concerned with how language is interpreted in conversational contexts. Hymes (1972) stated that there exists "a structure of language that goes beyond the aspect of structure dealt with in grammars" (p. xxii). Pragmatics is context-specific; that is, contextual environments can influence language interactions and language can influence the environment. Pragmatics cannot be separated from what is happening with the speaker and listener. Therefore, pragmatics is the study of speaker-listener interactions. In addition, Hertel (2003) stated that "some research has suggested that discourse factors may be more difficult to acquire than grammatical ones" (p. 280).

A complete understanding of student pragmatics is necessary in order to understand the true nature of classroom interactions. Pragmatics consists of intentions to communicate, messages that are conveyed, and understanding on behalf of the listener. In essence, pragmatics incorporates all aspects of language because sounds are produced (phonology), word inflections are used (morphology), words are spoken (semantics), and sentences are created (syntax).

Pragmatics development in bilingual students may be an effective indicator of second-language learning. Damico, Oller, and Storey (1983) reported that the criteria for measuring pragmatics were more effective than the surface language criteria of morphological and syntactic structures in identifying language difficulties versus language disorders. They reported that the typically used traditional criteria (e.g., norm-referenced tests, morphology analysis) did not differentiate between bilingual language disorders and normal second-language acquisition differences. Damico, Oller, and Storey's (1983) pragmatic categories consisted of nonfluencies, revisions, inordinate delays, nonspecific referential terms, inappropriate responses, poor topic maintenance, and the need for multiple repetitions. These categories were applied to language samples gathered in both English and Spanish by speech-language pathologists. The language samples were then analyzed using the traditional (surface-oriented) methods, such as morphology, and then by using the pragmatic criteria. Results indicated that the pragmatic criteria were more effective with the bilingual children in identifying students with language disorders. Furthermore, the students identified as having language disorders by the pragmatic criteria failed to make substantial academic gains seven months later. Some of the students identified by the traditional criteria (i.e., use of standardized, norm-referenced tests) made normal gains in school achievement. This would indicate that the traditional criteria were more likely to misidentify students, while the pragmatic criteria may have been more effective.

Brice (1992) developed a pragmatics scale (*the Adolescent Pragmatics Screening Scale [APSS]*) to investigate student pragmatics performance in various classroom contexts at a prereferral (i.e., pre-evaluation) level (see this chapter's Appendix A). He used this scale to study the pragmatics performance of students from three adolescent groups: monolingual language disordered, bilingual (e.g. Spanish-English-speaking), and monolingual general-education students. The findings of Brice and Montgomery's (1996) study, using the APSS, indicated that the language disordered students had difficulties in expressing themselves, establishing greetings, initiating and maintaining conversations, and listening to a speaker. These difficulties placed the language disordered students at risk for following and completing classroom lessons and participating in classroom discussions. The language disordered students displayed difficulties with oral (i.e., spoken) language particularly if it involved more grammatical and semantic aspects of language (e.g., describing personal feelings in an acceptable manner). Apparently, the language disordered students generalized their general language deficit into pragmatic behaviors, which adversely affected their interactions.

The bilingual students also displayed difficulties, particularly in making requests of others and in listening to a speaker. The bilingual students' pragmatic difficulties placed them at risk for cooperative learning situations in the classroom. Brice (1992) recommended that the teacher coach, model, and possibly instruct the behaviors for how to make requests and actively listen (to increase listening comprehension and follow-through on tasks). The speech-language pathologist (SLP) may offer suggestions about how to focus on listening actively. This knowledge may assist in learning the behaviors of making requests. Because many classroom behaviors may be affected by an inadequate control of English grammatical structures, Brice recommended that SLPs and teachers also focus on the grammatical aspects of language, including syntax, semantics, and morphology, is improving students' pragmatic skills.

Pragmatics in the school classroom is often viewed in an even broader context (Wong-Fillmore, 1992). For example, Wong-Fillmore (1992) notes that the teacher's use of oral directions, written directions, and classroom groupings is often culturally based and can have a profound effect on some students' academic success. SLPs may need to present rules of classroom interaction and use of strategies to the bilingual, Spanish-English-speaking students enrolled for language therapy.

The speech-language pathologist or special educator can encourage bilingual students to ask questions. The bilingual students receiving language therapy in initial learning stages should be allowed to make mistakes. SLPs and special education teachers can also employ more pauses and wait time for responses to allow these students to monitor and reflect on their language, especially because they may need additional processing time when compared to normal bilingual or monolingual students (Goldstein, 2000; Simon, 1985). SLPs and teachers can ask open-ended clarification questions, that is, questions that allow for expansion and elaboration to encourage heuristic (i.e., information-seeking) language. The use of grammar drills and direct instruction, that is, teaching specific skills such as note taking, is beneficial for bilingual students (Brice, Mastin, & Perkins, 1997). A naturalistic approach can be used later to reinforce learned skills (Nye, Foster, & Seaman, 1987). The use of case studies has been noted to facilitate understanding of complex subject matter. Hence, the two case studies in this chapter illustrate the overlapping and complex factors that affect bilingual language development.

CASE STUDY PERSPECTIVES

Case Study One presents a normal second-language learner's difficulties, while Case Study Two presents a child who has severe language impairments in both her first and second languages. Both students show difficulties associated with learning English as a second language and living in a bilingual environment.

Case Study One Background: Norma

Norma was born in Colombia, South America. Her parents were both native Spanish-speaking Colombians. She spoke Spanish exclusively until she was 4 years old. Norma was typical in her language development; that is, she has had no language acquisition difficulties. She was enrolled in preschool in Colombia when she was 2 years old and was reported to have learned basic vocabulary concepts in Spanish. Her family moved to Florida when she was 3 and a half. For the first 6 months she was not exposed to English. However, at 4 years of age, she was enrolled in an all-English preschool. All the students in this class, with the exception of her cousin, spoke only English. According to her mother, Norma's English development proceeded well; however, her Spanish development slowed tremendously. It was reported that when Norma wanted to play with other children at the preschool, they refused to play with her because of her limited English. At this time, her mother started speaking only English to her at home. Her father, not being very proficient in English, continued to speak only Spanish to her. Norma continued to be a sequential bilingual. However, her Spanish exposure decreased, while her English exposure increased at this time.

After kindergarten (two years of English exposure at school and from her mother), Norma's teachers reported that she was speaking English well. Note that this is in agreement with Cummins's (1984) theory that an oral proficiency of language [Cummins uses the term basic interpersonal communication skills (BICS)] can be acquired in approximately two or three years.

Norma returned to Colombia for two summers when she was 6 and 7 years old. Her mother reported that Norma was "having a hard time speaking Spanish" during these visits. When asked a question in Spanish, she would respond in English. This has been noted when children experience shifts in language environments. Norma's mother decided to resume speaking Spanish in the home.

At the beginning of second grade, Norma was experiencing difficulties with math word problems. Math word problems require good academic language comprehension. The fact that Norma was experiencing problems in school at this time is a normal phenomenon for second-language learners and is described by Cummins (1984). He states that in acquisition of academic language [Cummins uses the term cognitive academic language proficiency (CALP)], it may take a student five to seven years to achieve a level of native peer proficiency. At this time, Norma had had less than two and a half years of school English exposure. Norma never received any special English-language instruction. It should be mentioned that Norma was enrolled in a private school and that a 10–1 student/teacher ratio was employed. The amount of individual attention she received from her teacher was expected to be fairly high. According to Norma's mother, her daughter's English was age-appropriate; however, her Spanish was below age-appropriate levels. When Norma was in second grade, Norma's mother was speaking Spanish in the home.

Case Study One Comments: Norma

Norma's observed deceleration of Spanish acquisition when English was introduced is anecdotal evidence of subtractive bilingual education as reported by Westby (1991). Norma's Spanish was deteriorating when concentrated English was in place in both the home and the school. This subtractive bilingualism may have turned into Spanish attrition had not Norma's mother intervened at a later point by reintroducing exclusive use of Spanish in the home.

Norma's difficulties with math word problems indicated that strong language skills are a prerequisite for success across the entire school curriculum and that academic language (or CALP) takes a bilingual student longer to acquire than most teachers and speech-language pathologists may recognize. If Norma had experienced more difficulties in school, she may have been referred for language or special education testing. Her surface oral English-language skills appeared intact; however, she was still experiencing subtle problems. The referring teacher may have looked only at her oral skills and may not have consciously considered the different requirements of written academic language skills.

Case Study Two Background: Carlita

Carlita was referred to the University Communication Disorders Clinic because it was reported by her parents that she was not talking or communicating. Carlita was 3 years 2 months old at the time of the referral and evaluation. Her parents were concerned about Carlita's undeveloped Spanish-language skills. Her pediatrician recommended that Carlita receive language instruction in Spanish. Carlita's mother contacted several speech-language pathologists. They all recommended that language instruction be given solely in English. Most research indicates that children with disabilities or disorders can benefit from receiving therapy and instruction in both languages (Brice, 2002; de la Paz, 2001; Patterson, 1999; Roseberry-McKibbin, 1995). The parents both felt strongly that Spanish-language instruction was needed and sought services elsewhere.

From the case history information, it was reported that Carlita was born at home, the result of a full-term pregnancy. Carlita swallowed amniotic fluid during birth and as a result, she had difficulty breathing. She was admitted to the hospital for a week and was treated with antibiotics. Her birth history was otherwise unremarkable. Developmental milestones were within the normal range, with the exception of language developmental milestones being delayed (e.g., saying her first words, learning two-word combinations, combining multiple words).

Carlita was reported to be a responsive infant. However, she did not start using words until she was 2 years old. The majority of words reported were in Spanish, with a few English words. At the time of the evaluation, Carlita was saying words spontaneously, but she required imitation and clinician prompting.

Carlita lived in a home where Spanish was reportedly spoken approximately 60% of the time, while English was spoken 40% of the time. Carlita's mother reported that she spoke only Spanish to her. Carlita heard some English from her older brother and from the television.

Based on the results of the evaluation, Carlita appeared to be functioning well below her chronological age, with receptive Spanish language slightly better than her expressive Spanish language. Her vocabulary consisted of approximately 10 words. The majority of Carlita's expressive words were in Spanish. She was speaking in unintelligible jargon using a variety of vowel combinations, consonant combinations, and intonational patterns.

Carlita was enrolled in remedial language instruction at the university clinic. The student clinicians addressed Carlita's Spanish receptive and expressive language skills. Initial therapy objectives were to increase use of basic language skills such as prepositions (e.g. *adentro/afuera*), articles (e.g. *ese/esos*), and vocabulary.

Case Study Two Comments: Carlita

Carlita did not have a well-developed first language. To introduce English at this time would not have been beneficial because her mother (who spent most time with her) was not English-proficient. Carlita needed considerable interaction, modeling, and communicative exchanges with her primary caregiver (i.e., her mother). Carlita's parents were Spanish-dominant. The father was very proficient in English, yet Spanish was his first language. The mother was definitely more proficient in Spanish. Carlita would get more comprehensible input in Spanish, including varied uses of language (pragmatics) and preliteracy or emergent literacy. The parents felt very strongly about instruction in Spanish in order to maintain her cultural heritage. Carlita did not enter public school for another two years after this intervention due to her language deficits.

One issue to consider was the recommendation that Carlita enter a preschool to benefit from social interaction with children her age. If Carlita were English-dominant, she would most likely have benefited from the language stimulation that would have been occurring around her. However, because of Carlita's Spanish dominance, the university supervisors were hesitant to encourage the English-only preschool recommendation. They knew that Carlita would have future opportunities to learn English, but that instruction in Spanish and intensive use of Spanish in the home may have been the only opportunity to ensure that she developed a good Spanish base. Thus, the university supervisors felt that Carlita would benefit from one to two more years of intensive Spanish instruction before being introduced to an all-English school environment. Fradd (1987) said, "Hurrying students to function only in English may be counterproductive to their development of English proficiency" (p. 27). The opportunities for receiving Spanish instruction in school are minimal because most bilingual education programs across the country are in essence English as a second language (ESL) programs (Fradd, 1987) where English is typically the medium of instruction.

The University Communication Disorders Clinic supervisors suggested various alternatives to an English-only preschool environment: (1) having the mother be present at the preschool and provide conversation in Spanish, (2) having a play group situation where

Spanish-speaking children could interact with Carlita, and/or (3) trying to find a church preschool where some Spanish may be spoken at least some of the time. The major obstacle in implementing Spanish as the language of choice for instruction was the fact that the outside environment was not conducive to the Spanish-language needs of this child.

INSTRUCTIONAL STRATEGIES

Strategies for Spanish-English-Speaking Students

What is the role of native-language influence on learning English for children of elementary school age? Brice, Mastin, and Perkins (1997) suggested some sound pedagogical strategies for Hispanic students. Some conditions for English learning are suggested as strategies for speech-language pathologists (SLPs) and special education teachers to consider. Strategies for teachers to implement that allow for instances of bilingual communication to occur were taken from ESL and general education classrooms.

Auditory Processing and Attention Skills. The student should be seated in a quiet section of the classroom, that is, away from noise and distractors such as high traffic areas, open windows, pencil sharpeners, air conditioners, heaters, telephones, the overhead, etc. The student needs to concentrate on what is being said and what is being asked. The student should sit in the front row or near where the teacher spends most of her or his time to facilitate auditory processing of information. The student should be in a location where she or he can see and hear the teacher at all times.

The student may benefit from having a quiet study carrel or low-stimuli study area. This carrel or area can be called the office or the study space. It should be made available to all students so the student in need will not feel singled out.

Information in the classroom should be presented visually as well as auditorally (Roseberry-McKibbin, 1995). Important instructions should be written on the board as well as stated verbally. School professionals should check and make sure that the student understands and comprehends tasks or assignments before continuing. The teacher or SLP should use language to check understanding, comprehension, or knowledge of certain lesson-specific vocabulary (Brice, Mastin, & Perkins, 1997).

The student may profit and benefit from a peer buddy. The teacher or SLP should try to seat together students who speak the same language, especially when one student's English is more advanced. The more advanced student can then explain complicated directions and other information in the primary language. The English-language-learning student should be made to feel comfortable when asking for assistance from the teacher. Students should not be expected to remember more than two directions at a time. Teachers and SLPs should remember that directions may need to be repeated or reiterated because students may need more time to process another language (Brice, Mastin, & Perkins, 1997). Directions should be given slowly, and they should be repeated to ensure maximum comprehension and retention in memory.

When reading, it is helpful for students to see or draw pictures to add contextualization (Figueroa & Ruiz, 1997). The student should be asked frequent questions in

(continued)

order to keep her or him focused or to redirect the student to the task (Brice, Mastin, & Perkins, 1997). Additional time should be given for students to process questions. The student who is off-task may need to be redirected to the appointed task. The following examples illustrate this issue.

EXAMPLE

1. From a mathematics lesson, the paraprofessional redirects the student to the lesson: "How many tulips did you see? Count them. Mira ('look') Josefina. How many tulips did we see?"

Classroom Organization Strategies for All Bilingual Learners. This group includes ELL students and monolingual or bilingual students with LLD. The SLP or teacher may use preparatory sets to start lessons, such as lead statements (Brice, Mastin, & Perkins, 1997). Canagarajah (1995) identifies a **lead statement** as the action of opening the class to prepare students for preclass instructions or lessons. The lead statement is found at the beginning of a lesson. It distinctively cues the listener about what is to occur (Brice, Mastin, & Perkins, 1997). The teacher or paraprofessional proceeds in a verbal cuing, with the students following the directions. The five examples below provide the first step, which would lead to the next statement or step. To be able to follow the teacher's lead, children who are acquiring English will need more elaborate lead statements and explanations than the examples provided here.

EXAMPLES

1. Teacher: "First grade, let's get started."
2. Paraprofessional: "Okay, let's go. You ready?"
3. Teacher: "Here we go. *Little Bear and Owl* [the name of the book they will read]."
4. Paraprofessional: "Okay, lets go do a little bit of math and then you can look at this M."
5. Teacher: "Josefina, let's work on your reading."

Content Lesson Strategies. The following should assist the SLP, special-education teacher, or general-education classroom teacher with content lessons. The teacher or SLP should give instructions during quiet times. He or she should also allow extra language processing time. Lessons should be broken down into shorter components, and lessons should be scaffolded to assist understanding.

Scaffolding involves leading students through content information with the use of organized and planned steps. Specifically, the speech-language pathologist, special-education teacher, or classroom teacher should scaffold lessons with the following in mind: (1) relate the information to the student's previous knowledge (Figueroa & Ruiz, 1997); (2) use multiple examples in a multimodal approach to teaching; (3) encourage students to answer questions; (4) use a variety of questioning strategies (Brice, Mastin, & Perkins, 1997); and (5) avoid rhetorical questions, ambiguous questions, and run-on questions (Roseberry-McKibbin, 1995).

Assess Student's Comprehension. The SLP or teacher should assess the Hispanic student's comprehension of classroom assignments. She or he should occasionally ask for a brief summary of what was said. In addition, the teacher or SLP should ask the student's opinion of the material. In asking for an opinion, the SLP or teacher should make an attempt to ask for higher-order thinking skills, including application, analysis, synthesis, and evaluation questions (Bloom, 1956). Below are several examples.

EXAMPLES

1. An analysis question by the teacher: 'They said, my dad like to watch football games' [the teacher is reading from the overhead]. Okay, what is one thing that needs to be changed in the sentence? Okay, Mario?"

2. Asking student opinions: "José, what do you think of that?" or "What was your favorite thing about . . . ?" or "What didn't you like about . . . ?"

3. Seeking student opinions: After the teacher has read a story, he or she seeks to elicit the problem in the story: "Do you think she needs help or do you think she can do it by herself?"

The special education teacher, speech-language pathologist, or teacher should try to make input more comprehensible to students. For example, he or she may slow down his or her rate of speech, pause more frequently to allow more comprehension time, use shorter sentences and phrases, emphasize key words through increased volume, and slightly exaggerate rising intonations or variations in pitch. The example below illustrates the latter point.

EXAMPLE

1. The teacher raises her pitch to emphasize the point: "Okay, our first problem is 12 take away 4 and 12 take away 8." She then returns to her normal pitch and says, "What is our fact family for that problem?"

In addition, concepts should be taught in authentic communication situations (Figueroa & Ruiz, 1997) using the child's own language experiences. Students should be allowed to interject their own experiences into learning situations (language experience approach).

Strategies for Adolescent Spanish-English-Speaking Students

Strategies for teaching adolescent bilingual students also have a basis in scientifically based research (Brice, 2002; Brice, Mastin, & Perkins, 1997; Cook, 1996; Swain, 1985; Pica, 2002; Pica & Doughty, 1985; Wong-Fillmore, 1992). These conditions provide a basis for modifying instruction to enhance English learning with Hispanic adolescents (those with and without communication disorders). These strategies include:

1. *Teacher negotiation.* Brice, Mastin, and Perkins (1997); Cook (1996); Pica (2002); and Pica, Young, and Doughty (1987) reported that when students are encouraged to negotiate with teachers (i.e., seek clarification, confirm, or ask for repetition of teacher utterances that they do not understand), then better comprehension in English is noted. Teacher strategies such as repetition and rephrasing are encouraged to increase listener comprehension. In addition, encouraging students to ask questions seems to have a positive impact on students' understanding of classroom lectures.

2. *Learner opportunities.* Learners need opportunities to modify their language output beyond just hearing comprehensible input (Brice, 2000; Swain, 1985). Beginning learners of English may have limited opportunities to modify their output because teachers tend to model correct productions and not allow for student mistakes. The student then only has to acknowledge the correct model. Thus, SLPs and teachers need to model less and allow for students to practice their speaking skills.

The SLP or teacher should also allow for a greater wait time when expecting a response and allow the student to monitor and reflect on her or his spoken utterance.

3. *Functional conditions.* Wong-Fillmore (1992) identified several functional conditions for learning a second language: (1) a need to communicate; (2) access to the language from speakers of that language (peers, teachers, community members); (3) interaction, support, and feedback from others; and (4) close and continued interaction with others lasting three or four years. Teachers and speech-language pathologists should encourage these opportunities.

4. *Classroom interactions.* In classes where the majority of students are Hispanic, greater English proficiency was obtained with student-to-teacher interactions than with student-to-student interactions (Brice, 2000; Brice, Mastin, & Perkins, 1997; Chester-field, Chesterfield, Hayes-Latimer, & Chavez, 1983).

5. *Classroom sharing.* Discussions and giving opinions in class do not necessarily lead to increased English acquisition. Pica (2002) and Pica and Doughty (1985) found that discussion and opinion-giving tasks offered limited opportunities for English learning in group activities. However, sharing information with other students did have a positive impact (Pica, 2002; Pica & Doughty, 1985; Swain, 1985).

6. *Actions and open-ended questions.* Students talked more if they performed an action first (Brice & Montgomery, 1996). Also, when teachers used open-ended requests for clarification versus confirmation checks, (e.g., "What did you mean?" versus "Did you mean _____?"), then students made more linguistic adjustments.

7. *Direct instruction.* The use of direct instruction (directly teaching the specific micro skills) diminished with the introduction of more naturalistic language instruction (Krashen, 1985). However, researchers have found that the use of skilled practice played a significant role in adult learning of a second language because the adult was capable of being attentive to the L2 grammatical feature being highlighted when practicing specific skills (Nye, Foster, & Seaman, 1987; Schmidt & Frota, 1986). Thus, older learners, including adolescents, may benefit from drill-and-practice language lessons followed by a naturalistic approach to reinforce learned skills. Hakansson, Pienemann, and Sayehli (2002) and Pienemann (1984) found that direct grammatical instruction facilitates learning when the student is developmentally ready for moving to the next stage. Students who were not taught the next developmental stage rules did acquire them, but at a slower rate than those who were directly taught.

8. *Peer grouping, formal practice.* Some other factors also influence English acquisition, particularly peer grouping and formal practice. Allwright (1980) and Pica (2002) found that quieter students who were at similar English-proficiency levels as their classmates benefited from their more interactive peers. Thus, research calls for similar ability grouping.

CONCLUDING REMARKS

Speech-language pathologists, special education teachers, and general education classroom teachers will continue to work with bilingual populations. In addition, there still exists a need for information regarding bilingual instructional methods and strategies. The number of bilingual speech-language pathologists in the United States is inadequate to serve the growing bilingual school population (Brice, 2002; Kayser, 1995). In addition, the shortage of exceptional education teachers, particularly those from minority backgrounds, has also been documented (Office of Policy Research and Improvement, 2003). Therefore, it is imperative to have more fully prepared and qualified monolingual SLPs and exceptional education teachers to serve Hispanic students with and without disabilities. This point is stated by the 2004 President of the American Speech-Language-Hearing Association (ASHA). Dr. Larry Higdon stated:

> The changes in the United States demographics certainly speak to our need to increase recruitment efforts to attract cultural and linguistic minorities to the professions. If we are to provide quality services to all our consumers we need to become more knowledgeable of the many cultures of people we serve (Uffen, 2004, p. 5).

This chapter has sought to inform readers about second-language acquisition variables. It is hoped that the reader will serve Hispanic students in an informed manner, based on the information that has been provided.

REFLECTION QUESTIONS

1. Refer to Case Study One. How can Norma's parents ensure that her language development in both languages develops normally and that she does not fall behind in Spanish or English?
2. What can Norma's parents do to help her develop academic language abilities, e.g., accurate comprehenson of math word problems?
3. Should Norma's mother have switched to English when Norma first started experiencing normal difficulties with her two languages? Explain.
4. If you encountered a parent like Carlita's mother in Case Study Two, what language therapy would you recommend for his or her child? Explain.
5. If the parent were more proficient in English, would your answer to Reflection Question 4 be different? Explain.
6. What factors are involved in the two case studies regarding choice of language for home use, instruction, and/or therapy?
7. Refer again to Case Study One. What factors may contribute to Norma receiving instruction in Spanish? In English?

REFERENCES

Aguirre, A. (1988). Code switching, intuitive knowledge, and the bilingual classroom. In H. Garcia & R. Chavez (Eds.), *Ethnolinguistic issues in education* (pp. 28–38). Lubbock: Texas Tech University.

Allwright, R. (1980). Turns, topics, and tasks: Patterns of participation in language learning and teaching. In D. Larsen-Freeman (Ed.), *Discourse analysis in second language research* (pp. 165–187). Rowley, MA: Newbury House.

Anderson, R. T. (1995). Spanish morphological and syntactic development. In H. Kayser (Ed.), *Bilingual speech-language pathology. An Hispanic focus* (pp. 41–74). San Diego, CA: Singular.

Anderson, R. T. (1996). Assessing the grammar of Spanish-speaking children: A comparison of two procedures. *Language, Speech and Hearing Services in Schools, 27*, 333–344.

Asher, J., & Garcia, R. (1969). The optimal age to learn a foreign language. *Modern Language Journal, 53*, 334–341.

Asher, J., & Price, B. (1967). The learning strategy of the total physical response: Some age differences. *Child Development, 38*, 1219–1227.

Baca, L. M., & Cervantes, H. T. (Eds.). (1998). *The bilingual special education interface.* (3rd ed.). Upper Saddle River, NJ: Merrill.

Bedore, L. (1999). The acquisition of Spanish. In O. Taylor & L. Leonard (Eds.), *Language acquisition in North America.* San Diego, CA: Singular Press.

Bernthal, J., & Bankson, N. (1998). *Articulation and phonological disorders.* Boston, MA: Allyn and Bacon.

Bland-Stewart, L., & Fitzgerald, S. (2001). Morphological development in bilingual Hispanic preschoolers: A pilot study. *Communication Disorders Quarterly, 22*(4), 171–186.

Bloom, B. (1956). *Taxonomy of educational objectives: The classification of educational goals by a committee of college and university examiners.* New York: McKay.

Brice, A. (1990). Pragmatic skills in limited English proficient/non-English speaking students, speech and language students, and regular education students. *Dissertation Abstracts International University Microfilms International, U.S. July 1991, 52*(1-A), 97–98.

Brice, A. (1992). The Adolescent Pragmatics Screening Scale: A comparison of language-impaired students, bilingual/Hispanic students, and regular education students. *Howard Journal of Communications, 4*, 143–156.

Brice, A. (2000). Code switching and code mixing in the ESL classroom: A study of pragmatic and syntactic features. *Advances in Speech Language Pathology: Journal of the Speech Pathology Association of Australia, 20*(1), 19–28.

Brice, A. (2002). *The Hispanic child: Speech, language, culture and education.* Boston, MA: Allyn and Bacon.

Brice, A., & de la Paz, A. (1997). Disordered Cuban Spanish and American English phonology. *Florida Journal of Communication Disorders, 17*, 20–24.

Brice, A., Mastin, M., & Perkins, C. (1997). English, Spanish, and code switching use in the ESL classroom: An ethnographic study. *Journal of Children's Communication Development, 19*(2), 11–20.

Brice, A., & Montgomery, J. (1996). Adolescent pragmatic skills: A comparison of Latino students in ESL and speech and language programs. *Language, Speech, and Hearing Services in Schools, 27*, 68–81.

Brice, A. & Rivero, Y. (1996). Language transfer: First (L1) and second (L2) proficiency of bilingual adolescent students. *Per Linguam: The Journal for Language Teaching and Learning, 12*(2), 1–16.

Brice, A., & Wertheim, E. (2004/2005). Language differentiation in young bilingual children. *Tejas: Texas Journal of Audiology and Speech Language Pathology, 28*, 24–31.

Brice, R. (2004a). Connecting oral and written language through applied writing strategies. *Intervention in School and Clinic, 40*(1), 38–47.

Brice, R. G. (2004b). Identification of phonemes and graphemes in Spanish-English and English speaking kindergarten students. Doctoral dissertation, University of Central Florida. (ProQuest Digital Dissertations AAT 3144882.)

Canagarajah, A. S. (1995). Functions of codeswitching in ESL classrooms: Socialising bilingualism in Jaffna. *Journal of Multilingual and Multicultural Development, 6*(3), 173–195.

Canfield, D. L. (1981). *Spanish pronunciation in the Americas.* Chicago, IL: Chicago University Press.

Carey, M. (2002). *An L1-specific CALL pedagogy for the instruction of pronunciation with Korean learners of English.* Unpublished doctoral dissertation, Macquarie University, Sydney, Australia.

Carson, J. E., Carrell, P. L., Silberstein, S., Kroll, B., & Kuehn, P. A. (1990). Reading-writing relationships in first and second language. *TESOL Quarterly, 24*, 245–265.

Cheng, L. R., & Butler, K. (1989). Code switching: A natural phenomenon versus language deficiency. *World Englishes, 8*, 293–309.

Chesterfield, R., Chesterfield, K. B., Hayes-Latimer, K., & Chavez, R. (1983). The influence of teachers and peers on second language acquisition in bilingual preschool programs. *TESOL Quarterly, 17*(3), 401–419.

Collentine, J. G. (2003). The development of subjunctive and complex-syntactic abilities among foreign language learners of Spanish. In B. A. Lafford & R. Salaberry (Eds.), *Spanish second language acquisition: State of the science* (pp. 74–97). Washington, DC: Georgetown University Press.

Collier, V. (1987). Age and rate of acquisition of second language for academic purposes. *TESOL Quarterly, 21*(4), 617–641.

Cook, V. (1996). *Second language learning and language teaching* (2nd ed.). New York: St. Martin's Press.

Cummins, J. (1979). Linguistic interdependence and the educational development of bilingual children. *Review of Educational Research, 49,* 222–251.

Cummins, J. (1984). *Bilingualism and special education: Issues in assessment and pedagogy.* San Diego, CA: College-Hill Press.

Cummins, J. (1999). *BICS and CALP: Clarifying the distinction.* (ERIC Document Reproduction Service No. ED 438551).

Damico, J., Oller, J., Jr., & Storey, M. (1983). The diagnosis of language disorders in bilingual children: Surface-oriented and pragmatic criteria. *Journal of Speech and Hearing Disorders, 48,* 385–394.

De Houwer, A. (1990). *The acquisition of two languages from birth: A case study.* Cambridge, UK: Cambridge University Press.

De Houwer, A. (1995). Parental input language patterns and bilingual children's use. *Applied Psycholinguistics, 28*(3), 411–424.

de la Paz, A. (2001, November). *Bilingual pediatric assessment and treatment approaches. T-BAM and T-BIT methodology.* Paper presented at the American Speech-Language-Hearing Association Annual Convention, Atlanta, GA.

Diamond, F. (1983). *Phonological analysis of Spanish utterances of normally-developing bilingual Mexican-American children.* Unpublished master's thesis, San Diego State University, San Diego, CA.

Döpke, S. (1992). *One parent, one language: An interactional approach.* Amsterdam The Netherlands: Benjamins.

Doyle, A. B., Champagne, M., & Segalowitz, N. (1978). Some issues in the assessment of the consequences of early bilingualism. In M. Paradis (Ed.), *Aspects of bilingualism* (pp. 13–20). Columbia, SC: Hornbeam Press.

Eblen, R. E. (1982). A study of the acquisition of fricatives by three-year-old children learning Mexican Spanish. *Language and Speech, 25*(3), 201–220.

Ellis, R. (1987). *Second language acquisition in context.* Englewood Cliffs, NJ: Prentice Hall.

Faltis, C. J. (1989). Code-switching and bilingual schooling: An examination of Jacobson's new concurrent approach. *Journal of Multilingual and Multicultural Development, 10*(2), 117–127.

Fantini, A. (1985). *Language acquisition of a bilingual child: A sociolinguistic perspective.* San Diego, CA: College-Hill Press.

Figueroa, R. A., & Ruiz, N. T. (1997, January). *The optimal learning environment.* Paper presented at the Council for Exceptional Children Symposium on Culturally and Linguistically Diverse Exceptional Learners, New Orleans, LA.

Fradd, S. (1987). The changing focus of bilingual education. In S. Fradd & W. Tikinoff (Eds.), *Bilingual education and bilingual special education: A guide for administrators* (pp. 133–182). Boston, MA College Hill Press.

Garn-Nunn, P. G., & Lynn, J. M. (2004). *Calvert's descriptive phonetics* (3rd Ed.). New York: Thieme.

Genesee, F. (1989). Early bilingual development: One language or two. *Journal of Child Language, 16,* 161–179.

Genesee, F., Boivin, I., & Nicoladis, E. (1996). Talking with strangers: A study of bilingual children's communication competence. *Applied Psycholinguistics, 17,* 427–442.

Genesee, F., Nicoladis, E. & Paradis, J. (1995). Language differentiation in early bilingual development. *Journal of Child Language, 22,* 611–631.

Goldstein, B. (1995). Spanish phonological development. In H. Kayser (Ed.), *Bilingual speech-language pathology: An Hispanic focus* (pp. 17–39). San Diego, CA: Singular Publishing.

Goldstein, B. (2000). *Cultural and linguistic diversity resource guide for speech-language pathology.* San Diego, CA: Singular Publishing.

Goldstein, B., & Iglesias, A. (1996). Phonological patterns in normally developing Spanish-speaking 3- and 4-year olds of Puerto Rican descent. *Language, Speech, and Hearing Services in Schools, 27,* 82–89.

Gonzalez, A. (1981). *A descriptive study of phonological development in normal speaking Puerto Rican preschoolers.* Unpublished doctoral dissertation, Pennsylvania State University, State College, PA.

Greenburg, J. H. (1966). *Universals of language.* Cambridge, MA: MIT Press.

Grosjean, F. (1982). *Life with two languages: An introduction to bilingualism.* Cambridge, MA: Harvard University Press.

Gutierrez-Clellen, V. (1999). Language choice in intervention with bilingual children. *American Journal of Speech-Language Pathology, 8*(4), 291–302.

Hakansson, G., Pienemann, M., & Sayehli, S. (2002). Transfer and typological proximity in the context of second language processing. *Second Language Research, 18*(3), 250–273.

Hakuta, K. (1986). *Mirror of language. The debate on bilingualism.* New York: Basic Books.

Hamayan, E. V., & Damico J. S. (1991). *Limiting bias in the assessment of bilingual students.* Austin, TX: Pro-Ed.

Hammond, R. M. (1989). American Spanish dialectology and phonology from current theoretical perspectives. In P. C. Bjarkman & R. H. Hammond (Eds.), *American Spanish pronunciation* (pp. 137–169). Washington, DC: Georgetown University Press.

Hertel, T. J. (2003). Lexical and discourse factors in the second language acquisition of Spanish word order. *Second Language Research, 19*(4), 273–304.

Hodson, B. (1985). *Assessment of Phonological Processes—Spanish.* San Diego, CA: Los Amigos Research Associates.

Hymes, D. (1972). Preface. In C. Cazden, V. John, & D. Hymes (Eds.), *Functions of language in the classroom* (pp. xi–ivii). New York: Teachers College Press.

Jackson-Maldonado, D., & Bates, E. (1988*). Inventario del Desarrollo de las Habilidades Communicativas.* San Diego: University of California Center for Research in Language.

Jackson-Maldonado, D., Thal, D., Marchman, V., Bates, E., & Gutierrez-Clellen, V. (1993). Early lexical development in Spanish-speaking infants and toddlers. *Journal of Child Language, 20*, 523–549.

Jacobson, P. F., & Schwartz, R. G. (2002). Morphology in incipient bilingual Spanish-speaking preschool children with specific language impairment. *Applied Psycholinguistics, 23*, 23–41.

Jakobson, R., Fant, G., & Halle, M. (1952). *Preliminaries to Speech Analysis: Technical Report #13.* Cambridge, MA: MIT Acoustics Laboratory.

Johnson, J., & Newport, E. (1989). Critical period effects in second language learning: The influence of maturational state on the acquisition of English as a second language. *Cognitive Psychology, 21*, 60–99.

Kamwangamalu, N. M. (1992). Mixers and mixing: English across cultures. *World Englishes, 11*(2/3), 173–181.

Kayser, H. (1995). *Bilingual speech language pathology: An Hispanic focus.* San Diego, CA: Singular.

Krashen, S. (1985). *The input hypothesis: Issues and implications.* New York: Longman.

Krashen, S., Long, M., & Scarcella, R. (1992). Age, rate and eventual attainment in second language acquisition. *TESOL Quarterly, 13*, 573–582.

Kvaal, J. T., Shipstead-Cox, N., Nevitt, S. G., Hodson, B. W., & Launer, P. B. (1988). The acquisition of 10 Spanish morphemes by Spanish-speaking children. *Language, Speech, and Hearing Services in Schools, 19*, 384–394.

Lafford, B. A., & Salaberry, R. (2003). *Spanish second language acquisition: State of the science.* Washington, DC: Georgetown University Press.

Lambert, W. E. (1977). The effects of bilingualism on the individual: Cognitive and sociocultural consequences. In P. A. Hornby (Ed.), *Bilingualism: Psychological, social, and educational implications* (pp. 15–27). New York: Academic Press.

Lanza, E. (1992). Can bilingual two-year-olds code-switch? *Journal of Child Language, 19*, 633–658.

Lanza, E. (1997). *Language mixing in infant bilingualism: A sociolinguistic perspective.* New York: Oxford University Press.

Lenneberg, Eric H. (1967). *Biological foundations of language.* New York: Wiley.

Lindholm, K. J., & Padilla, A. M. (1978). Language mixing in bilingual children. *Journal of Child Language, 5*, 327–335.

Major, R. C. (1992). Losing English as a first language. *Modern Language Journal, 76*, 190–208.

Martinez, R. (1986). *Phonological analysis of Spanish utterances of normally developing Mexican-American Spanish-speaking 3-year-olds.* Unpublished master's project, San Diego State University, San Diego, CA.

McLaughlin, B. (1988). *Theories of second-language learning.* Baltimore, MD: Edward Arnold.

McLaughlin, B. (1995). *Fostering second language development in young children.* (Report No. EDO-FL-96–02). Washington, DC: Office of Educational Research and Improvement. (ERIC Document Reproduction Service No. ED 386 960).

Meisel, J. M. (1989). Early differentiation of languages in bilingual children. In K. Hyltenstam & L. K. Obler (Eds.), *Bilingualism across the lifespan: Aspects of acquisition, maturity, and loss* (pp. 13–40). Cambridge, UK: Cambridge University Press.

Miller, N. (1988). Language dominance in bilingual children. In M. J. Ball (Ed.), *Theoretical linguistics and disordered language* (pp. 235–256). San Diego, CA: College-Hill Press.

Moats, L. C. (1999). *Teaching reading is rocket science: What expert teachers of reading should know and be able to do.* Washington, DC: American Federation of Teachers.

National Research Council. (1998). Starting out right: A guide to promoting children's reading success.

Washington, DC: Committee on the Prevention of Reading Difficulties in Young Children.

Nye, C., Foster, S. H., & Seaman D. (1987). Effectiveness of language intervention with the language learning disabled. *Journal of Speech and Hearing Disorders, 52,* 348–357.

Office of Policy Research and Improvement. (2003). *Critical teacher shortage areas 2004–2005.* Tallahassee, FL: Florida Department of Education.

Oller, D. K., Eilers, R. E., Urbano, R., & Cobo-Lewis A. B. (1997). Development of precursors to speech in infants exposed to two languages. *Journal of Child Language, 24,* 407–425.

Olson, L., & Samuels, S. (1973). The relationship between age and accuracy of foreign language pronunciation. *Journal of Educational Research, 66,* 263–267.

Ortiz, A. (1991, September). *Guidelines for providing special education services for language minority students.* Paper presented at A Conference Assessing Limited English Proficiency, Culturally Diverse Exceptional Students, Phoenix, AZ.

Oyama, S. (1976). A sensitive period for the acquisition of a nonnative phonological system. *Journal of Psycholinguistic Research, 5,* 261–285.

Padolsky, D. (2002). How has the English language learner (ELL) student population changed in recent years? Retrieved November 10, 2003, from http://www.ncela.gwu.edu/askncela/08leps.htma.

Palloway, E. A., & Smith, T. E. C. (1992). *Language instruction for students with disabilities* (2nd ed.). Denver, CO: Love Publishing.

Patkowski, M. (1980). The sensitive period for the acquisition of syntax in a second language. *Language Learning, 30,* 449–472.

Patterson, J. L. (1998). Expressive vocabulary development and word combinations of Spanish-English bilingual toddlers. *American Journal of Speech-Language Pathology, 7,* 46–56.

Patterson, J. L. (1999). What bilingual toddlers hear and say: Language input and word combinations. *Communication Disorders Quarterly, 21*(1), 32–38.

Paulson, D. (1991). *Phonological systems of Spanish-speaking Texas preschoolers.* Unpublished master's thesis, Texas Christian University, Fort Worth, TX.

Pearson, B., & Fernandez, S. C. (1994). Patterns of interaction in the lexical growth in two languages of bilingual infants and toddlers. *Language Learning, 44,* 617–653.

Pearson, B., Fernandez, S. C., Lewedeg, V., & Oller, D. K. (1997). The relation of input factors to lexical learning by bilingual infants. *Applied Psycholinguistics, 18,* 41–58.

Pearson, B., Fernandez, S., & Oller, D. K. (1993). Lexical development in bilingual infants and toddlers: Comparison to monolingual norms. *Language Learning, 43,* 93–120.

Pearson, B., Fernandez, S., & Oller, D. K. (1995). Cross-language synonyms in the lexicons of bilingual infants: One language or two? *Journal of Child Language, 22,* 345–368.

Pica, T. (1994). Questions from the language classroom: Research perspectives. *TESOL Quarterly, 28,* 49–79.

Pica, T. (2002). Subject matter content: How does it assist the interactional and linguistic needs of classroom language learners? *Modern Language Journal, 86*(1), 1–19.

Pica, T., & Doughty, C. (1985). The role of group work in classroom second language acquisition. *Studies in Second Language Acquisition, 7*(2), 233–248.

Pica, T., Young, R., & Doughty, C. (1987). The impact of interaction on comprehension. *TESOL Quarterly, 21*(4), 737–758.

Pienemann, M. (1984). Psychological constraints on the teachability of languages. *Studies in Second Language Acquisition, 6*(2), 186–214.

Quay, S. (1995). The bilingual lexicon: Implications for studies of language choice. *Journal of Child Language, 22,* 369–387.

Redlinger, W. E., & Park, T. (1980). Language mixing in young bilinguals. *Journal of Child Language, 7,* 337–352.

Restrepo, M. A. (1998). Identifiers of predominantly Spanish-speaking children with language impairment. *Journal of Speech, Language, and Hearing Research, 41,* 1398–1412.

Restrepo, M. A., & Gutierrez-Clellen, V. F. (2001). Article use in Spanish-speaking children with SLI. *Journal of Child Language, 28*(2), 433–452.

Restrepo, M. A., & Kruth, K. (2000). Grammatical characteristics of a Spanish-English bilingual child with specific language impairment. *Communication Disorders Quarterly, 21*(2), 66–76.

Reyes, B. A. (1995). Considerations in the assessment and treatment of neurogenic disorders in bilingual adults. In H. Kayser (Ed.), *Bilingual speech language pathology: An Hispanic focus* (pp. 153–182). San Diego, CA: Singular Publishing.

Rivera-Umpierre, E. (1988). *Phonological analysis of 3- and 4-year old monolingual Puerto Rican Spanish-speaking children's utterances.* Unpublished master's thesis, San Diego State University, San Diego, CA.

Roseberry-McKibbin, C. (1995). *Multicultural students with special language needs: Practical strategies for assessment and intervention.* Oceanside, CA: Academic Communication Associates.

Schmidt, R. W., & Frota, S. N. (1986). Developing basic conversational ability in a second language: A case study of an adult learner of Portuguese. In R. R. Day (Ed.), *Talking to learn* (pp. 237–326). Rowley, MA: Newbury House.

Seliger, H., Krashen, S., & Ladefoged, P. (1975). Maturational constraints in the acquisition of a native-like accent in second language learning. *Language Sciences, 36,* 20–22.

Selinker, L. (1991). Along the way: Interlanguage systems in second language acquisition. In L. M. Malavé & G. Duquette (Eds.), *Language, culture and cognition* (pp. 23–35). Bristol, PA: Multilingual Matters.

Simon, C. (1985). *Communication skills and classroom success: Therapy methodologies for language-learning disabled students.* San Diego, CA: College-Hill Press.

Skutnabb-Kangas, T. (1981). *Bilingualism or not: The education of minorities.* Clevedon, UK: Multilingual Matters.

Snow, C. E., Burns, M. S., & Griffin, P. (Eds.) (1998). *Preventing reading difficulties in young children.* Washington, DC: National Academy Press.

Snow, C., & Hoefnagel-Hohle, M. (1977). Age differences in pronunciation of foreign sounds. *Language and Speech, 20,* 357–365.

Stockwell, R. P., & Bowen, J. D. (1965). *The sounds of English and Spanish.* Chicago, IL: University of Chicago Press.

Swain, M. (1985). Communicative competence: Some roles of comprehensible input and comprehensible output in its development. In S. Gass & C. Madden (Eds.), *Input in second language acquisition* (pp. 235–256). Rowley, MA: Newbury House.

Thomas, W. P., & Collier, V. P. (2002). *A national study of school effectiveness for language minority student's long term academic achievement.* Center for Research on Education, Diversity and Excellence and the Office of Educational Research Improvement. (ERIC Document Reproduction Service No. ED 475048).

Torres, L. (1989). Code-mixing and borrowing in a New York Puerto Rican community: A cross generational study. *World Englishes, 8*(3), 419–432.

Uffen, E. (2004, January 20). Larry Higdon: Advocate for the professions. *The ASHA Leader, 22,* 4–5.

U.S. Census Bureau. (2000). *Profile of general demographic characteristics.* Washington, DC: Author.

U.S. Census Bureau. (2001). *The Hispanic population in the United States: Population characteristics.* Washington, DC: Author.

U.S. Census Bureau. (2003). *The Hispanic population in the United States: Population characteristics.* Washington, DC: Author.

U.S. Department of Education. (2002). *No Child Left Behind: A desktop reference.* Washington, DC: Author.

Vihman, M. M. (1985). Language differentiation by the bilingual infant. *Journal of Child Language, 12,* 297–324.

Volterra, V., & Taeschner, T. (1978). The acquisition and development of language by bilingual children. *Journal of Child Language, 5,* 311–326.

Westby, C. (1991, October). *Standardized tests: Uses and abuses.* Paper presented at Adelante, National Forum on the Communication Needs of the Hispanic Population, Albuquerque, NM.

Whitely, S. M. (2002). *A course in Spanish linguistics: Spanish/English contrasts* (2nd ed.). Washington, DC: Georgetown University Press.

Wong-Fillmore, L. (1991). A question of early-childhood programs: English first or families first? *National Association of Bilingual Education News, 14*(7), 14–19.

Wong-Fillmore, L. W. (1992). *When does 1 + 1 = <2?* Paper presented at Bilingualism/Bilingüismo: A Clinical Forum, Miami, FL.

Wylie, E., & Ingram, D. E. (1999). *International second language proficiency ratings.* Brisbane, Australia: Griffith University.

Zygouris-Coe, V. (2001). *Literacy for limited English proficiency (LEP) students.* Orlando, FL: Family, Literacy and Reading Excellence Center.

CHAPTER APPENDIX

Adolescent Pragmatics Screening Scale (© 1990 Brice)

Student Information

Name _____ Age _____ Grade _____ School _____ Date _____

1. Indicate the student's first language background.
2. Indicate the student's home language background if different first language.
3. Indicate student's English language proficiency level from 1 to 5.
   (1 = nativelike, 2 = near-nativelike, 3 = medium, 4 = limited, 5 = very limited)
4. Indicate the student's cultural/ethnic background (e.g., Euro-American, African-American, Hispanic, Asian-American, Native American, or the student's specific cultural background).
5. Indicate the number of years the student has been in schools in the United States.

Teacher/Rater Information

Indicate your professional background (speech-language pathologist, bilingual teacher, ESL teacher, regular education teacher, special education teacher, special education–classroom).

7. Indicate your first language background.
8. Indicate your proficiency level from 1 to 5 in English.
   (1 = nativelike, 2 = near-nativelike, 3 = medium, 4 = limited, 5 = very limited)
9. Are you proficient in another language other than English (yes/no)?
10. If yes, indicate what language.
11. Indicate your proficiency level from 1 to 5 in your other language.
    (1 = nativelike, 2 = near-nativelike, 3 = medium, 4 = limited, 5 = very limited)
12. Are you culturally knowledgeable or aware about another culture?
13. Indicate your cultural knowledge/awareness level of the other culture from 1 to 5.
    (1 = nativelike, 2 = near-nativelike, 3 = medium, 4 = limited, 5 = very limited)
14. Indicate which culture or cultures.

Test Score Information

Scoring : Mean Topic Scores (M.T.S.)

Topic 1 sum of the individual behaviors __ divided by 11 = __ No. 1. **M.T.S.**

Topic 2 sum of the individual behaviors __ divided by 7 = __ No. 2. **M.T.S.**

Topic 3 sum of the individual behaviors __ divided by 4 = __ No. 3. **M.T.S.**

Topic 4 sum of the individual behaviors __ divided by 6 = __ No. 4. **M.T.S.**

Topic 5 sum of the individual behaviors __ divided by 7 = __ No. 5. **M.T.S.**

Topic 6 sum of the individual behaviors __ divided by 3 = __ No. 6. **M.T.S.**

Sum of ALL the individual behaviors __

Sum of ALL the individual behaviors __ divided by 39 = __ Total Score (T.S.)

15. Do you feel that this student's performance was influenced by the student's cultural background?
    _____ Yes _____No

If the answer is yes, please indicate which behaviors lead you to this conclusion by making a notation in the **Observation** section next to the corresponding behavior.

THE ADOLESCENT PRAGMATICS SCREENING SCALE (APSS)

Name: _____

Score: Please indicate the student's level using the scale below:

1. **Behavior is highly appropriate.**
2. **Behavior is moderately appropriate.**
3. **Behavior is borderline appropriate.**
4. **Behavior is moderately inappropriate.**
5. **Behavior is highly inappropriate.**

Observations: This section is reserved for performance observations that you feel are pertinent to your rating.

1. Affects listener's behavior through language

Behavior	Score	Observation
1. Asks for help (e.g., "I don't know how to do this problem," "Can you show me how to look up a word in the dictionary?" "How do you spell _____?")		
2. Asks questions (e.g., "How many times does 9 go into 72?" "How does a president get elected?")		
3. Attempts to persuade others (e.g., "I really think John is the best candidate because _____" "I don't think I should have to do this because _____.")		
4. Informs another of important information (e.g., "Teacher, someone wrote some bad words on the wall outside," "I saw a snake in the boy's bathroom down the hall.")		
5. Asks for a favor of a friend/ classmate (e.g., "Can you give me a ride to school?" "Will you ask Sally out for Friday night for me?")		
6. Asks for a favor of the teacher (e.g., "Can I redo the homework assignment?" "Can I get out of class five minutes early so I can catch the new bus?")		
7. Asks for teachers' and/or adults' permission (e.g., going to the bathroom, asking to get a drink of water, asking to sharpen a pencil.)		

Behavior	Score	Observation
8. Asks for other student's permission (e.g., "Can I invite John to go with us?" "Can I ask your girlfriend for her phone number?")		
9. Able to negotiate, give and take, in order to reach an agreement (e.g. "I'll give you a ride to school if you pay me five dollars a week for gas," "I'll help you with your Algebra homework if you help me paint the signs for homecoming.")		
10. Is able to give simple directions (e.g., telling how to find the Spanish teacher's classroom or how to find the bathroom.)		
11. Rephrases a statement (e.g., "You meant this, didn't you?" "Did you mean this _____?")		
Topic 1. Sum of Scores		

2. Expresses self

Behavior	Score	Observation
1. Describes personal feelings in an acceptable manner (e.g., says, "I wish that this English class wasn't so boring," "I'm feeling really frustrated by all the setbacks on my homework.")		
2. Shows feelings in acceptable manner (e.g., taking audible breaths to contain one's anger or smiling with enthusiasm to show pleasure.)		
3. Offers a contrary opinion in class discussions (e.g., "I don't believe that Columbus was the first to discover America; Leif Ericson was said to have reached Greenland and Nova Scotia before Columbus," "I don't believe that the two-party system really offers a choice to voters.")		

Behavior	Score	Observation
4. Gives logical reasons for opinions (e.g., "I believe that the two-party system offers a wider choice than the one-party system," "I think we should work on something else; we did something like this yesterday.")		
5. Says that they disagree in a conversation (e.g., "I don't agree with you," "We can't agree on this one.")		
6. Stays on topic for an appropriate amount of time.		
7. Switches response to another mode to suit the listener (e.g., speaks differently when addressing the principal than when addressing a friend, speaks differently to a younger child of 2–3 years than addressing peers of the same age.)		
Topic 2. Sum of Scores		

3. Establishes appropriate greetings

Behavior	Score	Observation
1. Establishes eye contact when saying hello or greeting.		
2. Smiles when meeting friends.		
3. Responds to an introduction by other similar greeting.		
4. Introduces self to others ("Hi, I'm _____", "My name is _____, what's yours?)		
Topic 3. Sum of Scores		

4. Initiates and maintains conversation

Behavior	Score	Observation
1. Displays appropriate response time.		
2. Asks for more time (e.g., "I'm still thinking," "Wait a second," "Give me some more time.")		
3. Notes that the listener is not following the conversation and needs clarification or more information (e.g., "There's a thing down there, down there, I mean there's a snake down in the boy's bathroom down the hall.")		
4. Talks to others with appropriate pitch and loudness levels of voice (e.g., uses appropriate levels for the classroom, physical education, the lunchroom, or after school.)		
5. Answers questions relevantly (e.g., "Nine goes into 72 8 times," "The president gets elected by the people.")		
6. Waits for appropriate pauses in conversation before speaking.		
Topic 4. Sum of Scores		

5. Listens actively

Behavior	Score	Observation
1. Asks to repeat what has been said for better understanding (e.g., "Could you say that again?" "What do you mean?")		
2. Looks at teacher when addressed (e.g., through occasional glances or maintained eye contact.)		
3. Listens to others in class (e.g., head is up, leaning toward the speaker, eyes on the speaker.)		
4. Changes activities when asked by the teacher (e.g., is able to put away his or her paper and pencil or close a book or pull out something different without having to be told personally.)		
5. Acknowledges the speaker verbally (e.g., says, "Uh-huh, yeah, what else?")		
6. Acknowledges the speaker nonverbally (e.g., looks at the speaker through occasional glances, maintained eye contact, or nodding.)		
7. Differentiates between literal and figurative language (e.g., the student knows that the expression "John is sharp as a tack" actually it means that John is very smart, or that if "Sally's leg is killing her" it does not mean that Sally will die.)		
Topic 5. Sum of Scores		

6. Cues the listener regarding topic shifts

Behavior	Score	Observation
1. Waits for a pause in the conversation before speaking about something else (e.g., waits for a pause of approximately 3–5 seconds at the end of a thought or sentence.)		
2. Looks away to indicate loss of interest in conversation (e.g., looks away and maintains this look for approximately 3–5 seconds.)		
3. Makes easy transitions between topics (e.g., the listener does not question what they are talking about.)		
Topic 6. Sum of Scores		

Chapter 5

School-Age Language Development

Terry Irvine Saenz

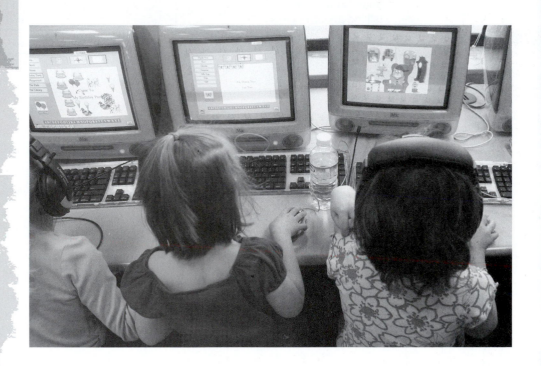

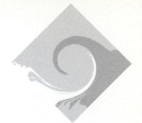

CHAPTER OUTLINE

HOME LANGUAGE VERSUS SCHOOL AND CLASSROOM LANGUAGE

Children face two challenges when they enter school: ". . . knowing what to say, and knowing the rules of interaction that allow one to say it." (Snow & Blum-Kulka, 2002, p. 328). Conversation with groups of family members has taught children rules about participation in conversation at home, including appropriate times to speak; opportunities to take turns in conversation; and, in bilingual families, rules for using each language with each family member in different contexts. To engage successfully in classroom discourse, children must learn the rules for classroom participation, which also may vary with different contexts. They need to learn when to respond to the teacher's questions by calling out answers or waiting to be called on (Peled & Blum-Kulka, 1997, cited in Snow & Blum-Kulka, 2002). Students must recognize when a teacher indicates approval or disapproval of their responses and decipher the hints that many teachers use to control students or to signal changes in activities (Snow & Blum-Kulka, 2002).

Students also need to recognize when teachers are genuinely requesting information that they do not know or merely asking children to display their knowledge (Snow & Blum-Kulka, 2002). Prior to school entry, some children have been exposed to parent-child routines in which they were expected to display their knowledge, as, for example, by naming pictures in books during book reading (DeTemple & Snow, 2003). These routines prepared children well for similar display routines in school. In contrast, some children may have had limited exposure to such parent-child routines (Beals & Snow, 1994) and may be confused by requests to provide information that the teacher already knows.

Students also need to learn how to participate in different types of verbal contexts in elementary school, such as book reports and sharing (Snow & Blum-Kulka, 2002). Teachers often exhibit a strong preference for factual knowledge that is relevant to the topic at hand presented in a specific format. Some children from higher socio-economic status families may have had greater opportunities to converse with family members before entering school and may therefore be more familiar with what is expected in the classroom. However, children unfamiliar with mainstream standards for narratives may produce narratives that differ in form from that expected by classroom teachers (Snow & Blum-Kulka, 2002).

For children who speak a language other than English, entry into school also may mark their first exposure to English. Their maintenance of their home language during the school years is influenced by their social environment, including their parents' language use (Kasuya, 2002; Wei, 1993). Bilingual children develop rules for using each of their languages in new contexts. They learn to be sensitive to the dominant languages of their conversational partners, often addressing listeners in their native languages (Kasuya, 2002). Conversely, bilingual children may answer in the language they are addressed in, whether or not that language is the speaker's native language.

Second-language acquisition continues throughout the elementary years for many bilingual children (refer to Chapter 4 on second-language acquisition issues). It has been estimated that children take approximately two years of exposure to acquire basic interpersonal communicative skills (BICS), or conversational skills, in a second language, but they take five to seven years to acquire cognitive/academic language proficiency (CALP), or the use of language in academic contexts (Cummins, 1984). However, students who are performing below their expected grade level in their first language take longer, that is, 7 to 10 years, to reach the 50th normal curve equivalent (NCE). The NCE is a standard score with a mean of 50 and a standard deviation of 21.06. Some never reach this norm (Thomas & Collier, 1997). As bilingual students grow in second-language proficiency during the school years, the gap in academic performance between monolingual and bilingual children in English should narrow (Cobo-Lewis, Pearson, Eilers, & Umbel, 2002a).

PHONOLOGICAL DEVELOPMENT IN THE PRIMARY SCHOOL YEARS

Children acquire a number of phonemes in the early elementary grades. The following phonemes are correctly produced by 75% of English-speaking school-age children at the following ages: age 5, /ʃ/ (*sh*), /s/, and /tʃ/ (*ch*); age 5 and one half, /ð/ (*th* in *this*); and age 6, *ng* in *ring*, *th* in *thumb*, /z/, /l/, and /r/ (Smit, Hand, Freilinger, Bernthal, & Bird, 1990). In addition, children at age 5 still may use the phonological processes of gliding of the liquid /r/, in which /w/ is substituted, and stopping on /ð/ (*th* in *this*) and /0/ (*th* in *thumb*) with substitutions of /d/ and /t/ (Grunwell, 1981, 1997).

Most research studies of bilingual phonological acquisition identify some **cross-linguistic effects** (Goldstein, Fabiano, & Iglesias, 2004, cited in Goldstein, Fabiano, & Washington, 2005; Goldstein et al., 2005), or the influence of one language's phonological system on another. Effects may be due to differences in the phonological systems of each language because one language may lack a phoneme that is included in another language (Goldstein & Iglesias, 2001). Differences in the distribution of sounds in two languages can also cause interfering cross-linguistic effects (Goldstein & Iglesias, 2001). Different phonotactic constraints, or a language's restrictions on the position of sounds or sequences of sounds in syllables or words, may be the cause of cross-linguistic effects in children's phonological development (Perez, 1994). For example, in Spanish, only /s, n, r, l, d/ appear in word-final position (Goldstein et al., 2005). In addition, bilingual Spanish-speaking children may add an /e/ at the beginning of a word, transforming *stop* into *estop*, because consonant blends cannot begin with /s/ in Spanish (Goldstein et al., 2005). However, the influence of cross-linguistic effects may be minimal. Studies of Spanish-English bilingual children in the early elementary grades have determined that less than 0.3% of all segments result from cross-linguistic effects (Goldstein et al., 2004, cited in Goldstein et al., 2005).

Bilingual children's phonological skills in each language may not be significantly related to the frequency with which they speak each language (Goldstein et al., 2005). Predominantly Spanish-speaking and bilingual 5-year-olds may produce Spanish phonemes with comparable accuracy, and the same pattern occurs with primarily English-speaking and bilingual 5-year-olds in English (Goldstein et al., 2005). Each group has an overall 90% accuracy rate, with cluster reduction the only phonological process produced with greater than 10% frequency.

MORPHOLOGICAL DEVELOPMENT IN THE PRIMARY SCHOOL YEARS

By school age, children have acquired a number of grammatical morphemes. By the time they are 5, children average 85% or above accuracy in producing plural -*s* (e.g., "socks"), third person singular -*s* (e.g., "He eats"), regular past tense -*ed* (e.g., "He walk*ed*"), *be* (e.g., "He *is* going," "He *is* hungry"), and *do* (e.g., "He *does* eat cookies") (Rice & Wexler, 1996; Rice, Wexler, & Cleave, 1995; Rice, Wexler, & Hershberger, 1998).

At age 6, children understand the suffixes of -*man* and -*er* and use many plural nouns (Owens, 2001). In addition, 8-year-olds use -*er* to indicate someone who initiates an action (e.g., bak*er*), and 11-year-olds use -*er* to indicate an instrument (e.g., *eraser*).

Students who initially are exposed to a second language in elementary school may present a somewhat different pattern of morphological development. Four-and-a-half to 7-year-olds recently exposed to English are still in the process of acquiring basic interpersonal communicative skills (Paradis, 2005). After 9 months, they average less than 40% accuracy for the following tenses: third person present tense -*s* (e.g., "He sit*s*"); regular past -*ed* (e.g., "He jump*ed*"); and irregular past tense (e.g., "He *ate*"). However, the bilingual children's accuracy is far higher for other verb forms, including *be* as an auxiliary or copula verb (e.g., "It *is* raining," "He *is* sick"), and *do* (e.g., "I *do* like it"). Noteworthy is the fact that the typical second-language learners' morphological errors may be similar to those of monolingual children with language disorders (Paradis, 2005; Paradis & Crago, 2000).

SEMANTIC DEVELOPMENT

A number of developments take place in the area of semantics during the school-age years. It is estimated that 5- to 6-year-olds know between 2,500 and 5,000 words (Beck & McKeown, 1991). It is also estimated that children learn approximately 9 or 10 new words each day (Carey, 1978), or 3,000 words per year (Beck & McKeown, 1991). However, this estimate of vocabulary growth refers to **fast mapping,** the initial representation of a new word after minimal exposure (McGregor, Friedman, Reilly, & Newman, 2002). The process of fast mapping marks the beginning of the **slow mapping** of a word, a process in which children compare the characteristics of an object or concept with other representations of words and use the new information to update the word's meaning (Carey, 1978).

Children in the early elementary school years, when attempting to identify objects, most often make **semantic errors,** in which they substitute the name of another related object (McGregor et al., 2002). These semantic errors may include **superordinate substitutions,** in which a category itself may be substituted for an object (e.g., *animal* for *cat*), and especially **coordinate substitutions** (e.g., *dog* for *cat*), in which another word of the same category is substituted. Many semantic errors arise from the fact that children have begun learning some of the attributes of an object but are in the process of learning the characteristics that differentiate it from other objects.

CASE STUDY PERSPECTIVES

This case study is presented to illustrate strategies that speech-language pathologists (SLPs), classroom teachers, other school professionals, and parents may use with their students or children.

Case Study One Background: Mark

Mark (not his real name) is an 8-year-old monolingual English-speaking boy in third grade. His father, who reported that Mark had difficulty with word finding and problems remembering even common words, referred him for assessment. Mark was reported to have no social or academic difficulties in school. He had received therapy for stuttering in early elementary school, but he had protested so much that therapy was discontinued after two years.

Mark was extremely cooperative during testing. He performed well on a number of measures. Audiological screening and articulation testing indicated that his hearing and articulation were within normal limits.

In a language sample, Mark's mean length of utterance (MLU), his average number of morphemes per utterance, was 8.95, within normal limits. He produced a variety of simple, compound, and complex sentences and a number of pronouns, infinitives, negatives, and conjunctions correctly. He also produced several verb tenses correctly, including the present tenses, regular past tenses, irregular past tenses, and modals (e.g., *did*, *do*, *would*, and *could*). His only verb errors were *catched* for the irregular past form *caught*, and the omission of *do* in a sentence with a question.

For a narrative about the story *Little Red Riding Hood*, Mark produced a well-formed narrative with events in the correct sequence and a complex episode. Mark's pragmatic skills were appropriate; he demonstrated appropriate turn taking and responses to questions.

However, Mark's standardized language testing results were extremely inconsistent. On the *Clinical Evaluation of Language Fundamentals—3 (CELF—3)*, a test measuring different language skills, Mark's performance was average or above on all of the subtests with the exception of formulated sentences, on which he scored at the 9th percentile. In this subtest, children are given a word and asked to make up a sentence using the word that describes a picture. Mark also performed at the 60th percentile on the *Peabody Picture Vocabulary Test (PPVT)*, a test in which children pointed to pictures when named, but only scored at the 40th percentile on the Expressive One Word Picture Vocabulary Test (EOWPVT), a test in which he had to label pictures. His errors on the EOWPVT were primarily of words that were related to the picture but that were less specific, such as *car* for *bus*. Most important, Mark scored at the second percentile on the Test of Word Finding, a test that included tasks in which he had to name pictures of a variety of types of concepts.

When tested for fluency, Mark had a 6.5% disfluency rate. Almost 1% of his speech consisted of revisions of his sentences, and he often forcefully initiated speech without stuttering. At these times, he demonstrated considerable tension in his neck and shoulders and sometimes swallowed hard before speaking.

Case Study One Comments: Mark

Mark has a combination of a fluency and a language disorder. He clearly has problems with stuttering, which he is aware of and which he is trying to control. At the same time, he has word-finding problems in terms of naming and describing pictures and concepts. There may be a relationship between his word-finding difficulties and attempts to control his disfluency. By avoiding certain words or revising his sentences, he may be trying to avoid stuttering.

Speech-language therapy should include therapy for his disfluency that includes techniques to enhance fluency and to not avoid words. At the same time, he can receive therapy for word finding that involves reinforcing vocabulary using thematic units, preferably using themes that are being taught in his classroom. Such vocabulary is easier to remember when it is taught together with other vocabulary words that address the same theme. In addition, Mark can be taught one or more **mnemonic strategies** for remembering words (Scruggs & Mastropieri, 2000). In the **keyword method,** the word being learned is recoded into a keyword that is easy to picture, is familiar to the child, and sounds similar to the word being learned. For example, to teach *alliance*, *lions* can be selected as the keyword, and the child can be taught to visualize a circle of lions making an agreement not to fight, or an alliance (Scruggs & Mastropieri, 1989). In the **pegword method,** children are taught words that rhyme with numbers to help them remember numbered information (Scruggs & Mastropieri, 2000). For example, a child is taught to remember that insects have six legs by picturing insects on *sticks,* a word that rhymes with *six.* For **letter strategies,** children are taught acronyms or acrostics, verses in which the initial or final letters of the lines taken in order form a word or phrase. For example, HOMES is an acronym for the first initials of the Great Lakes. Mnemonic strategies have been found to be highly effective in teaching students with learning disabilities vocabulary and other information and can be used in classroom contexts (Mastropieri, Scruggs, Levin, Gaffney, & McLoone, 1985; Mastropieri, Sweda, & Scruggs, 2000; Scruggs & Mastropieri, 2000).

Students' comprehension of figurative language increases during the school years. **Metaphors** and **similes** are figures of speech that involve a comparison of an actual object to a description of an image (Owens, 2001). Metaphors include an implied comparison, such as "he has a *soaring* imagination." Similes have an explicit comparison that includes the words *like* or *as,* as in "he is *as slow as* molasses." **Proverbs** are short sayings that convey advice or a generally accepted thought, such as "a penny saved is a penny earned" (Owens, 2001), and are often literally interpreted by young school-age children.

Students also grow in their comprehension of **idioms,** or figurative expressions that cannot be analyzed grammatically, such as "it's raining cats and dogs" or "don't look a gift horse in the mouth," (Nippold, Moran, & Schwarz, 2001; Owens, 2001). Idioms can vary in their familiarity (how often children have read or heard an idiom) and **transparency** (how closely the literal meaning relates to the nonliteral meaning of the expression). Children often find familiar idioms easier to produce than unfamiliar ones (Levorato & Cacciari, 1992). With a transparent idiom, the nonliteral meaning is similar to its literal meaning, as in "the coast is clear" to state that a person does not need to hide (Gibbs, 1987). In contrast, an **opaque** idiom has a nonliteral meaning that is substantially different from its literal meaning, as in "don't pull my leg" to tell a listener not to attempt to fool the speaker. Children often use the context in which an idiom is spoken to determine what the idiom actually means (Levorato & Cacciari, 1992). For further discussion of idioms and figurative language in adolescents, please refer to Chapter 2.

Initially, elementary students find idioms confusing. First-graders experience great difficulty in explaining idioms (Johnson & Anglin, 1995), but fifth-graders are more successful at the task (Nippold & Rudzinski, 1993). When given a choice of definitions of idioms, children in upper elementary school perform better at selecting the definitions of the most transparent idioms (Nippold & Taylor, 1995, 2002).

Preadolescents also vary in their ability to infer meaning from idioms presented in a written story format (Nippold et al., 2001). Good comprehenders are able to interpret idioms that they are familiar with and to utilize contextual cues from stories to interpret unfamiliar ones. In contrast, poor comprehenders, typically students with poor reading and listening comprehension, have trouble interpreting both familiar and unfamiliar idioms.

In developing semantic skills in two languages, bilingual children appear to fast map vocabulary in their second language as well as their first language, later filling in the characteristics of words (Poulisse, 1997). Many bilingual children also demonstrate a shift toward greater English vocabulary with increased exposure to the language (Kohnert & Bates, 2002; Kohnert, Bates, & Hernandez, 1999). In Spanish and English, children who begin to learn English between 4 and 6 years of age perform comparably in the two languages in nonverbally identifying whether common pictured objects and spoken labels match by ages 5 to 7 (Kohnert & Bates, 2002). Their performance improves in both languages, but it is superior in English by ages 11 to 13. In terms of naming pictures, the performance of children aged 5 to 7 is consistently stronger in Spanish, mixed by ages 8 to 10, and relatively equal by 11 to 13 (Kohnert, Bates, & Hernandez, 1999). While the acquisition of Spanish vocabulary slows relative to English, skills may plateau rather than decrease (Kohnert, 2000).

Formal Definitions: A Metalinguistic Skill

Producing a formal definition is an evolving **metalinguistic skill** that develops during the elementary school years. Metalinguistic skills allow language users to conceptualize language apart from their own behavior, and they involve speakers' ability to consciously evaluate language behavior (McLaughlin, 1998; Owens, 2001).

Definitions of objects in the early elementary school years often involve descriptions of the physical properties of objects and their functions (Benelli, Arcuri, & Marchesini, 1988; McGregor et al., 2002). Students from the early through middle elementary school years have less difficulty in defining compound nouns and root nouns without prefixes or suffixes than in defining nouns with prefixes or suffixes, verbs, or adjectives (Johnson & Anglin, 1995). The majority of their errors may involve definitions that are too narrow in scope and are tied to a particular experience or context (e.g., "An apple is something you eat for lunch"). However, children also may produce definitions that are too broad in scope and that do not differentiate words from other related concepts (e.g., "A cat is a pet"). The content of students' definitions generally is superior to the form throughout the middle elementary years.

As students grow older, however, they become more adept at providing what are called **Aristotelian, formal, or dictionary definitions** (Marinellie & Johnson, 2003; Nippold, 1995). These types of definitions include a **superordinate category** in conjunction with specific characteristics (e.g., "A chair is a piece of furniture that you sit on"). This development of formal definitions includes both changes in grammatical form (e.g., "A is a type of B that is C") and in content with the use of superordinate terms (Marinellie & Johnson, 2003; Nippold, Hegel, Sohlberg, & Schwarz, 1999). Other, less formal types of definitions include negation, in which a concept is described by what it is not (e.g., "When something is *quick*, it is not slow"), example (e.g., "For example, Siamese is a popular *breed* of cat"); comparison, in which a concept is compared to a familiar concept (e.g., "A *hamster* is like a big mouse"); and operational, in which a concept's definition is related to the purpose or function of the concept in a specific situation (e.g., "*Cheering* is when people yell at a football game") (Makau, 1990; Nippold et al., 1999).

Students in late childhood are able to define concrete nouns using Aristotelian definitions, although abstract nouns are more difficult to define, and their development continues into adolescence (McGhee-Bidlack, 1991). Twelve-year-olds' errors in describing abstract nouns are likely to consist of the analysis of a word into its constituent parts to come up with an inaccurate but reasonable definition (e.g., analyzing *misreading* into *mis-* and *reading*) or the interpretation of an unfamiliar word based on a similar-sounding word (e.g., defining *parrot* for *merit*) (Nippold et al., 1999). Alternatively, 12-year-olds' definitions may consist of a short description of a word with an omission of a superordinate category. Definitions seldom include a superordinate category alone or in conjunction with an inaccurate description (Nippold et al., 1999).

However, even students in the upper elementary grades (sixth grade) define adjectives in a variety of ways (Marinellie & Johnson, 2003). They may provide a near-synonym (e.g., *beautiful*: "pretty"), a synonym (e.g., *beautiful*: "lovely"), or a negation in which they use a negative with an antonym or opposite (e.g., *beautiful*: "not ugly"). Students also may produce an explanation that uses a related concept with additional specific information (e.g., *beautiful*: "something that is very nice") or an illustration/association (e.g., *beautiful*: "everyone likes to look at them"). Sixth-graders are most likely to define adjectives by using a near-synonym, possibly with the addition of a negation or an association. They are less likely to provide superordinate categories in their adjective definitions than are adults. In addition, they, along with adults, are more effective in defining words that are used more frequently in English.

Translation Skills in Bilingual Students

Bilingual children may be able to perform some language functions in their second language without translation relatively early in their exposure to a second language (Cummins, 2000; Mägiste, 1992). With increased exposure to a second language, bilingual students' relative processing speed changes in their first and second languages (Mägiste, 1992). Elementary school students can name objects as quickly in their second language as their first after four years of exposure (Mägiste, 1992). This increased naming speed may be an indication that, at least in terms of everyday conversational tasks, students no longer need to translate common words. In addition, Cummins's (2000) concept of basic interpersonal communication skills, typically acquired after a few years of exposure to the second language, also presupposes the ability to communicate in conversational contexts without extensive translation.

Bilingual children may use their translation skills strategically as they become more proficient in the second language. Many students take on the role of language brokers, orally interpreting important conversations and translating written documents for their families (Morales & Hanson, 2005; Weisskirch & Alva, 2002). The majority of immigrant children may become language brokers, starting to interpret and to translate within one to five years after arriving in the United States, and frequently beginning as young as age 8 or 9 (Morales & Hanson, 2005). Language brokers interpret for their parents, other relatives, and school administrators in a variety of settings, and they can translate sophisticated written documents such as notes from school, bank statements, job applications, and immigration forms.

Bilingualism and Cognitive Development

The ability to acquire basic interpersonal communicative skills, at least at the elementary level, appears to be relatively unaffected by measures of general intelligence (Genesee, 1976, 1987; Genesee, Paradis, & Crago, 2004). However, cognitive academic language proficiency tends to vary with intelligence. Children who are second-language learners and score high or low in their first language on tests of general intelligence and related reading, writing, and spelling skills tend to score similarly in their second language on the same skills (Genesee, Paradis, & Crago, 2004). Introduction of a second language also does not appear to harm students' cognitive academic language proficiency in their first or second languages. The second-language performance in reading and writing of children who participate in well-constructed second-language immersion programs, in which instruction is provided in the second language, is comparable to the performance of similar students being educated and tested in their first language. Their performance in their first language on tests of language arts and mathematics may also be comparable to that of similar monolingual students in their first language (Caldas & Boudreaux, 1999; Jacobs & Cross, 2001).

Bilingualism does not affect children's mathematical problem solving, although calculations in the weaker language may be made at a slower speed (Bialystok, 2001). In addition, young bilinguals with higher levels of bilingualism are better at paying selective attention to tasks. Consequently, children do not suffer academic disadvantages if at least one language is at a level that is appropriate for their age (Bialystok, 2001).

Cummins (2000) has gone further in proposing the **interdependence hypothesis,** or a positive relationship between children's cognitive academic language proficiency in their first and second languages (see Figure 5–1). This interdependence is based primarily on the cognitive and personality attributes of a bilingual individual when languages are dissimilar, such as Japanese and English, but is also based on linguistic similarities when languages are similar, such as Spanish and English. Cummins (2000) has hypothesized that the continued development of cognitive academic language

FIGURE 5–1
Cummins's Cognitive and Contextual Demands

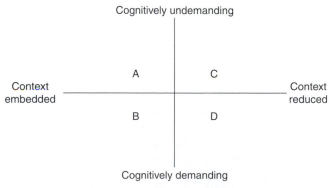

Source: From *Language, power, and pedagogy: Bilingual children in the crossfire* by J. Cummins (2000), page 68. Copyright © 2000 by Multilingual Matters. Reprinted with permission of the author.

proficiency in a bilingual's two languages is associated with increased metalinguistic, cognitive, and academic skills.

There is some support for the interdependence hypothesis (Cobo-Lewis, Pearson, Eilers, & Umbel, 2002b). There is a strong relationship between literacy skills in Spanish and English, although oral language abilities may not be strongly related in the two languages (Cobo-Lewis et al., 2002b). However, there is no tendency for competence in one language to harm competence in another. Furthermore, English test scores of children in bilingual classes initially lag behind bilingual children in English immersion classes, but they may later catch up and even surpass the other children in some academic tests in English (Cobo-Lewis et al., 2002b). In addition, children who act as language brokers can develop high levels of cognitive ability because of the complexity of the documents that they translate, and there may be a positive relationship between language brokering and academic performance (Morales & Hanson, 2005). Consequently, it may be cognitively advantageous to bilingual children to continue to develop proficiency in their first language after initial exposure to their second language.

SYNTACTIC DEVELOPMENT: NOUN AND VERB PHRASE DEVELOPMENT

During the elementary years, children's noun phrase development includes important changes in terms of pronouns and adjectives (Owens, 2001). Less than 50% of children in first grade can use correct pronouns (Owens, 2001). However, children become better able to distinguish between subject pronouns, such as *we, they, he, she,* and *I,* and object pronouns, such as *us, them, him, her,* and *me.* Children also begin to use reflexives, such as *ourselves, himself, herself,* and *myself.* They learn to use pronouns to refer to nouns in prior sentences (e.g., "The wind was blowing. *It* swept up the leaves").

Children also begin adding postnoun modifiers (e.g., The girl *with the basket* sat down") and ordering strings of adjectives correctly based on the adjectives' properties. They also distinguish between mass nouns, such as *corn,* and count nouns, such as *cookies* (Miller, 1991).

Children's verb phrases become more complex as they advance through the school years and increase their use of perfect verb tenses (e.g., "He *has jumped* into the mud puddle," "He *had jumped* into the mud puddle," and "The mud puddle *had been jumped* into") and modal auxiliaries such as *could, might,* and *should* (e.g., "She *could* run around the barn'") (Owens, 2001; Scott & Stokes, 1995). By school age, the *-ed* of the past participle used in producing short passive sentences is well established (e.g., "The boy *was kicked*") (Redmond, 2003). In addition, about 80% of students between 7-and-a-half and 8 produce full passive sentences, which include *be* or *got* with a past tense maker and a preposition that is followed by a noun phrase (e.g., "The cake was baked by the girl") (Owens, 2001).

In terms of sentence types, the types of wh- questions asked by children increase during the school years. While preschool children can ask *who* or *what* questions, by age 8, students can consistently produce *how, when,* and *why* questions (Wallach, 1984, cited in McLaughlin, 1998).

As children reach school age, their sentence structures increase in complexity (Nippold, 1998). They produce a variety of clauses, or grammatical structures that include a subject and a verb (e.g., "The boy tripped"), and phrases, structures without a subject and verb (e.g., "The ball fell *into the pond*"). Children continue to produce **simple sentences** that consist of one **independent,** or **main, clause** that can stand alone as a sentence and any attached phrases (e.g., "The girl went to the mall"). They additionally produce larger numbers of **compound sentences** that consist of two or more independent clauses connected by **coordinating conjunctions** such as *and* or *but* (e.g., "The student ran quickly, but his best friend sat down"). Also increasing is the use of **complex sentences** that consist of an independent clause and one or more **dependent,** or **subordinate, clauses** that cannot stand alone as sentences. **Subordinating conjunctions,** such as *because* or *if,* connect the clauses of complex sentences (e.g., "She is upset because she missed the movie") (Nippold, 1998). Complex sentences also include sentences with an independent clause and an infinitive (e.g., "I want *to sing* a song"); a gerund, which functions as a noun (e.g., "*Swimming* is fun"); or a participle, which functions as an adjective (e.g., "*Running*, she stumbled"). Finally, **compound-complex sentences** include a minimum of two independent clauses and one or more dependent clauses (e.g., "The girl jumped and the boy started when they saw a large bug"). The percentage of complex sentences rises to between 20% and 30% in children's narratives during the school years (Scott, 1984, cited in Owens, 2001).

Dependent clauses can be included, or embedded, in the center or the end of sentences. The inclusion of a dependent clause in the center of a sentence is especially difficult for school-age children to understand (e.g., "The boy, *who sat down*, was tired") (Owens, 2001). There is also a hierarchy of difficulty of comprehension of embedded sentences (Abrahamsen & Rigrodsky, 1984; Owens, 2001), ranging from the easiest to the most difficult. Parallel central embedding, where the independent and dependent clauses have the same subjects, is the easiest to understand (e.g., "The *girl who* is jumping is happy"). Parallel ending embedding shares the same object for the independent and dependent clauses (e.g., "She handed him the *paper that* he needed"). Nonparallel ending embedding has the object of the independent clause as the subject of the dependent clause (e.g., "The girl saw the *plate that* was on the floor"). Finally, nonparallel central embedding has the subject of the independent clause as the object of the dependent clause (e.g., "The *girl that* was frightened by the boy was scared") and is the most difficult to comprehend.

In terms of conjunctions, *and* is used in 50% to 80% of compound sentences (Scott, 1988a) and remains the most common conjunction into adulthood (Scott, 1984, cited in Scott, 1988a). In addition, *because* and *when* are most often used to join clauses up to age 12, with *in order to* and *if* used frequently as well. However, children may not consistently comprehend the meaning of *because* until age 10 and *if* and *though* until age 11 (Owens, 2001).

Children also use relative pronouns to produce relative clauses, embedded clauses that modify subjects or objects (e.g., "The girl *who* fell ran on"). Additional relative pronouns acquired during the school years include *whose, whom,* and *in which* (Scott, 1988a).

Sentence length and **clausal density,** or **subordination index,** are two important measures of older children's syntactic development (Nippold, Hesketh,

Duthie, & Mansfield, 2005). As children move into the school years, their sentence length is often measured in terms of **terminable units,** or **T-units** (Scott, 1988b), which consist of a main clause and any attached or embedded subordinate clauses or nonclausal structures (Hunt, 1970). **Communication units,** or **C-units,** are another measure of sentence length and include all T-units as well as responses to questions that do not include an independent clause (Loban, 1976). Sentence length consists of the mean number of words per T-unit and is obtained by summing the number of words in a language sample and dividing the sum by the number of T-units. Clausal density is defined as the mean number of clauses, including independent and dependent clauses, per T-unit (Nippold et al., 2005). It is obtained by summing the number of clauses in a language sample, both main and subordinate, and dividing by the number of C-units or T-units (Nippold et al., 2005). Of the two measures, sentence length may be the more sensitive indicator of syntactic development (Nippold et al., 2005; Hunt, 1970).

Students' clausal density and mean length of T-unit in words continue to slowly grow through the school years (Nippold et al., 2005; Scott & Stokes, 1995; Scott & Windsor, 2000). Scott and Windsor studied 8- and 11-year-olds producing narratives and expository discourse that described factual information. The 8-year-olds and 11-year-olds produced a mean of 9.5 and 10.3 words per T-unit, respectively, for narratives, compared to means of 10.5 and 11.4 for expository discourse. In terms of the number of clauses produced per T-unit, the 8-year-olds and 11-year-olds produced means of 1.78 and 1.90 for narratives and 1.67 and 1.75 for expository discourse. Nippold and colleagues (2005) also studied 8- and 11-year-olds in conversation and using expository discourse to talk about a favorite sport. The mean number of words per T-unit was 6.74 for 8-year-olds and 7.31 for 11-year-olds for conversation, and 8.59 and 9.27, respectively, for expository discourse. Similarly, clausal density was 1.18 for 8-year-olds and 1.25 for 11-year-olds for conversation and 1.42 and 1.45 for expository discourse. Consequently, for these studies, narratives had the greatest number of clauses per T-unit, but expository discourse had the most words per T-unit.

CLASSROOM DISCOURSE OR PRAGMATIC DEMANDS

An integral part of school-age children's pragmatic abilities involves **classroom discourse,** or the types of speech acts involved in classroom interactions. These may involve interactions between teachers and students or between students.

Researchers have discovered a traditional classroom discourse pattern in lessons of **teacher initiation, student response,** and **teacher evaluation** (IRE) (Mehan, 1979) or **teacher follow-up** (IRF) (Wells, 1993). There are many types of teacher initiations, including closed questions, in which there is only one correct answer, and open questions, in which there are a variety of correct answers. Teachers may also ask **metacognitive questions,** in which students are asked to reflect on their own thinking and knowledge (Duckworth, 1981, cited in Cazden & Beck, 2003).

There are a number of criteria for the evaluation of students' answers, including the following (Snow & Blum-Kulka, 2002): (1) quantity, providing sufficient information; (2) quality, providing accurate information; (3) relevance, providing information pertaining to the question; and (4) manner, providing responses that conform to the form preferred by the teacher. Teacher evaluations may be explicit, such as "right" or "not quite," or implicit (McHoul, 1990; Snow & Blum-Kulka, 2002). For example, teachers may respond to an answer with silence, change the topic, or repeat the answer, any of which may serve as an acceptance or rejection of students' responses. In addition, teachers often provide clues or reformulate questions (McHoul, 1990), which allows students to self-correct their answers. Teacher follow-up may be used to expand on students' answers, to help students make connections between other experiences and the task, or to emphasize the significance of responses (Wells, 1993).

In addition, teachers wait for periods of time after their initiations for students to respond and following students' responses to react, time periods that are referred to as **wait time** (Rowe, 1986). When teachers' wait time extends beyond 2.7 seconds, there are several positive consequences: students are more likely to respond to questions, to participate in discussions, to ask questions, and to produce longer responses, and teachers are more likely to elaborate on students' responses.

Teachers select different ways in which students may participate and respond in the classroom (Jones & Thornbarrow, 2004). The ways in which teachers and students participate are called **floors** (Mehan, 1982). In a whole-class floor, the teacher addresses the entire class and selects which pupils may speak (Jones & Thornbarrow, 2004; Philips, 1972). At times, students can participate simultaneously in a whole-class floor by **chorusing,** or producing the same utterance at the same time, or by using **utterance completion,** in which teachers pause in the middle of utterances and allow students to complete them. In an overlapping floor, children's talk overlaps, while teachers interact with individual students in a one-to-one floor (Jones & Thornbarrow, 2004).

Classroom discourse also has its **critical moments,** times in which teachers' utterances support or hinder children's understanding or miss chances to build on children's responses (Myhill & Warren, 2005). There are three types of critical moments produced by teachers: (1) moments that cause confusion for students, (2) moments that continue classroom interaction on a predetermined path, and (3) moments that respond to students' needs. These critical moments can benefit students by allowing them less formal opportunities to verbalize and think through their ideas than the highly structured teacher-student interactions often characteristic of classroom instruction. Teachers can also help students comprehend instruction by building on the responses of students who are articulating concepts.

Classroom discourse may vary in terms of the cognitive and contextual demands of different types of communicative tasks (Cummins, 2000). Cummins (2000) classifies tasks by their degree of cognitive involvement into cognitively undemanding or cognitively demanding. A cognitively undemanding task is an automatic or rote task such as reciting the alphabet, while a cognitively demanding task is not automatic and necessitates active cognitive involvement, such as persuading fellow students of a particular point of view. Tasks also vary in their degree of contextual support. Context-embedded tasks include tasks in which students can actively negotiate meaning by asking questions, and situational and interpersonal cues are provided by teachers, such as overheads, notes on the blackboard, and other visual cues. One context-embedded task is a classroom discussion that involves a number of contextual cues. Context-reduced tasks almost exclusively rely on the linguistic message for understanding, as in essay writing.

In classroom discourse, rules are established to open and close lessons, change topics, take turns, and clarify meanings (Leinhardt & Steele, 2005). Brice, Mastin, and Perkins (1997) have identified a total of 50 **classroom language functions** that describe pragmatic uses of language in classrooms. One language function is **questioning,** in which questions are used for a variety of purposes, including to implicitly direct students to perform tasks, to elicit answers, and to ask permission. **Commands** function as types of requests that elicit responses from others, involving direct and indirect requests for action and requests for a fill-in answer (or cloze, e.g., "Five minus three is _____."). The **informative** category comprises functions that provide information and are most often used by teachers and aides. In **feedback/reinforcement,** different methods are used to provide reinforcement and feedback, including a variety of types of reinforcement and correction or reprimands and examples. **Answering/responding** comprises different ways in which students can respond to questions.

Some of Brice, Mastin, and Perkins' (1997) classroom language functions include language functions directly related to the beginning and ending of lessons. In **starting a lesson,** devices are used to ready students for instruction, including statements that cue students to the beginning of a new topic, shifts in topic, and fillers that alert students that important information is about to be given. Teachers provide cues that it is time to leave or to finish a lesson in **ending a lesson.**

Other classroom language functions (Brice, Mastin, & Perkins, 1997) delineate additional categories. **Seeking clarification** represents ways for students to obtain assistance with activities, ways for teachers and aides to clarify what is requested of them, and translation. In **speaking out loud,** students talk to themselves or practice responses aloud. Finally, **other code moves** involve a variety of other language functions, including reading and writing and language functions involving the alternation between languages.

NARRATIVE DEVELOPMENT

Narratives become an increasingly important type of discourse during the school years in the classroom. The school years also mark important developments in narrative production.

Four Basic Narrative Types

There are four basic types of **narratives** (Brice-Heath, 1986; Owens, 2004). **Recounts** consist of the retelling of a past experience that usually has been shared with listeners and requested by them. Parents often elicit recounts from their children about past shared experiences. **Eventcasts** are replays or explanations of activities that are currently occurring or are being planned for a future occasion. Children often use eventcasts during cooperative play, as when playing house together. Teachers, parents, and other authority figures can also elicit eventcasts. **Accounts** are narratives of past experiences that speakers spontaneously share with listeners. Finally, **stories** are not based on speakers' experiences but on their imagination and are not believed to be real by listeners.

Development of Narratives

Stein and Glenn (1979, 1982) developed **story grammar analysis** to describe the elements of children's stories. They define a story as a **setting** plus an **episode** system. The setting serves two purposes in the story. It describes the physical, social, or temporal context in which the story occurs and introduces the main characters. Setting statements usually occur at the beginning of a story, but they may occur whenever a new character or physical or social context is introduced. Settings typically present the habitual states or actions of characters or the environment:

> *Once there were these three pigs, and their mom didn't have enough money so they had to go make their own houses.*

The rest of a story consists of an episode system that can include one or more episodes (Owens, 2004; Stein & Glenn, 1979, 1982). An episode can include an **initiating event** whose purpose is to cause a response in a character or characters. It may include an environmental event, such as a storm; an action by another character, such as a mother scolding her child; the perception of an external event, such as a child seeing a cookie; or an internal event, such as a child feeling hunger. The initiating event represents a change in state in the environment or in the characters:

> *The third little pig came running to tell them something. He told them the fox was coming.*

An **internal response** is the psychological state of the characters after the initiating event (Owens, 2004; Stein & Glenn, 1979, 1982). It includes the characters' emotional responses, thoughts, and desires or intentions:

> *The three pigs were scared.*

An **internal plan** describes the characters' strategy for changing the situation and directs the characters' later behavior (Owens, 2004; Stein & Glenn, 1979, 1982). Children usually omit this component:

> *The pigs decided to trick the fox.*

An **attempt** includes information that refers to the characters' actions to reach a goal (Owens, 2004; Stein & Glenn, 1979, 1982):

> *The three little pigs put a pot with burning hot water under the chimney.*

A **direct consequence** involves the success or failure of the characters to attain their goals and is the cause of the characters' reaction (Owens, 2004; Stein & Glenn, 1979, 1982):

When the fox came down, he landed in it. And then he ran straight out the door, and he never came back again.

A **reaction** is the final category of an episode and includes emotions, thoughts, and actions following the direct consequence (Owens, 2004; Stein & Glenn, 1979, 1982):

The three pigs played and singed in their house.

Children who do not tell stories using all of the components of an episode may tell stories using three types of structures (Stein & Glenn, 1982). A **descriptive sequence** includes traits, states, and actions of a main character with no specific sequencing. These stories consist of a series of setting statements. An **action sequence** involves the typical everyday actions of the main characters arranged in chronological order. However, there are no causal connections between events. The story has a setting statement and attempts (Owens, 2004). A **reaction sequence** has a beginning and an end, with causal relations between events (Owens, 2004; Stein & Glenn, 1982). The main characters, however, never develop a goal or plan, and their welfare depends on other people or circumstances. The reaction sequence includes a setting, an initiating event, and attempts (Owens, 2004).

As children mature, they produce narratives that are more complete (Owens, 2004). **Abbreviated episodes** have a tacit or explicit goal and may contain either a direct consequence and an initiating event or an internal response. Characters typically have purposeful but not premeditated behavior. **Complete episodes** include a behavioral sequence that is oriented toward a goal and is comprised of a direct consequence and two of the following: initiating event, attempt, and internal response. **Complex episodes** involve expansions of complete episodes or multiple episodes. **Interactive episodes** have two characters whose separate goals and actions influence one another.

Half of kindergarteners and approximately three quarters of third- and sixth-graders tell stories with a basic episodic structure (Stein & Glenn, 1982). Children as young as 5 may have the basic concept of a story. However, older children construct stories that conform more closely to narrative expectations. Students also recall story grammar components best in the following order: setting statements about characters, initiating events and direct consequences, attempts, internal responses, and other types of setting statements (Stein & Glenn, 1979). Eighty percent of kindergarteners include an attempt, but 50% of kindergarteners and nearly 40% of older children do not include a reaction (Stein & Glenn, 1982). In addition, the only category significantly more frequently recalled by fifth- than by first-graders is the internal response category (Stein & Glenn, 1979). Children also sometimes invert the order of the story grammar categories (Stein & Glenn, 1982).

Children in the early elementary years are more likely to tell stories in the third person and to include characters that are fictional (Sutton-Smith, 1986). Story length increases dramatically with the inclusion of conjunctions, locatives (e.g., *around*), dialogue, adjectives, comparatives (e.g., *faster than*), and possessives (e.g., *their*), and stories become more chronological.

CROSS-CULTURAL NARRATIVE SIMILARITIES AND DIFFERENCES

Children from other cultures are often brought up to use different types of narrative styles. They may enter school with their own narrative traditions.

Narratives of Hispanic Children

In some Hispanic homes, the dinner table is not a location where children typically speak (Silva & McCabe, 1996). In contrast, much storytelling can occur when families are preparing food together. Stories may center on family experiences, religious stories, or stories used to discipline or to instill fear in children.

Hispanic children may be more likely to tell a story in the present tense (e.g., "They *sit* in the living room") or a progressive tense (e.g., "They *are eating* the cookies") to describe habitual actions than in the past tense (Sebastian & Slobin, 1994). They may not follow a linear model in telling narratives (Silva & McCabe, 1996). Narratives may include a great deal of descriptive detail, especially of extended family members and their characteristics, which may be interpreted as not "sticking to the plot" (Silva & McCabe, 1996, p. 128). Narrators also often overlap in their telling of stories.

Bilingual Hispanic children are more likely to include an initiating event and an attempt in Spanish narratives and to include a consequence in English narratives (Fiestas & Peña, 2004). Children learning English may have better narrative skills in one language than in the other. However, even students who appear limited in one language may have sufficient grammar, narrative quality, and narrative structure to produce a narrative (Gutiérrez-Clellen, 2002), although they may have less control over formal grammatical elements than monolinguals (Oller & Eilers, 2002; Pearson, 2002). Children learning English may have greater difficulty recalling a story than in spontaneously producing one.

CASE STUDY PERSPECTIVES

This case study is presented to illustrate strategies that speech-language pathologists, classroom teachers, other school professionals, and parents may use with their students or children.

Case Study Two Background: Yvonne

Yvonne is 6 years old and in first grade. She has grown up in a bilingual English- and Spanish-speaking home and began to talk when she was 3. When Yvonne was a preschooler, her mother asked her pediatrician to have her hearing tested, but the pediatrician refused, stating that Yvonne's hearing was normal.

Yvonne was placed in a bilingual kindergarten, but she failed the kindergarten hearing screening. Further audiological testing at the end of kindergarten revealed that Yvonne had a hearing loss that was slightly below normal in the lower frequencies most important for speech but more severe at higher frequencies. Yvonne was immediately fitted for hearing aids in both ears.

An assessment in English one month after she was fitted for hearing aids found that she produced incomplete sentences and had limited vocabulary in English. She also demonstrated problems with basic concepts. Yvonne had particular difficulties with articulation/phonology; she was only 60 to 65% intelligible in English. Yvonne demonstrated omissions, distortions, and substitutions of other sounds for stops (such as /t/ and /k/), fricatives (such as /f/, /s/, and /z/), affricates (such as /tʃ/, or *ch*, and *j* in *judge*), liquids (/l/ and /r/), and nasals (such as /n/). In addition, she tended to omit one sound in a consonant cluster (e.g., /m/ for /sm/) or substitute sounds (e.g., /fw/ for /sw/).

Yvonne was enrolled in speech-language therapy in first grade, and Yvonne's parents moved her to a monolingual English classroom in December of the same year. Nine months after her English evaluation and ten months after her being fitted with hearing aids, Yvonne was tested in Spanish.

It quickly became apparent during the evaluation that Yvonne now preferred English in her interactions, at least in certain contexts. When a bilingual interpreter tried to talk to her in Spanish, she initially turned to the monolingual English-speaking evaluator and conversed with her in English. Yvonne, however, eventually was willing to interact in Spanish. Her preference for speaking in English may have been pragmatically appropriate for the situation because she correctly deduced that the interpreter was bilingual but that the evaluator spoke only English.

Standardized testing in Spanish was attempted but was discontinued due to poor performance. Instead, a language sample was taken. In Spanish, Yvonne produced prepositions (e.g., "*abajo* de la silla," "*under* the chair"), the present progressive (e.g., "El niño *está corriendo* en la calle," "The boy *is running* in the street"), the present tense with a modal (e.g., "El no *quiere hacer* nada," "He *doesn't want* to do anything"), and a form of Spanish past tense (e.g., "La mamá *dijó*, 'Yo no sé,'" "The mother *said*, 'I don't know' "). However, Yvonne also produced a number of errors, especially in terms of articles, pronouns, and plurals. Sentences were up to eight words long.

In English, Yvonne produced the same grammatical structures. At times, she produced sentences with semantic errors (e.g., "Everybody get away a Piglet and because they gonna get 'Happy Birthday to Piglet'"). She additionally omitted the third person singular *-s* (e.g., "And then everybody *go* in his house.") At the same time, her sentences were up to 15 words in length, and some sentences were quite sophisticated (e.g., "I don't know what it is").

Yvonne's production of a narrative contained a generally correct sequence of events. However, she occasionally used pronouns to refer to unclear referents, thereby making the sequence of events somewhat confusing.

In terms of her phonology/articulation in Spanish, Yvonne omitted some initial consonants of words (e.g., "inero" for *dinero*). She at times produced front consonants for back consonants (e.g., /t/ for /k/), and produced /l/ for /r/. Overall, her intelligibility in Spanish and English had greatly improved since her initial evaluation in English.

Case Study Two Comments: Yvonne

Yvonne unquestionably has made considerable progress in her speech and language skills in the 10 months since she has been fitted for hearing aids and has begun speech and language therapy. She continues to be a candidate for speech and language therapy; however, her progress in therapy is now more rapid because her hearing has greatly improved. In addition, she now appears to have stronger skills in English and prefers to speak it in at least some bilingual situations, making speech and language therapy in English appropriate.

Because the introduction of aids clearly has made a marked difference in Yvonne's speech and language skills, it is recommended that Yvonne's English skills be completely reevaluated in the near future. In addition, a number of modifications in Yvonne's classroom can help her better comprehend instruction. Seating her in the front and center of the class will enable her to hear the instructions of the teacher more clearly. Having the teacher turn toward Yvonne whenever she speaks also will help Yvonne's comprehension. Finally, the teacher should be encouraged to write down homework assignments and other important information on the board.

In terms of speech-language therapy, Yvonne will benefit from an emphasis on both articulation/phonological and language therapy. Based on her Spanish and English evaluations, it is appropriate to remediate her replacement of back consonants by front consonants, a phonological process that is usually extinguished by 4 years of age (Grunwell, 1997). More current testing in English also should indicate other appropriate objectives.

In terms of language therapy, systematic teaching of basic vocabulary, such as prepositions, and work on the third person singular -*s* and possibly plural -*s* is appropriate, particularly because /s/ is difficult to hear with her high-frequency hearing loss. Yvonne can also practice producing narratives because narratives are a common and important form of communication in the classroom. Her frequent use of ambiguous pronouns in narratives makes the sequence of events somewhat unclear.

Narratives of African American Children

African American children may tell what are termed classic European North American narratives even more often than European North American children (Champion, 1998, cited in Craddock-Willis & McCabe, 1996). African American children are also encouraged to talk extensively on a number of topics. There is a tradition of a "performed narrative" (Michaels & Foster, 1985, cited in Craddock-Willis & McCabe, 1996, p. 100), in which the narrator is dramatic, improvisational, interactive, and animated. Narratives often include a great deal of evaluation (Hicks, 1991; Labov, 1972). Some of the devices used to indicate evaluation include gestures, the lengthening of vowels, the use of quantifiers such as *all*, and the repetition of phrases (Labov, 1972).

African American children may start with a true event and improvise upon it (Craddock-Willis & McCabe, 1996). Events may be presented in a way that emphasizes characters' internal motivations and conflicts (Hicks, 1991). African American children also may link together events from different times and places that have a common theme. They may begin and end with the theme and improvise on events in between (Craddock-Willis & McCabe, 1996). Narratives may also involve four sentences per subtopic and use refrains, the repetition of a phrase or sentence throughout the narrative.

Narratives of Asian American Children

Children from Asian cultures differ from children in mainstream American culture in the themes of their narratives (Wang & Leichtman, 2000). Chinese children may include more references to group cooperation, demonstrate a greater concern for doing correct or moral actions, make more references to the feelings of characters, and demonstrate more concern for authority. In addition, Japanese and Chinese American children often talk about multiple experiences in one narrative, unlike European North American children. Japanese children also may exhibit a preference for nonverbal, implicit, and intuitive communication (Lebra, 1986, cited in Minami & McCabe, 1996). Emotional reactions may not be voiced because the listener is expected to empathize with the speaker (Minami & McCabe, 1996). Japanese 5-year-olds have proportionally more action statements and less orientation statements than do adults, but, like adults, they have more statements of evaluation than 4-year-olds (Minami, 1996). Narratives may be of three lines per subtopic in imitation of haiku (Minami & McCabe, 1996).

Narratives of Native American Children

Native American students may initially be hesitant to produce narratives when they enter school, due to some groups' tradition of children observing while elders tell stories (Roseberry-McKibbin, 2002). Native American students from middle to upper elementary school grades may produce narratives that are descriptive or are simple action sequences of behavior in their second language (Westby, Moore, & Roman, (2002). In these stories, characters may have desires or intentions but may infrequently produce plans to achieve them, and their goals may be achieved by outside forces or events. Native American children's narratives may include an orientation, action, and evaluation (Pesco, Crago, & McCabe, 1996); a number of events that focus on the same theme; and dialogue.

THE ENGLISH-AS-A-SECOND-LANGUAGE CLASSROOM VERSUS THE GENERAL EDUCATION CLASSROOM

There are different types of English-as-a-second-language classrooms (refer to Chapter 12 on school language programs available for bilingual children). Sheltered English programs are explicitly designed to teach English and subject matter to bilingual students during their initial exposure to English. The term comes from the time when English-language learners were taught in separate classrooms and sheltered from academically competing with English monolingual students (Freeman & Freeman, 1988). Transitional bilingual programs are designed to shift instruction from predominantly the home language in kindergarten to primarily English for up to three years (Genesee et al., 2004; Snow & Blum-Kulka, 2002). Maintenance or developmental bilingual programs help students retain and develop their first language while learning a second language, and often include some degree of bilingual instruction through the elementary and sometimes secondary grades (Genesee et al., 2004; Oller & Pearson, 2002). Two-way bilingual programs include instruction in English and in another language, with typically half of the children speaking English and half the other language as their native languages (Genesee et al., 2004; Oller & Pearson, 2002).

Language use in English-as-a-second-language classrooms typically includes code switching and code mixing (also refer to Chapter 4 on second-language acquisition). **Code switching** occurs whenever individuals produce complete sentences in a single language yet alternate between languages (e.g., "Quiero la galleta. I want ice cream, too"). **Code mixing** involves the alternation between two languages within a single sentence (e.g., "Dame la doll") (Kamwangamalu, 1992). In most cases, each part of an utterance or each utterance is well formed according to the rules of the respective language (Genesee et al., 2004). Although there is some disagreement as to whether they constitute two different phenomena or one and the same (D'Souza, 1992), code switching and code mixing are generally regarded as the same phenomenon (Brice, 2002). They should not be regarded as deficient phenomena, but instead as complex forms of communication (Kamwangamalu, 1992; MacSwan, 2004; Reyes, 1995; Zentella, 1997). With proficient bilingual speakers, code switching and code mixing are an indication of their comprehension of the syntactic, morphological, semantic, and pragmatic aspects of both languages (Brice & Perkins, 1997). Code switching and code mixing are also common in English-as-a-second-language classrooms. In Brice and Perkins' study of an English-as-a-second-language classroom, 17.4% of utterances involved code switching and code mixing.

In a study of an English-as-a-second-language classroom using Brice and colleagues' language functions (Brice, Mastin, & Perkins, 1997), the use of language functions in the English-as-a-second-language classroom did not appear to be very different from their use in general education classes. The top general categories used in the English-as-a-second-language classroom were teacher-directed and included questioning, commands, giving information, giving feedback, and answering and responding. Certain specific language functions appeared to be associated with learning English as a second language, including vocabulary questions, reiterations (repetitions for emphasis), comprehension questions, and translating a response, in which a response previously stated by another person is translated. Similarly, the general-education class had the top general categories of commands, informative, questioning, feedback, and starting a lesson (Brice & Perkins, 1997). The general-education classroom used more explaining, indirect requests, declarations, one-line cues to finish statements, and one-line statements to change topics (Brice & Perkins, 1997).

CONCLUDING REMARKS

The elementary years are a time for consolidating language skills and learning new ones in a new environment, the elementary classroom. In the areas of phonology, semantics, and syntax, much of the groundwork has been laid and children further develop their skills in the production of longer and more complex utterances. In the area of semantics, students' vocabulary grows at a rapid rate, and more formal definitions become the norm. The pragmatics of classroom discourse involves learning a new set of interaction rules for classroom settings and deciphering the often subtle clues and hints of teachers. Narratives show development in the increasingly skilled use of story grammar components.

Children whose families of origin speak languages other than English may have their first exposure to the English language in kindergarten. Although they take only a few years to attain basic conversational fluency in English, it may be several years before their performance on academic tasks in English matches that of their monolingual peers. In addition, they may bring with them rich traditions of family discourse, pragmatics, and narratives that are, nonetheless, sometimes substantially different from those of the mainstream culture. Consequently, bilingual students may need time to adapt to classroom expectations if those expectations differ substantially from those of their own culture. In addition, they greatly benefit from teachers' sensitivity to their cultural traditions as they learn to adapt to the classroom setting.

INSTRUCTIONAL/CLINICAL STRATEGIES

The following instructional and clinical strategies can be applied to the general education classroom or speech-language therapy, with special reference to the language skills of school-age children.

1. Explain the purpose of school routines that may be unfamiliar to children entering school for the first time, such as the importance of answering questions that the teacher already knows the answer to (Snow & Blum-Kulka, 2002).

2. Monitor students for evidence that they are experiencing breakdowns in understanding (Merritt & Culatta, 1998). Some students, especially culturally diverse students, may be hesitant to tell you that they are confused.

3. Carefully monitor tasks for their degree of cognitive demand and contextual support, especially when working with children who speak English as a second language (Cummins, 2000). Cummins advocates beginning with context-embedded and cognitively undemanding activities, then moving to context-embedded and cognitively demanding activities before working on context-reduced and cognitively demanding activities. Teach new skills using context-embedded strategies, allowing for questions and providing visual cues and translation as needed. Occasionally, context-reduced and cognitively undemanding activities can be included to reinforce or practice skills (Cummins, 2000).

4. Allow bilingual children to code-switch and code-mix (Kamwangamalu, 1992; Reyes, 1995) in the classroom and in therapy because they are not deficient phenomena and may actually help children understand lessons better (Brice, Mastin, & Perkins 1997; Brice & Perkins, 1997).

5. Use mnemonic strategies to help students remember vocabulary and course content (see Case Study One Comments). The keyword method, pegword method, or letter strategies may be used to help students remember concepts (Mastropieri, Scruggs, Levin, Gaffney, & McLoone, 1985; Mastropieri, Sweda, & Scruggs, 2000; Scruggs & Mastropieri, 2000).

6. Teach students idioms and give them practice in figuring out unfamiliar idioms with varying degrees of transparency (Nippold, Moran, & Schwarz, 2001).

7. Teach students the form of formal definitions (Marinellie & Johnson, 2003; Nippold, 1995) and give them practice in developing them. Start with concrete definitions and move to more abstract definitions as children grow older.

8. Focus on helping children to develop their use of longer and more complex sentences by practicing the linking together of short, simple sentences with different types of conjunctions.

9. Teach students the form of narratives used in the public schools by introducing the elements of story grammar (Owens, 2004; Stein & Glenn, 1979, 1982) and having them produce narratives. However, emphasize that other cultural traditions of narratives are not wrong; they are just different.

REFLECTION QUESTIONS

1. Refer to Case Study One. How would you prepare a lesson plan for Mark's word-finding difficulties? What strategies would you use to assist him in remembering information?

2. Refer to Case Study Two. How would you prepare a lesson plan to help Yvonne produce better narratives? Assume that she is more familiar with Latino traditions for narratives than with mainstream narratives. How would you introduce the mainstream format for narratives to her, while respecting her culture's traditions for narratives?

3. How would you introduce children from nonmainstream homes to classroom rules of discourse? What might you need to teach them?

4. Five-year-old Ashley produces a number of sounds incorrectly, including /ʃ/ (sh), /tʃ/ (ch), /z/, and /l/. In addition, she uses gliding for /r/, substituting /w/ instead. You are a speech-language pathologist. Which sounds and phonological processes, if any, would you work on in therapy at her current age? Which ones would you wait to work on until she is older? Why?

5. Eight-year-old Antonio started learning English in kindergarten and is now in third grade. His conversational skills in English are fine, but his formal testing results on English tests of language skills and reading and writing are at the seventh percentile for his age. Should he be placed in speech-language therapy? Why or why not?

6. You are a speech-language pathologist or special education teacher. You want to teach formal definitions to children who are in the upper elementary grades. How would you prepare a lesson plan to teach them?

7. An 8-year-old child you are testing produces the following sentences in conversation:

   a. I like baseball games on sunny days.
   b. I like the teams, and I enjoy the excitement.
   c. The Allstars should win if they play hard enough.

   How many T-units are in the three sentences? What is the mean length of T-units in words (divide the total number of words by the number of T-units)? How does the child's mean length of T-units in words compare with the research results in the chapter for 8-year-olds speaking in conversation? What is the subordination index or clausal density (divide the total number of main and subordinate clauses by the number of T-units)? How does the child's clausal density compare with the research results in the chapter for 8-year-olds speaking in conversation?

8. You are a special education teacher or a speech-language pathologist who wants to improve your lessons. What are some strategies you can use to start a lesson? To indicate the ending of a lesson? What are some different kinds of questions you can use during lessons or therapy? What are some different comments you can make to reinforce or correct children's answers?

REFERENCES

Abrahamsen, E., & Rigrodsky, S. (1984). Comprehension of complex sentences in children at three levels of cognitive development. *Journal of Psycholinguistic Research, 13*, 333–350.

Beals, D., & Snow, C. (1994). "Thunder is when the angels are upstairs bowling": Narratives and explanations at the dinner table. *Journal of Narrative and Life History, 4*, 331–352.

Beck, I., & McKeown, M. (1991). Conditions of vocabulary acquisition. In R. Barr, M. Kamil, P. Mosenthal, & P. Pearson (Eds.), *Handbook of reading research* (Vol. 2). White Plains, NY: Longman.

Benelli, B., Arcuri, L., & Marchesini, G. (1988). Cognitive and linguistic factors in the development of word definitions. *Journal of Child Language, 15*, 619–635.

Bialystok, E. (2001). *Bilingualism in development: Language, literacy, and cognition.* Cambridge, UK: Cambridge University Press.

Brice, A. (2002). *The Hispanic child: Speech, language, culture and education.* Boston, MA: Allyn and Bacon.

Brice, A., Mastin, M., & Perkins, C. (1997). English, Spanish, and code switching use in the ESL classroom: An ethnographic study. *Journal of Children's Communication Development, 19*, 11–20.

Brice, A., & Perkins, C. (1997). What is required for transition from the ESL classroom to the general education classroom? A case study of two classrooms. *Journal of Children's Communication Development, 19*, 13–22.

Brice-Heath, S. (1986). Sociocultural contexts of language development. In D. Holt (Ed.), *Beyond language: Social and cultural factors in schooling language minority students* (pp. 142–186). Los Angeles: Evaluation, Dissemination, and Assessment Center.

Caldas, S., & Boudreaux, N. (1999). Poverty, race, and foreign language immersion: Predictors of math and English language arts performance. *Learning Languages, 5*, 4–15.

Carey, S. (1978). The child as word learner. In M. Halle, J. Bresnan, & G. Miller (Eds.), *Linguistic theory and psychological reality* (pp. 264–297). Cambridge, MA: MIT Press.

Cazden, C., & Beck, S. (2003). Classroom discourse. In A. Graesser, M. Gernsbacher, & S. Goldman (Eds.), *Handbook of discourse processes.* Mahwah, NJ: Lawrence Erlbaum.

Champion, T. (1998). "Tell me somethin' good": A description of narrative structures among African American children. *Linguistics and Education, 9*, 251–286.

Cobo-Lewis, A., Pearson, B., Eilers, R., & Umbel, V. (2002a). Effects of bilingualism and bilingual education on oral and written language skills: A multifactor study of standardized test outcomes. In L. Wei (Series Ed.) & D. Oller & R. Eilers (Vol. Eds.), *Child language and child development 2: Language and literacy in bilingual children* (pp. 64–97). Clevedon, UK: Multilingual Matters.

Cobo-Lewis, A., Pearson, B., Eilers, R., & Umbel, V. (2002b). Interdependence of Spanish and English knowledge in language and literacy among bilingual children. In L. Wei (Series Ed.) & D. Oller & R. Eilers (Vol. Eds.), *Child language and child development 2: Language and literacy in bilingual children* (pp. 118–132). Clevedon, UK: Multilingual Matters.

Craddock-Willis, K., & McCabe, A. (1996). Improvising on a theme: Some African American traditions. In A. McCabe (Ed.), *Chameleon readers: Teaching children to appreciate all kinds of good stories* (pp. 98–115). New York: McGraw-Hill.

Cummins, J. (1984). *Bilingualism and special education: Issues in assessment and pedagogy.* San Diego, CA: College-Hill Press.

Cummins, J. (2000). *Language, power, and pedagogy: Bilingual children in the crossfire.* Clevedon, UK: Multilingual Matters.

DeTemple, J., & Snow, C. (2003). Learning words from books. In A. van Kleeck, S. Stahl, & E. Bauer (Eds.), *On reading books to children: Teachers and parents.* Mahwah, NJ: Lawrence Erlbaum.

D'Souza, J. (1992). The relationship between code-mixing and the new varieties of English: Issues and implications. *World Englishes, 11,* 217–233.

Duckworth, K. (1981). *Linking educational policy and management with student achievement.* Eugene, OR: Eugene Center for Educational Policy and Management, University of Oregon.

Fiestas, C., & Peña, E. (2004). Narrative discourse in bilingual children: Language and task effects. *Language, Speech, and Hearing Services in Schools, 35,* 155–168.

Freeman, D., & Freeman, Y. (1988). Sheltered English instruction (ERIC Digest ED301070). Retrieved February 9, 2007, from http://thememoryhole.org/edu/eric/ed301070.html.

Genesee, F. (1976). The role of intelligence in second language learning. *Language Learning, 26,* 267–280.

Genesee, F., Paradis, J., & Crago, M. (2004). *Dual language development and disorders: A handbook on bilingualism and second language learning (Vol. 11. Communication and language intervention series).* Baltimore, MD: Paul H. Brookes.

Gibbs, R. (1987). Linguistic factors in children's understanding of idioms. *Journal of Child Language, 14,* 569–586.

Goldstein, B., Fabiano, L., & Iglesias, A. (2004). Spontaneous and imitated productions in Spanish-speaking children with phonological disorders. *Language, Speech, and Hearing Services in Schools, 35,* 5–15.

Goldstein, B., Fabiano, L., & Washington, P. (2005). Phonological skills in predominantly English-speaking, predominantly Spanish-speaking, and Spanish-English bilingual children. *Language, Speech, and Hearing Services in Schools, 36,* 301–318.

Goldstein, B., & Iglesias, A. (2001). The effect of dialect on phonological analysis: Evidence from Spanish-speaking children. *American Journal of Speech-Language Pathology, 10,* 394–406.

Grunwell, P. (1981). The development of phonology: A descriptive profile. *First Language, 1,* 161–191.

Grunwell, P. (1997). Natural phonology. In M. Ball & R. Kent (Eds.), *The new phonologies: Developments in clinical linguistics* (pp. 35–75). San Diego, CA: Singular.

Gutiérrez-Clellen, V. (2002). Narratives in two languages: Assessing performance of bilingual children. *Linguistics and Education, 13,* 175–197.

Hicks, D. (1991). Kinds of narrative: Genre skills among first graders from two communities. In A. McCabe & C. Peterson (Eds.), *Developing narrative structure* (pp. 55–87). Hillsdale, NJ: Lawrence Erlbaum.

Hunt, K. (1970). Syntactic maturity in school children and adults. *Monographs of the Society for Research in Child Development, 35* (Serial No. 134, No. 1).

Jacobs, K., & Cross, A. (2001). The seventh generation of Kahnawàke: Phoenix or dinosaur. In J. Burton (Series Ed.) & D. Christian & F. Genesee (Vol. Eds.), *Case studies in TESOL practice series: Bilingual education* (pp. 109–121). Alexandria, VA: Teachers of English to Speakers of Other Languages, Inc.

Johnson, C., & Anglin, J. (1995). Qualitative developments in the content and form of children's definitions. *Journal of Speech and Hearing Research, 38,* 612–629.

Jones, R., & Thornborrow, J. (2004). Floors, talk, and the organization of classroom activities. *Language in Society, 33,* 399–423.

Kamwangamalu, N. (1992). 'Mixers' and 'mixing': English across cultures. *World Englishes, 11,* 173–181.

Kasuya, H. (2002). Bilingual context for language development. In S. Blum-Kulka & C. Snow (Eds.), *Talking to adults: The contribution of multiparty discourse to language acquisition* (pp. 295–325). Mahwah, NJ: Lawrence Erlbaum.

Kohnert, K. (2000). *Lexical skills in bilingual school-age children: Cross-sectional studies in Spanish and English.* Unpublished doctoral dissertation, University of California, San Diego, and San Diego State University.

Kohnert, K., & Bates, E. (2002). Balancing bilinguals II: Lexical comprehension and cognitive processing in children learning English and Spanish. *Journal of Speech, Language, and Hearing Research, 45,* 347–359.

Kohnert, K., Bates, E., & Hernandez, A. (1999). Balancing bilinguals: Lexical-semantic production and cognitive processing in children learning Spanish and English. *Journal of Speech, Language, and Hearing Research, 42,* 1400–1413.

Labov, W. (1972). *Language in the inner city: Studies in the Black English vernacular.* Philadelphia: University of Pennsylvania Press.

Lebra, T. S. (1986). Self-reconstruction in Japanese religious pyschotherapy. In T. S. Lebra & W. P. Lebra (Eds.), *Japanese culture and behavior* (pp. 354–368). Honolulu: University of Hawaii Press.

Leinhardt, G., & Steele, M. (2005). Seeing the complexity of standing to the side: Instructional dialogues. *Cognition and Instruction, 23,* 87–163.

Levorato, M., & Cacciari, C. (1992). Children's comprehension and production of idioms: The role of context and familiarity. *Journal of Child Language, 19,* 415–433.

Loban, W. (1976). *Language development: Kindergarten through grade twelve.* Urbana, IL: National Council of Teachers of English.

MacSwan, J. (2004). Code switching and grammatical theory. In T. Bhatia & W. Ritchie (Eds.), *The handbook of bilingualism* (pp. 283–311). Malden, MA: Blackwell.

Mägiste, E. (1992). Second language learning in elementary and high school students. *The European Journal of Cognitive Psychology, 4,* 355–365.

Makau, J. (1990). *Reasoning and communication: Thinking critically about arguments.* Belmont, CA: Wadsworth.

Marinellie, S., & Johnson, C. (2003). Adjective definitions and the influence of word frequency. *Journal of Speech, Language, and Hearing Research, 46,* 1061–1076.

Mastropieri, M., Scruggs, T., Levin, J., Gaffney, J., & McLoone (1985). Mnemonic vocabulary instruction for learning disabled students. *Learning Disability Quarterly, 8,* 57–63.

Mastropieri, M., Sweda, J., & Scruggs, T. (2000). Putting mnemonic strategies to work in an inclusive classroom. *Learning Disabilities Research and Practice, 15,* 69–74.

McGhee-Bidlack, B. (1991). The development of noun definitions: A metalinguistic analysis. *Journal of Child Language, 18,* 417–434.

McGregor, K., Friedman, R., Reilly, R., & Newman, R. (2002). Semantic representation and naming in young children. *Journal of Speech, Language, and Hearing Research, 45,* 998–1014.

McHoul, A. (1990). The organization of repair in classroom talk. *Language in Society, 19,* 349–377.

McLaughlin, S. (1998). *Introduction to language development.* San Diego, CA: Singular Publishing Group.

Mehan, H. (1979). *Learning lessons.* Cambridge, MA: Harvard University Press.

Mehan, H. (1982). The structure of classroom events and their consequences for students' performance. In P. Gilmore & A. Glatthorn (Eds.), *Children in and out of school: Ethnography and education* (pp. 59–87). Washington, DC: Center for Applied Linguistics.

Merritt, D., & Culatta, B. (1998). *Language intervention in the classroom.* San Diego, CA: Singular Publishing Group.

Michaels, S., & Foster, M. (1985). Peer-peer learning: Evidence from a student-run sharing. In A. Jaggar & M. Smith Burke (Eds.), *Observing the language learner* (pp. 143–158). Newark, DE: International Reading Association.

Miller, J. F. (1991). *Assessing language production in children: Experimental procedures.* Boston, MA: Allyn and Bacon.

Minami, M. (1996). Japanese preschool children's language development. *First Language, 16,* 339–363.

Minami, M., & McCabe, A. (1996). Compressed collections of experiences: Some Asian American traditions. In A. McCabe (Ed.), *Chameleon readers: Teaching children to appreciate all kinds of good stories* (pp. 72–97). New York: McGraw-Hill.

Morales, A., & Hanson, W. (2005). Language brokering: An integrative review of the literature. *Hispanic Journal of Behavioral Sciences, 27,* 471–503.

Myhill, D., & Warren, P. (2005). Scaffolds or straitjackets? Critical moments in classroom discourse. *Educational Review, 57,* 55–69.

Nippold, M. (1995). School-age children and adolescents: Norms for word definition. *Language, Speech, and Hearing Services in Schools, 26,* 320–325.

Nippold, M. (1998). Later language development: *The school-age and adolescent years* (2nd ed.). Austin, TX: Pro-Ed.

Nippold, M., Hegel, S., Sohlberg, M., & Schwarz, I. (1999). Defining abstract entities: Development in preadolescents, adolescents, and young adults. *Journal of Speech, Language, and Hearing Research, 42*, 473–481.

Nippold, M., Hesketh, L., Duthie, J., & Mansfield, T. (2005). Conversational versus expository discourse: A study of syntactic development in children, adolescents, and adults. *Journal of Speech, Language, and Hearing Research, 48*, 1048–1064.

Nippold, M., Moran, C., Schwarz, L. (2001). Idiom understanding in preadolescents: Synergy in action. *American Journal of Speech-Language Pathology, 10*, 169–179.

Nippold, M., & Rudzinski, M. (1993). Familiarity and transparency in idiom explanation: A developmental study of children and adolescents. *Journal of Speech and Hearing Research, 36*, 728–737.

Nippold, M., & Taylor, C. (1995). Idioms understanding in youth: Further examination of familiarity and transparency. *Journal of Speech and Hearing Research, 38*, 426–433.

Nippold, M., & Taylor, C. (2002). Judgments of idiom familiarity and transparency: A comparison of children and adolescents. *Journal of Speech, Language, and Hearing Research, 45*, 384–391.

Oller, D., & Eilers, R. (2002). Balancing interpretations regarding effects of bilingualism: Empirical outcomes and theoretical possibilities. In L. Wei (Series Ed.) & D. Oller & R. Eilers (Vol. Eds.), *Child language and child development 2: Language and literacy in bilingual children* (pp. 281–292). Clevedon, UK: Multilingual Matters.

Oller, D., & Pearson, B. (2002). Assessing the effects of bilingualism: A background. In L. Wei (Series Ed.) & D. Oller & R. Eilers (Vol. Eds.), *Child language and child development 2: Language and literacy in bilingual children* (pp. 3–21). Clevedon, UK: Multilingual Matters.

Owens, R. (2001). *Language development: An introduction* (5th ed.). Boston: Allyn and Bacon.

Owens, R. (2004). *Language disorders: A functional approach to assessment and intervention* (4th ed.). Boston, MA: Pearson Education.

Paradis, J. (2005). Grammatical morphology in children learning English as a second language: Implications of similarities with specific language impairment. *Language, Speech, and Hearing Services in Schools, 36*, 172–187.

Paradis, J., & Crago, M. (2000). Tense and temporality: A comparison between children learning a second language and children with SLI. *Journal of Speech, Language, and Hearing Research, 43*, 834–847.

Pearson, B. (2002). Narrative competence among monolingual and bilingual school children in Miami. In L. Wei (Series Ed.) & D. Oller & R. Eilers (Vol. Eds.), *Child language and child development 2: Language and literacy in bilingual children* (pp. 135–174). Clevedon, UK: Multilingual Matters.

Peled, N., & Blum-Kula, S. (1997). Dialogue in the Israeli classroom. *Xelkat Lashon 24 Seminar.* Tel Aviv: Levinsky Publishers.

Perez, E. (1994) Phonological differences among speakers of Spanish-influenced English. In J. Bernthal & N. Bankson (Eds.), *Child phonology: Characteristics, assessment, and intervention with special populations* (pp. 245–254). New York: Thieme Medical.

Pesco, D., Crago, M., & McCabe, A. (1996). Context and structure: Some North American Indian and aboriginal traditions. In A. McCabe (Ed.), *Chameleon readers: Teaching children to appreciate all kinds of good stories* (pp. 137–154). New York: McGraw-Hill.

Philips, S. (1972). Participant structures and communicative competence: Warm Springs children in community and classroom. In C. Cazden, V. John, & D. Hymes (Eds.), *Functions of language in the classroom* (pp. 370–394). New York: Teachers College Press.

Poulisse, N. (1997). Language production in bilinguals. In A. de Groot & J. Kroll (Eds.), *Tutorials in bilingualism: Psycholinguistic perspectives* (pp. 201–224). Mahwah, NJ: Lawrence Erlbaum.

Redmond, S. (2003). Children's productions of the affix -ed in past tense and past participle contexts. *Journal of Speech, Language, and Hearing Research, 46*, 1095–1109.

Reyes, B. (1995). Considerations in the assessment and treatment of neurogenic communication disorders in bilingual adults. In H. Kayser (Ed.), *Bilingual speech-language pathology: An Hispanic focus.* San Diego, CA: Singular Publishing Group.

Rice, M., & Wexler, K. (1996). Toward tense as a clinical marker of specific language impairment in English-speaking children. *Journal of Speech and Hearing Research, 39*, 1239–1257.

Rice, M., Wexler, K., & Cleave, P. (1995). Specific language impairment as a period of extended optional infinitive. *Journal of Speech and Hearing Research, 38*, 850–863.

Rice, M., Wexler, K., & Hershberger, S. (1998). Tense over time: The longitudinal course of tense acquisition in children with specific language impairment. *Journal of Speech, Language, and Hearing Research, 41*, 1412–1431.

Roseberry-McKibbin, C. (2002). *Multicultural students with special language needs: Practical strategies for assessment and intervention* (2nd ed.). Oceanside, CA: Academic Communication Associates.

Rowe, M. (1986). Wait time: Slowing down may be a way of speeding up! *Journal of Teacher Education, 37*, 43–50.

Scott, C. M. (1984). Abverbial connectivity in conversations of children 6 to 12. *Journal of Child Language, 11*, 423–452.

Scott, C. (1988a). Producing complex sentences. *Topics in Language Disorders, 8*, 44–62.

Scott, C. (1988b). Spoken and written syntax. In M. Nippold (Ed.), *Later language development: Ages nine through nineteen* (pp. 49–95). Austin, TX: Pro-Ed.

Scott, C., & Stokes, S. (1995). Measures of syntax in school-age children and adolescents. *Language, Speech, and Hearing Services in Schools, 26*, 301–319.

Scott, C., & Windsor, J. (2000). General language performance measures in spoken and written narrative and expository discourse of school-age children with language learning disabilities. *Journal of Speech, Language, and Hearing Research, 43*, 324–339.

Scruggs, T., & Mastropieri, M. (1989). Mnemonic instruction of LD students: A field-based evaluation. *Learning Disability Quarterly, 12*, 119–125.

Scruggs, T., & Mastropieri, M. (2000). The effectiveness of mnemonic instruction for students with learning and behavior problems: An update and research synthesis. *Journal of Behavioral Education, 10*, 163–173.

Sebastian, E., & Slobin, D. (1994). Development of linguistic forms: Spanish. In R. Berman & D. Slobin (Eds.), *Relating events in narrative: A crosslinguistic developmental study* (pp. 239–284). Hillsdale, NJ: Erlbaum.

Silva, M., & McCabe, A. (1996). Vignettes of the continuous and family ties: Some Latino American traditions. In A. McCabe (Ed.), *Chameleon readers: Teaching children to appreciate all kinds of good stories* (pp. 116–136). New York: McGraw-Hill.

Smit, A., Hand, L., Freilinger, J., Bernthal, J., & Bird, A. (1990). The Iowa articulation norms project and its Nebraska replication. *Journal of Speech and Language Disorders, 55*, 779–798.

Snow, C., & Blum-Kulka, S. (2002). From home to school: School-age children talking with adults. In S. Blum-Kulka & C. Snow (Eds.), *Talking to adults: The contribution of multiparty discourse to language acquisition* (pp. 327–341). Mahwah, NJ: Lawrence Erlbaum.

Stein, N., & Glenn, C. (1979). An analysis of story comprehension in elementary school children. In R. Freedle (Ed.), *Advances in discourse processes: Vol. 2. New directions in discourse processing* (pp. 53–120). Norwood, NJ: Ablex.

Stein, N., & Glenn, C. (1982). Children's concept of time: The development of a story schema. In W. Friedman (Ed.), *The developmental psychology of time* (pp. 255–282). New York: Academic Press.

Sutton-Smith, B. (1986). The development of fictional narrative performances. *Topics in Language Disorders, 7*, 1–10.

Thomas, W. P., & Collier, V. (1997). *School effectiveness for language minority students.* Washington, DC: National Clearinghouse for Bilingual Education.

Wallach, G. P. (1984). Later language learning: Syntactic structures and strategies. In G. P. Wallach & K. G. Butler (Eds.), *Language learning disabilities in school-age children* (pp. 82–102). Baltimore, MD: Williams & Wilkins.

Wang, Q., & Leichtman, M. (2000). Same beginnings, different stories: A comparison of American and Chinese children's narratives. *Child Development, 71*, 1329–1346.

Wei, L. (1993). Mother tongue maintenance in a Chinese community school in Newcastle upon Tyne: Developing a social network perspective. *Language and Education, 7*, 199–215.

Weisskirch, R., & Alva, S. (2002). Language brokering and the acculturation of Latino children.

Hispanic Journal of Behavioral Sciences, 24, 369–378.

Wells, G. (1993). Reevaluating the IRF sequence: A proposal for the articulation of theories of activity and discourse for the analysis of teaching and learning in the classroom. *Linguistics and Education, 5,* 1–37.

Westby, C., Moore, C., & Roman, R. (2002). Reinventing the enemy's language: Developing narratives in Native American children. *Linguistics and Education, 13,* 235–269.

Zentella, A. (1997). *Growing up bilingual: Puerto Rican children in New York.* Malden, MA: Blackwell.

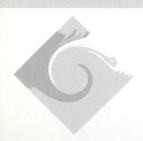

Chapter 6

Adolescent Language Development

Toya A. Wyatt

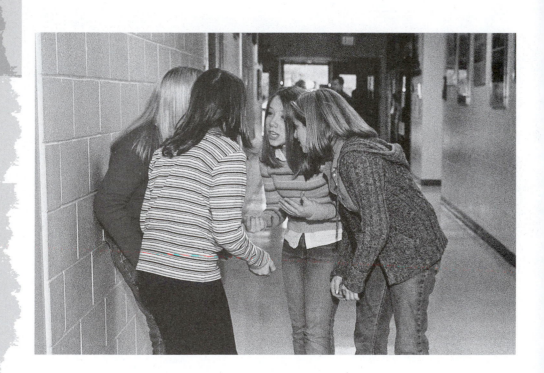

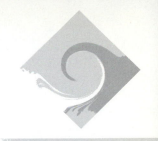

CHAPTER OUTLINE

INTRODUCTION

Until recently, research on children's language development has primarily focused on the language development of younger children, with little attention to that of school-age and adolescent children. With the increased emphasis on school curriculum standards, state-mandated standardized testing, high school exit examinations, and literacy, however, educators and speech-language professionals have begun to pay closer attention to the language development of older students (Ehren, 2002). The focus on the academic language needs of this population has also been prompted by national statistics that suggest fairly large numbers of students are reading at "below basic levels" (Whitmire, 2005). Studies of the language skills of older school-age and adolescent children provide evidence of ongoing language development into adolescence and adulthood (Ehren, 2002).

Much of the recent attention to the development of adolescent language skills has centered on what children need in order to be academically successful in the general education classroom setting and what children who have underlying language weaknesses need in terms of academic language support to access the curriculum of the classroom setting. In addition to mastering the language of the classroom, adolescents also have to learn how to become successful communicators in daily social interactions with others, particularly their peers. During adolescence children begin to acquire an understanding of who they are as people, what they enjoy doing most, and with whom they enjoy spending time. Adolescence is also a period of development where individuals learn how to use communication to negotiate the process of dating, establish friendships, and affiliate with certain social or peer groups. Some students, particularly those who are entering a different type of school environment than what they have been used to, will also have to acquire new ways of interacting with peers if the peer groups within their new school setting are different from those in their old educational setting. As adolescents move out of the teenage years, they will also begin to master the vocabulary and social communication skills necessary for successful entry into the workplace and a chosen job, career, or profession.

THE NATURE OF ADOLESCENCE

Everyone who has gone through adolescence remembers what it was like to be an adolescent. It is perhaps one of the most difficult periods of development for individuals in every cultural community. Whitmire (2000) describes adolescence as a period of transition. During this period of transition, adolescents are often described in terms of their defiance, moodiness, and unconventional tastes in music, hairstyles, and dress. Although adolescence is often described as a period of turbulence and rebellion, it is a period that can also be more positively defined as an important period of complex cognitive and social growth (Whitmire, 2000). Refer to Chapter 1 for discussion of some of the later developing aspects of the brain.

There are slightly different interpretations as to what constitutes adolescence, but according to Whitmire (2000), adolescence can be divided into at least three different stages: (1) early adolescence (10 to 13 years for girls, 12 to 15 for boys), (2) middle adolescence (13 to 16 years for girls, 14 to 17 years for boys), and (3) later adolescence (16 or 17 years to mid-twenties). One hallmark of early adolescence is the increased yearning for the approval of peers. Middle adolescence is a period that is typically marked by various types of rebellion (e.g., as displayed through dress styles, hairstyles, the use of slang, and certain types of music). **Slang** can be defined as an informal/colloquial/casual speech that is used by members of social groups as a form of social and in some cases political solidarity (Munro, 2002). Slang is one means for identifying with a particular group and/or excluding others from that same group. It is a very important language development during the adolescent years.

Later adolescence (according to Whitmire, 2000) is characterized by a greater reliance on friends versus family. It is also a key period for the development of specialized friendships with members of the opposite sex.

Throughout the adolescent years, peer relationships (e.g., cliques) become increasingly important and begin to replace a child's previous psychological dependence on adult family members (e.g., parents or caregivers). Adolescence is also a period where teenagers strive for autonomy from their parents and begin to see themselves as equals to their parents (Damon, 1983, as cited in Whitmire, 2000). As a result of this change, teenagers often begin to challenge once-accepted adult rules and expectations. However, research studies reported by Whitmire (2000) still indicate that the majority of adolescents respect their parents, want to be like them, and maintain harmonious relationships with them.

Many of these developments that occur during adolescence are the result of co-occurring physical and psychological changes as well as key cognitive developments that are crucial to an understanding of self within the context of human relationships. These cognitive changes are important to the future attainment of academic pursuits, knowledge, skills, and learning strategies considered essential for life-long learning (Whitmire, 2000).

According to Larson and McKinley (2003), adolescence is also a period where individuals begin to have an established **self-concept** (a notion of who one is as a person) and developing **self-esteem** (how one feels about him- or herself). As children mature, they grow from viewing themselves in terms of their possessions, self/body image, and territoriality (where they live) to viewing themselves in terms of internal belief systems, standards, and stable personality traits (Suls, 1989, as cited in Larson & McKinley, 2003).

ADOLESCENT SPOKEN-LANGUAGE DEVELOPMENT

Phonological Development

Although children have generally mastered the basic language skills and knowledge of their home communities before they enter their adolescent years, key linguistic developments continue into adolescence and beyond. The following is a summary of key phonological developments that continue to occur past the elementary school-age years.

According to most normative studies of children's phonological development, typically developing English-speaking children have mastered the phonemic system of English by 8 years of age. In addition, early developing phonological process errors such as stopping, fronting, and gliding have generally faded by the end of the preschool-age period for most sounds.

As children enter the school-age years, however, there are some phonological developments that still occur, with some continuing into adulthood. These include developments such as changes in temporal coordination of speech production, with a gradual change in speech rate and articulation with age. There are also developmental changes in the durations of certain consonants such as the /l/ consonant in consonant clusters, which becomes shorter in duration. These changes are evidence of the fact that older children are still continuing to develop fluency in the planning and production of complex sequences of sounds into adulthood (Vihman, 1998).

As older students become exposed to literacy in the classroom setting and begin to understand the rules for spelling new words and the types of vowel and syllable stress changes that occur in related word pairs such as *divine-divinity, retain-retention, promise-promissory,* there appears to be some influence on speech/sound production and perception of sounds within newly learned words. Ehri (as cited in Vihman, 1998) suggests that knowledge of spelling helps children detect and accurately segment sounds embedded in words. Older students are still in the process of abstracting patterns in the pronunciation of new words into grade 10, according to several research studies cited by Vihman (1998).

Other changes involve strategies for lexical retrieval based on the phonetic structure of words. For example, in a study of children and adults' **malapropisms** (mistakes involving the substitution of one word for another, such as *monuments* for *condiments*), Aitchinson and Straf (cited in Vihman, 1998) found that adults are more likely to retain the initial sound in their substituted productions while children are more likely to retain the final sound. Vihman (1998) suggests that this trend is the result of schooling and dictionary/library work.

One last form of phonetic and phonological change that can persist past early childhood is the acquisition of a second dialect pronunciation when speakers move from one dialect area or region to another. In studies of linguistic change within a small middle-class community on the outskirts of Philadelphia, Payne (cited in Vihman, 1998) found that younger speakers between the ages of 4 and 14 years, which is a period of great peer-group influence, are more likely to acquire new patterns of speaking associated with a new dialect region than those outside the peer-group influence years.

Of course, adolescents who have grown up in a community that speaks a non-standard dialect of English different from **Mainstream American English (MAE)** (the dialect spoken by individuals perceived to represent the primary code of mainstream American culture and upward social/economic mobility) will generally continue to display speech pronunciation patterns that differ from MAE well into adolescence in at least some speaking situations, depending on their degree of dialect exposure, social peer-networks, and attitudes toward their native dialect.

For adolescents who are predominant speakers of **African American English (AAE),** a nonmainstream English dialect that is spoken at least some of the time by a large number of but not all African Americans, possible pronunciation differences can include absence of final postvocalic /l, r/, final /m/, devoicing of final voiced sounds, and deletion of initial unstressed syllables, all features associated with normal AAE (Wyatt, 1995). Differing word syllable stress patterns can also be seen in words like *Detroit* and *police,* which may be produced as "DE troit" (instead of "de TROIT") and "PO lice" (instead of "po LICE").

For adolescent bilingual speakers who are still in the early stages of learning English as a second language (e.g., only one to two years of exposure), it is not uncommon to still see the existence of cross-linguistic influences in both languages spoken, with some sounds in a student's native language being influenced by the newly developing second language and some sounds in the second language being influenced by the first language (also known as interference; refer to Chapter 4 on second-language acquisition issues). These patterns are sometimes predictable when taking speech/sound differences between the two languages into account (i.e., **contrastive analysis**) (Goldstein, Fabiano, & Washington, 2005; Iglesias & Goldstein, 1998). Like younger children and older adult second-language learners, adolescents who are still in the early stages of acquiring a second-language phonology can also make second-language pronunciation errors that are associated with an emerging interlanguage system (a transitional stage of second-language acquisition where speakers make errors in their production of target second-language sounds that are the result of unsuccessful attempts at those sounds). Errors that are the result of interlanguage influences can change in nature over time.

Morphological Development

Very little has been written about the types of morphological developments associated with the adolescent years. Most of the references to children's morphological development have focused on the acquisition of early developing morphemes such as the plural *-s*, past tense *-ed*, present progressive *-ing,* and third person singular *-s* markers during the preschool years and the mastery of later-developing **derivational morphemes** (morphological markers that, when added to a word, change the grammatical status of the word) such as the **agentive -er** (morphological marker that conveys the meaning of a "person who . . ." in words like *dancer*) and **instrumental -er** (morphological marker that conveys the meaning of "an instrument that. . . ." in words like *eraser*), as well as the *-y* and *-ly* **suffixes** (morphological markers occurring at the ends of words) that develop in later school-age years (Owens, 2005).

The continued development of morphological knowledge, including morphological marker use and comprehension, is important to ongoing word-learning abilities. Nippold (1998) cites several studies showing that older children's abilities to decipher the meaning of newly encountered words during the school-age and adolescent years is at least partly based on children's abilities to analyze the different components of words. These components include the base or root part of a word, which provides the primary meaning, and any attached **inflectional morphemes** (word endings and beginnings that, when added to a base or root word form, add additional meaning), including derivational morphemes (morphological markers that, when added to a word, change its grammatical status). Examples include the word *cats*, which contains the lexical root word *cat* plus the inflectional plural *-s* suffix to convey the meaning of plurality; the word *walked*, which contains the lexical verb form *walk* plus the inflectional past tense *-ed* suffix; the word *unpleasant*, which contains the lexical item *pleasant* plus the **affix** (word beginning) *un-*, which conveys the opposite of *pleasant*; and the word *sadly*, which contains the lexical item *sad* (an adjective) plus the derivational *-ly* suffix, which changes the word to an adverb.

Researchers who have investigated children's learning of new words have found that as children get older and progress through the later elementary grades, they become more proficient at being able to use both morphological analysis and context clues to decipher the meanings of these new words (Anglin, 1993; Wysocki & Jenkins, 1987, as cited in Nippold, 1998). Studies by Nagy and Windsor (as cited in Nippold, 1998) have also revealed that the understanding of certain derivational morphemes, including the suffixes *-ette, -ize, -ify,* and *-ful,* increases during school-age and adolescent years.

There is very little research on the morphological development of bilingual and nonstandard English (NSE) adolescent speakers. However, in a study of preschool and school-age early ESL children (children who have been learning English for less than two years), Paradis (2005) found that children in the early stages of learning English as a second language made errors in their production of English grammatical morphemes similar to those made by typically developing monolingual English-speaking children. Grammatical morphemes/forms that were investigated by Paradis (2005) and found to be either omitted or produced incorrectly included third person singular -s; regular past tense -ed; copula be; prepositions, such as in and on; articles; and plural -s. The primary factor that determines the type and number of errors made is not a child's age but instead the number of years that a child is exposed to a second language.

Similar to younger children who have been exposed to English only a couple of years, bilingual adolescent speakers are likely to display problems with English morphology in both their spoken and written language. These errors are the result of normal second-language learning difficulties rather than disorder-based processes.

Adolescents who are primary speakers of dialects other than MAE, such as AAE, are also going to display patterns of English language morphology in spoken, and in some cases written, language that can be attributed to normal dialect influences. While some of these grammatical differences may look similar to those seen in MAE-speaking students who have underlying language disorders, they can be attributed in most cases to normal dialect differences. Examples of morphological markers that might be produced differently include omission of the past tense -ed, present progressive -ing, third person singular -s, and plural -s markers.

There are also some aspects of AAE morphology that do not differ from MAE and that should be used in the same manner as in MAE. For example, there are some morphological forms, such as articles a and the and prepositions like in, with, and on, that are used in the same manner in both AAE and MAE. These morphological forms are considered to be **nondialect-specific** or **noncontrastive** (meaning that they occur similarly 100% of the time in the same sentence contexts across all dialects of English). It is important to note, however, that there can be some regional variations in terms of certain morphological forms, such as how prepositions are expressed and used. One example includes the types of prepositions that are used across English dialects to convey the notion of being sick, as in "sick to one's stomach," "sick at one's stomach," "sick in one's stomach," and "sick on one's stomach" (Wolfram & Schilling-Estes, 2006). Understanding what is normal versus abnormal language use can, therefore, be complicated when dealing with students who are not native speakers of MAE.

Semantic Development

One important aspect of semantic development that continues to improve through adolescence and adulthood is the ability to define words. Over time, older speakers display both qualitative and quantitative changes in their word definitions.

Quantitative changes involve vocabulary size. As older students move through adolescence into the adult years, their vocabulary, as would be expected, increases in size. Upon graduating from high school, the average adolescent has learned the meaning of at least 800,000 words (Larson & McKinley, 2003).

There are also qualitative changes. For example, according to research cited by Nippold (1998), older speakers are more likely to use specific versus general categorical terms in their word definitions (e.g., "a horse is an *animal* that runs" versus "a horse is *something* that runs"). Adolescents are also more likely to use synonyms (e.g., "a wife is the spouse of a husband") and explanations (e.g., "expensive means something that costs a lot of money") in their definitions, while younger children have a tendency to use more descriptives ("a straw is yellow"), demonstrations (e.g., pointing to an eyelash when asked to define eyelash), and/or repetitions of words that they are asked to define. As would be expected, younger children are also less accurate than older children in their ability to explain the meanings of words. The ability to define words improves, according to Nippold (2000), as students become more exposed to conventional dictionary meanings during formal classroom instructional activities.

As adolescents move into adulthood and begin to pursue some form of occupation, vocation, or career, they also begin the process of acquiring specialized technical words, or **jargon** (defined by Munro [2002] as the specialized vocabulary of a particular profession or avocation), that are associated with that occupation, vocation, or career. These differences are among the many that occur as older students learn how to shift into different **registers** (different styles of talking required for different social communication situations or group interactions). (A more detailed discussion of language registers can be found in the section on pragmatics.)

As previously mentioned, adolescence is also a period where students are beginning to master the slang vocabulary that is spoken within their affiliated peer groups. Adolescents in every language community speak some form of slang; however, the type of slang that is understood and used in some speech communities can be different from that used in others (Munro, 2002). The differences in slang items can occur as a function of ethnic-cultural identity. Examples of White versus African American college and high school students' use and understanding of ethnic-group slang, along with racial lines, are discussed in Green (2002) and Munro (2002).

With bilingual students, as in every other aspect of language development, English vocabulary skills are not likely to be as strong as first-language vocabulary skills until students become proficient in the second language. Until that period of time, it is typical for bilingual adolescent speakers to have greater vocabulary in one language than in the other. Bedore et al. (2005) found that children scored best on a bilingual test of semantic development when conceptual vocabulary scoring versus monolingual vocabulary scoring was used. Participants included 4- to 8-year-old children exposed to Spanish in the home who were (1) predominantly English-speaking, (2) predominantly Spanish speaking, and (3) Spanish-English bilingual. Under the total scoring condition, all responses (both Spanish and English) were accepted if correct. Under the monolingual scoring condition, separate scores were generated in each of the two languages. Findings from this study support what is already known about bilingual children's vocabulary development: the fact that vocabulary skills can be distributed across two languages, sometimes with overlap (terms known for the same item in both languages) but also sometimes with no overlap (with terms known in only one language). The same is likely to be true for bilingual adolescents. As a result, it is clear that some bilingual adolescents display less knowledge of academic classroom vocabulary compared to their monolingual peers if English is the only language in which classroom instruction and/or assessment is done.

In the last few years, a number of educational programs and initiatives have focused on improving the "limited" vocabulary skills of minority and bilingual youth. Many minority youth, particularly if they are predominant speakers of dialects other than MAE, use differing vocabulary from that used in mainstream communities in the school academic setting. Unfortunately, these differences, as evident from the poorer performance of minority students on standardized measures of school-based, academic vocabulary, are described as being "deficient" when in fact, they are simply "different." Part of the differences in school vocabulary knowledge can be attributed to limited exposure to vocabulary used within mainstream American classrooms, daily social interactions, and textbooks.

In reality, the vocabulary of students from nonmainstream communities is generally very rich. Consider for example, the slang used by African American teenagers and adults. Much of the vocabulary used within the African American community, can potentially have two levels of meanings, "one black, one white" (Smitherman, 1977), that are used flexibly depending on the speaking context and condition (e.g., to whom one is speaking and where the talking is occurring). For example, the term *bad*, which was frequently used within the African American community during the 1970s, could convey something that is negative from the Mainstream English community perspective or something good from an AAE community perspective. The intended meanings of words within the AAE speech community can also vary depending on the tone or prosodic manner in which they are produced (Smitherman, 1977; Spears, 2001). Furthermore, the strong vocabulary abilities of African American teenagers can be captured in the dynamic and ever-changing slang used. As stated in Smitherman (1977), whenever the linguistic currency of the African American community is adopted by mainstream American speakers, it loses its value, and terms are replaced by newer terms with the same meanings. Consider the example of the word *bad*, which was used in the 1970s to convey the meaning of *good* but which has been systematically replaced within the African American speech community, over the last 30 years, with terms such as *fresh, dope, down, phat, def, the bomb, jammin', slammin', tight, sweet,* and *off the hook*.

Although the vocabulary skills of students from nonmainstream backgrounds fail to look rich when compared to academic measures of school-based vocabulary developed for and derived based on the vocabulary valued most in other communities, educators need to be careful in drawing conclusions about true vocabulary ability from these measures. However, there is a way for educators to address the issue effectively, as long as they recognize that the primary issue is to transition students into the academic, curriculum-based vocabulary of the classroom setting while building on existing culturally based vocabulary strengths. With typically developing adolescents, differences can be overcome with repeated exposure to vocabulary that is necessary for success in the general education classroom setting. For bilingual adolescents, mastery of English vocabulary essential to academic success will also occur over time as students naturally transition from their first language to their second language and become more proficient with the vocabulary of the second language. This process can take years; however, it is basically no different from that of monolingual students, who take years to master the vocabulary of the language to which they have been primarily exposed.

Syntactic Development

With age, children's sentences become even more complex and elaborate, with multiple embedded and/or conjoined phrases and clauses often occurring within the same sentence, as in "We went to the movies and saw a movie with Spider Man" and "I know somebody who can get me a doll that's big." The changes in sentence length and complexity that occur during the school-age years are best measured through the use of **C-units** (communication units) and **T-units** (terminable units). C-units, as defined by Loban (1976), are sentences that consist of an **independent clause** (a main clause that can stand alone) and any additional modifiers, including an attached **dependent clause** (a clause that modifies some aspect of the main clause in a sentence and cannot stand alone). The only difference between the C-unit and the T-unit measure is that C-units include incomplete sentences produced when responding to questions. When analyzing language productions according to T-units, however, incomplete sentences are excluded (Nippold, 1998).

As typically developing children move through their school-age and adolescent years, they continue to display small but regular increases in sentence length, as determined by mean number of words per C-unit and T-unit, in both spoken and written discourse. Loban (1976) tracked these changes in terms of average number of words per C-unit and average number of dependent clauses per C-unit in the oral as well as written productions of low- to high-ability students (rated as high or low by participating teachers) in kindergarten through twelfth grade.

In a 1979 study of written compositions produced by sixth- and tenth-graders, Crowhurst and Piche (as cited in Nippold, 1998) found evidence of differences in average T-unit length based on the written discourse mode where they were elicited. The mean number of words per T-unit was highest in the persuasive mode (written samples where students were asked to take and defend their position about a given controversy), lowest in the narrative mode (written samples where students were asked to write an exciting story), and intermediate in the descriptive mode (written samples where students were asked to describe a picture). In all three conditions, older students produced sentences that contained a greater number of words per T-unit.

In addition to changes in sentence length, school-age and adolescent children also begin to use an increased variety of **intra-sentential cohesion** forms (linguistic forms that help to join ideas within sentences) such as subordinating, coordinating, and correlative conjunctions (Nippold, 1998). **Subordinating conjunctions** (conjunctions that introduce dependent clauses) include words such as *after, although, as, before, if, since, unless, when,* and *whenever* in sentences like "We are going to the store *after* we get home"). **Coordinating conjunctions** (conjunctions that join two independent clauses) include words like *and, but, or,* and *so* in a sentence like "He hit him *and* then he ran over there" **Correlative conjunctions** (conjunctions that are used to indicate a symmetrical relationship between ideas, individuals, or events) include words pairs like *both/and, either/or, neither/nor* and *not only/but also* in sentences like "*Neither* Sarah *nor* Tiffany want to go to the dance tonight." Many of these conjunctions are frequently found in older grade level and high school texts. Mastery of these varied syntactic forms is therefore important to school success.

Studies of school-age, adolescent, and/or adult speakers, as reported in Nippold (1998), reveal that students become increasingly accurate in their use and comprehension of these conjunctions with age. Results from studies have also revealed increased use of certain types of conjunctions in oral narratives. The research of McClure and Steffensen (as cited in Nippold, 1998), however, found that certain conjunctions, such as *but, and,* and *because,* plateau by grade 6, while others, such as *even though,* continue to improve into adolescence and adulthood and are still sometimes difficult for students in the older grades (e.g., grade 9).

Although there is little research on the comprehension and use of conjunctions in bilingual children or children from monolingual non-native English-speaking backgrounds, the research that does exist suggests similar patterns of development in the comprehension and/or use of these syntactic forms in their native languages. For example, Flores d'Arcais (as cited in Nippold, 1998), who studied the comprehension of conjunctions in school-age Dutch speakers, found that Dutch-speaking children still have not achieved a full understanding of conjunctions in Dutch, which continues to develop beyond age 12 years.

Teachers and clinicians need to remember that when they are instructing adolescents who are still in the early stages of acquiring English as a second language, the school professionals are likely to see less elaborate syntactic constructions in bilingual speakers who have had limited exposure to English. However, comparative analyses of native-language-speaking abilities (and writing abilities, if children have had formal written language instruction and education in their native language) should reveal grammatical structures that are more complex and elaborate in the native language compared to English if the child is typically developing. The types of observed syntactic structures will differ, of course, depending on the types of syntactic structures that exist within the grammar of that child's first language.

In children who are speakers of dialects other than English, age-related increases and changes in sentence complexity should be observed as for MAE speakers. The only potential difference is that certain complex constructions, such as relative clauses, may be produced differently from those produced by MAE speakers. For example, the relative pronouns *who* and *that,* which are generally used in MAE to head relative clauses in sentences like "You are the one *who* told me" and "He's the one *that* I've been seeing," can be optional in AAE grammar (Green, 2002; Rickford, 1999). This can result in sentences like "You the one [who] told me" and "He the one [that] I've been seein'". In spite of these differences, these sentences would still be considered as complex in terms of syntactic structure, even though they deviate from the rules of MAE.

Another key aspect of adolescent student language development involves emerging use of **intersentential cohesion** forms (grammatical forms used to join sentences in a cohesive manner). **Adverbial conjuncts** (cohesive devices that link clauses or sentences on the basis of some logical relationship) are one type of intersentential cohesive form described by Quirk and Greenbaum (as cited in Nippold, 1998). These words are frequently used within textbooks, essay writing assignments, lectures, and high school as well as college-level classrooms (Nippold, 1998). Some, such as *by the way,* are used to signal transitions into new or related topics (Mentis, 1994, as cited in Nippold, 1998). Others, such as *on the other hand*, are used to express a difference in opinion and also occur in less formal contexts, including casual conversation. Additional examples of both types of adverbial conjunctions include *fortunately, hence, nevertheless, coincidentally, furthermore, however, overall,* *consequently,* and *therefore* (Nippold, 1998). Similar to previously described conjunctions, older children become more proficient in the use and understanding of these syntactic devices with age, but as adults still continue to be less than 100% accurate in their use and/or comprehension. Students have greater difficulty using these forms during written tasks than during reading tasks.

Nippold (1998) suggests that competence in the use of adverbial conjuncts is closely related to the amount of meaningful exposure that a student receives during formal academic instruction. Nippold also suggests that some adolescents and adults may never fully master such forms if their formal education is limited to high school. This has significant implications for minority adolescents, who have been found to be consistently more at risk for early high school dropout. In a recent report released by the Harvard University Civil Rights Project, as reported in the *Los Angeles Times* (Helfand, 2005), only 57% of African Americans and 60% of Latinos attending California high schools graduated, in comparison to 78% of Whites and 84% of Asians. In the Los Angeles Unified School District, data collected by researchers from the University of California at Los Angeles (UCLA) found that most students who drop out leave high school between the ninth and tenth grades. Findings also revealed that less that one-third of ninth-graders graduated on time. These statistics have obvious implications for the development of higher-level academic literate language.

Data from Colorado's Department of Education in 2004 revealed similar discrepancies in reading ability between Latino and White elementary school-age students in Colorado's schools. According to recent Department of Education data (Stainburn, 2004), only 44% of Latino fourth-graders read at a basic level or better, with only 15% reading at a proficient or advanced level. In contrast, 75% of White students at the same grade level read at a basic level or better, with 41% being proficient or advanced. Again, these figures have obvious implications for these students as they continue on to middle school and high school.

For many African American, Hispanic, and Native American students, the lingering effects of prejudice, desegregation, deferred economic opportunity, poverty, and disparities in the quality of education provided to students in lower-income communities and schools continue to result in an academic achievement gap compared to their Asian American and European American counterparts (Edelman, 2006; Gordon, 2006). The additional impact of language differences related to dialect differences and second-language learning issues also contributes to unequal schooling experiences for minority versus nonminority students and the corresponding lack of academic success with academic language skills.

One additional aspect of syntactic development that has been studied in older child and adolescent students is the use of **mazes** (revisions), false starts, and hesitations in spoken sentences. As Nippold (1998) points out, while the use of excessive maze behavior can potentially signal language-formulation difficulties in older students, mazes are also common in the speech of typically developing speakers, especially the speech of adolescent girls. A research study of teenage-girl discourse by Eckert (cited in Nippold, 1998) revealed frequent use of maze phrases such as the following: ". . . like November . . . like was it . . . late about . . . late October . . . ."

Loban's (1976) study investigated grade-related changes in student's maze behavior and revealed only slight changes in the number of words produced per maze, with fluctuating increases and decreases noted from kindergarten through grade 12 for both high-ability and low-ability students. Low-ability students, however, generally produced more frequent maze behavior (more words per maze). Overall, however, the number of words per maze across grade levels and ability groups was around two words per maze.

The outcomes from Loban's (1976) research suggest that students who display more than two words per maze may be displaying evidence of underlying language difficulties in expression and/or formulation. Once again, however, caution needs to be taken when evaluating the English-language productions of adolescent second-language learners who are still emerging English-language learners. With such learners, non-normal fluency associated with normal second-language learning processes is not unusual (Wyatt, 2002). It is normal for second-language learners to display speaker phrase revisions, hesitations, and interjections in a second language that are associated with normal language patterns until they become fully proficient in that language. Therefore, caution must be exercised in viewing such difficulties as evidence of disorder-based language-formulation problems in non-native adolescent bilingual speakers.

In addition, clinicians and educators need to be mindful of the cross-cultural variations in discourse style that can occur during conversation and narrative retell tasks, even among monolingual English speakers. False starts, hesitations, pauses, pacing, repetition, and redundancy can sometimes be used as stylistic devices for organizing and contextualizing information within narratives in some cultural speaker groups (Gutierrez-Clellen & Quinn, 1993). It is also possible in some parts of the country to see maze behavior that is associated with stylistic regional speech variations, as in "up-talk" or "valley girl talk."

Pragmatic Conversation

As previously stated, adolescence is a time when social interactions with peers increase. As a result, conversation with peers also increases, with girls spending about twice as much time talking and socializing with friends by phone and in person than boys by grade 9 (Raffaelli & Duckett, as cited in Nippold, 2000). The types of topics that adolescents engage in with age peers also differ from those they engage in with other family members, with much of their peer conversation focusing on personal topics such as relationships and teenage social activities (e.g., parties).

The way that conversation is constructed and organized also changes. Research conducted by Larson and McKinley (as cited in Larson & McKinley, 2003, and Nippold, 2000) on adolescents in grades 7 and 12 revealed that as grade levels increase, the number of abrupt topic shifts in conversation begin to decrease. The number of interruptions, however, also begin to increase. No significant gender differences were noted between boys and girls with respect to these conversational variables. When conversations with peers were compared to those with adults, results also revealed that adolescents did the following more often when communicating with their peers than they did when communicating with adults: (1) asked questions, (2) used conversation to obtain information, (3) shifted to new topics, (4) returned to old topics, (5) used figurative expressions, and (6) made attempts to entertain their partner.

There are nonverbal changes that occur as well with age during conversational exchanges. For example, according to Larson and McKinley (2003), there is an increase in older students' ability, after fifth grade, to provide nonverbal feedback and acknowledgments, such as head nods, to let the listener know that they are listening to them. Part of the basis for these conversational changes is the fact that adolescents are more effective at reading others' feelings and emotions, taking the perspective of others, and understanding their listeners' needs and adjusting spoken as well as written communication accordingly (Larson & McKinley, 2003). These cognitive changes contribute to overall communicative effectiveness with respect to several different conversational parameters, including topic maintenance and shift, **discourse cohesion** (connectedness and flow between messages), **semantic contingency** (relevant, related responses), requests for clarification, and conversational repairs during conversational breakdowns. However, these pragmatic attributes may be influenced by learning to speak English as a second language and also acculturation to U.S. classrooms. For example, Hispanic/Latino adolescent students may experience normal second-language pragmatic difficulties.

As adolescents improve their overall conversational skills, they will also better master the culture-specific discourse rules of their communities. This includes mastering culturally based rules for initiating discourse, sustaining discourse, turn-taking, providing verbal as well as nonverbal acknowledgments, and determining the most appropriate topics for discussion in public versus private settings.

Language Function and Use: Persuasion and Negotiation Skills

One important aspect of effective communication is the ability to use language effectively in both spoken and written discourse. Although children have already mastered several different aspects of language use during the early preschool and school-age years, they continue to refine various functions of language in later social and academic language exchanges.

Two key uses of language that have been studied in adolescents are the abilities to persuade and negotiate with others. **Persuasion,** as defined by Freeley (cited in Nippold, 1998), is the use of communication to "influence the acts, beliefs, attitudes, and values of others." Key elements of persuasion include being able to provide listeners with the stated advantages for complying with a given request; adjusting persuasive strategies to match listener background based on background personal characteristics, such as age, authority, and familiarity; generating varied arguments to support a given request; anticipating and replying to counterarguments; and being able to use strategies such as politeness and bargaining as tools of persuasion. Although children begin to master persuasive speech as early as third grade, the ability to use persuasive speech improves significantly in both spoken and written discourse after third grade and into adolescence and adulthood.

Negotiation, as defined by Nippold (1998), involves the ability to reason with words and use cooperative, collaborative strategies; mutual agreement; and compromise to resolve conflict. According to research cited by Nippold (1998), with age, children are able to use a greater percentage of high-level negotiation strategies and demonstrate greater awareness of others' needs. Older adolescents are most concerned about the long-term consequences of a given conflict and are most interested in resolving it through compromise and mutual agreement. There is also increased use of cooperative, collaborative strategies.

Although there has not really been any significant research on cross-cultural differences in adolescents' use of persuasion and negotiation strategies, it is important to recognize that this is another area of communication where there is a possibility for cross-cultural communication style issues to occur inside and outside the normal classroom setting. For example, in his analysis of the communication exchanges between African American and White students in his university classroom setting, Kochman (1981) noticed definite differences in the styles used by his students during classroom debates and arguments. For example, Kochman found that there were distinct differences between the types of argument used by African American students to express an opinion and to vent anger. The primary intention behind the first type was to foster an open, honest discussion of issues so that a unified group resolution could be achieved. White students, however, had some difficulty perceiving the difference between the two different styles of argument and almost always attributed both the first type and the second type to an expression of anger and hostility with the ultimate goal of creating divisiveness.

Kochman (1981) also noted differences between the two student groups in their degree of verbal participation and their interpretation of participation during group debate. For example, his White students were more likely to display more active listening versus participation, in contrast to the African American students, who viewed lack of active verbal participation during group debate as a deliberate attempt to conceal one's true position on a given issue.

One additional difference was the contrasting beliefs of the two groups as to what was the most appropriate style to use during debates of key issues. While African American students felt it was important and appropriate to take a strong stance toward a debated discussion issue and to advocate one's position through passionate appeal to listeners, White students preferred to use a more neutral style of interaction that was somewhat more detached from emotion. Kochman's interpretation of this stance was that the use of emotion during debate was viewed as interfering with the rational process of debate.

These differences, along with other aspects of communication style such as degree of verbal directness in African American discourse (Spears, 2001), can make it difficult for the persuasion and negotiation styles used by some African American adolescents to be viewed accurately by others. It also suggests that African American adolescents who engage in these styles of conversational exchange may have to learn new ways of negotiating and persuading, according to a different set of cultural discourse rules.

Figurative Language

As adolescents refine their ability to use interpersonal conversational functions such as persuasion and negotiation, they also refine the use and interpretation of various **figurative language** (nonliteral language) expressions such as **metaphors,** which are literary comparisons between items that are typically viewed as distinct on the basis of one or more shared items, as in "the fog crept in on cat-like feet." This sentence compares fog and a cat in terms of movement. **Similes** are literary comparisons between items using the word *like* or *as,* as in the sentence "He is as excited *as a* kid in a candy store." Similes are also figurative expressions that are refined in understanding and use during the school-age and adolescent years. Nippold (1998) reports, as one would expect, steady age-related improvement in children's comprehension of metaphors and similes. Key factors in the development of metaphors and similes are the changes in cognitive flexibility that occur in older stages of childhood that enable children to understand multiple aspects of word and sentence meaning. Nippold (1998) also suggests that exposure to metaphoric language in formal classroom writing assignments helps to increase comprehension and appropriate use of these forms.

Idioms and proverbs represent two other aspects of language use that improve with time. **Idioms,** as defined by Nippold (1998), are expressions such as "read between the lines" that have both a literal and figurative interpretation, with meaning depending on the linguistic context. According to studies cited by Nippold, children learn idioms at least partially through teacher-directed speech in the classroom. As with metaphors and similes, comprehension of idioms improve with age, with interpretation being easier when presented in context versus isolation. Studies of idiom comprehension have revealed that, while accuracy in interpretation improves throughout adolescence and adulthood, idioms are not completely understood by even the oldest subjects (adults) involved in these studies. Some idioms are easier to interpret than others by individuals at all ages, based on degree of **transparency** (how closely they match their intended meaning) and familiarity. Similar findings have been observed with adolescents from rural backgrounds (Qualls, O'Brien, Blood, & Hammer, 2003), with idioms presented in enriched context being comprehended best.

Proverbs (cultural expressions of wisdom, warning, encouragement, and/or advice, such as "Don't count your chickens before they hatch" and "Every cloud has a silver lining") are one other type of figurative language that continues to develop throughout adolescence (Nippold, 2000). Some studies indicate that proverbs are much more difficult for younger children to understand than idioms and metaphors; however, Nippold (1998) asserts that this position is not supported by clear and convincing evidence. As with all other forms of figurative language, accuracy increases with age, with some proverbs continuing to be difficult for some adults. Proverbs are also comprehended differently, depending on factors such as degree of familiarity associated with frequency of exposure and level of concreteness (Nippold, 1998). Knowledge of words contained within proverbs can also play a role in how well they are interpreted (Nippold, 2000). Although proverbs are listed in this chapter as being associated with a form of pragmatic competence, Nippold (2000) lists them as being associated with the dimension of semantics because of the strong meaning relationships conveyed by proverbs.

From a cross-cultural perspective, there are many opportunities for cross-cultural misunderstandings of certain figurative language forms such as idioms and proverbs because these forms are strongly culturally determined, based and passed on through sociocultural interactions. For these reasons, there are many expressions that adolescents from **nonmainstream cultural backgrounds** (cultural or social communities that have norms for behavior that differ from a perceived dominant cultural community) understand and use in certain social contexts outside school. An example from the African American cultural experience is "The eagle flies on Friday," which one is most likely to hear from older adult language users (it refers to "payday"). Another example is that the same idiom can have two different meanings in two different cultures. In mainstream American culture, the idiom of "A rolling stone gathers no moss" indicates that one should keep moving because gathering moss is perceived as a negative feature. However, in Japanese culture, this expression means that one should plant oneself because gathering moss is perceived as positive and valued in Japanese gardening. The connotation of moss differs between these two cultures. Every cultural community has such differences.

Research by Qualls and Harris (1999) provides evidence of cross-cultural differences in the use and interpretation of idioms when examining the comprehension of idioms by African American and White fifth-graders. Findings from their study revealed that idioms that were rated as being highly familiar in one race-ethnic group were not necessarily always so for the other group. Qualls et al. (2003) conducted research on the comprehension of idioms by adolescents residing in rural areas and suggested that cross-cultural differences in perceived familiarity may have also affected the results from their research study. Specifically, they found that rural adolescents comprehended moderate-familiarity idioms better than those preclassified as having high familiarity. They suggest that what might have been preclassified as being highly familiar according to research on other adolescent populations may not have been as familiar to the population researched in their study.

These differences are important for both teachers and clinicians to keep in mind when using or assessing figurative language expressions in adolescents from diverse cultural backgrounds. Figurative language also has obvious relevance for student success with academic curricula (e.g., written literary texts) that use figurative language.

Expository Language

In addition to refining uses of language for everyday social interactions and narratives, adolescents need to refine their use and understanding of expository language. **Expository language** is used to instruct and is required for both oral and written classroom language tasks. It also informs, in contrast to narratives, which are designed to entertain (Larson & McKinley, 2003). Students entering high school are required to engage in a variety of oral expository language activities, such as using language through classroom presentations and discussions, for various purposes, such as to inform, explain, and/or debate. They need to learn how to use expository language in written assignments as well. See the discussion of written language development. Students are also refining their knowledge of the differences in style and expectation between everyday language use and language required in the classroom setting.

Registers

One additional aspect of social communicative competence and language use that is developed and refined in adolescence is the ability to shift between different registers or styles of talking depending on the communication situation and/or group with whom someone is interacting. Some of the registers that adolescents begin to use more effectively are (1) polite versus impolite register; (2) group-related registers based on affiliations and developing social networks with various religious, professional, fraternal, and recreational groups; (3) intimate versus nonintimate registers; (4) gender-based registers; and (5) registers associated with cultural group identity and sexual orientation (McLaughlin, 1998; Owens, 2005).

Narratives

The ability to tell stories according to the cultural norms and standards of a given language community is generally mastered by children in the early school-age years. However, as with every other aspect of language development, the ability to tell stories continues to develop and be refined in adolescence into adulthood. By the early school-age years, children have learned to construct narratives with complete causal-chain episodes and several **story grammar** (story structure) components, such as settings, initiating events, attempts, consequences, and reactions. Throughout the school-age years, stories improve in length and complexity, with multiple conjoined and/or embedded episodes. In addition, stories become more goal-based, with character goals and intentions expressed more explicitly. Stories also begin to include obstacles that affect one or more character's attainments of these goals. Other changes include the use of more **appendages** (story beginnings and endings), with the nature of the appendages used becoming more varied and sophisticated. Stories contain more narrator **evaluations** (personally stated perspectives and reactions to events in the story). They also become more cohesive in flow, with the links between events and characters more clearly indicated. The types of cohesive devices that are used become more sophisticated and varied in nature. Stories also contain more **orientation** information, which includes background information about character actions, traits, relationships, and names, as well as where and when the story takes place (Lahey, 1988).

As individuals move into adolescence and adulthood, their stories continue to include increased references to character emotions, thoughts, and plans. Stories are also much longer in terms of clause length. Storytellers display increased awareness of character mental states, thoughts, plans, and actions. The number of embedded episodes increases, as does the number of complete episodes, although some are still incomplete (Nippold, 1998).

As with other aspects of adolescent language development, there can be cross-cultural differences in the ways in which narratives are produced by adolescents from different cultural backgrounds (Champion, 2003; Guttierez-Clellen & Quinn, 1993; Westby, 1994). Possible cross-cultural variations include (1) the amount of detail and elaboration used within stories, (2) how stories are organized, (3) the extent to which links between events and characters within stories are expressed, (4) what is emphasized or considered to be important when telling stories, (5) how evaluations are expressed, and (6) the channels through which story information is conveyed (e.g., primarily verbal or nonverbal).

ADOLESCENT LITERACY DEVELOPMENT

Reading

As children enter the school-age and adolescent years, there is an increased emphasis on reading and writing (refer to Chapters 8 and 9 on monolingual and bilingual reading development). Reading involves the decoding of words (recognizing printed words), the fluent ability to read, and reading comprehension (the understanding and processing of meaning). Successful reading requires the integration of several cognitive, metacognitive, linguistic, and metalinguistic abilities. Some of the most important metacognitive and metalinguistic aspects include (1) phonological and phonemic awareness; (2) the morphosyntactic rules and vocabulary of the language in which a text is produced and read; (3) figurative uses of language, such as idioms and metaphors; and (4) **text grammars** (how texts are organized and structured) found in academic texts. Achieving good reading skills also involves the development of good attention, auditory perceptual, visual perceptual, meta-cognitive and memory skills.

According to Chall (as cited in Larson & McKinley, 2003) and McLaughlin (1998), there are several different stages of reading that children go through during the early and later grade levels. Some of the skills that are typically acquired by children in earlier grades include being able to decode written words through phonological analysis and segmentation, and achieving automaticity and fluency during the reading process. In the middle school-age years, reading for various academic purposes, such as reading to learn, is highly emphasized. In grades 8 to 12, reading is used as a means for learning new ideas and pursuing knowledge. In the post–high school/college years, students learn to read for inquiry and critical analysis.

In addition to mastering reading for different purposes, school-age and adolescent students have to learn how to read and comprehend different types of expository, narrative, and persuasive text. Students also have to learn to adjust their reading depending on the varied demands and purposes of different texts. They must develop key metacognitive strategies that are important to good reading comprehension (Larson & McKinley, 2003).

According to Ehren (2005), good reading comprehension skills require good background knowledge (prior knowledge of information contained within written texts), world knowledge (knowledge of general world facts and information relevant to what is being read), vocabulary skills, and conceptual knowledge (knowledge of concepts relevant to what is being addressed within a given text).

Students also need to know how to recognize and interpret varied text grammars. As previously discussed, when students enter into the later academic years, they are exposed to a variety of different expository structures in classroom texts. Some of those expository structures, as noted in Westby (1994), include (1) descriptive texts (which describe what something is), (2) enumerative texts (which provide a list related to a topic), (3) sequential/procedural texts (which provide an overview of how to do something or a sequence of events that have occurred), (4) comparison-contrast texts (which provide a comparison of how two or more things are the same or different), (5) problem-solution texts (which state a problem and offer solutions), (6) persuasive texts (which take a position on some issue and justify it), and (7) cause-effect texts (which give reasons why something happened). Each of these texts is characterized by different organizational structures depending on their purpose and focus (Westby, 1994). The differences can be found, for example, in the varying types of signaling devices (visual cues that clue the reader to the type of structure being used) and cohesive ties (linking structures used to tie related ideas together both within and across sentences) (Ehren, 2006).

Adolescent students must be able to recognize the organization patterns that occur within academic texts. They must also be able to apply strategic text structure analysis procedures. Important text grammar analysis strategies include being able to (1) activate prior knowledge important to a given text, (2) predict what will be addressed within a text given that knowledge, (3) ask important questions about the text, (4) use active self-questioning techniques to make important inferences, (5) use visual imagery to enhance comprehension, (6) paraphrase as well as summarize what has just been read, (7) monitor and repair breakdowns in comprehension, and (8) integrate the use of these various strategies (Ehren, 2005). All these academic written language abilities continue to develop well into the high school–college years.

Although there are generally similar factors that contribute to effective reading comprehension in readers from different cultural and language backgrounds, some cultural factors can potentially influence reading comprehension and other aspects of reading performance in children from differing backgrounds. Several factors became apparent in the research of Bradford and Harris (2003), who studied the relationship between cultural knowledge and reading ability in fourth-, fifth-, and sixth-grade African American students across three different domains of content knowledge (arts, news events, history). Students' cultural knowledge of mainstream versus African American items in each of these domains was examined. Results revealed that, generally speaking, older students performed better than younger students across all domains, with an increase of both mainstream and African American cultural knowledge. The authors also found that the students displayed higher levels of African American history and news events knowledge than mainstream history and news events knowledge. The reverse was found, however, in the arts. In addition, the researchers observed that students from higher-income backgrounds outperformed those from middle-class backgrounds in all content domains. They attributed this difference to greater accessibility and quality of literate resources by this student group.

Based on their research findings, Bradford and Harris (2003) concluded that school-age African American students are fairly literate in their knowledge of information from their home cultural community as well as what is emphasized within the mainstream culture. The authors go further and state that these findings are likely to have strong implications for success with academic literacy (reading and writing skills) in the school setting. They also suggest that teachers should consider drawing upon the cultural capital and knowledge that their students bring to the classroom in improving students' overall academic performance.

There have also been some studies examining reading skill development in bilingual children. One such study by Swanson, Hodson, and Schommer-Aikens (2005) examined the relationship between the acquisition of phonological awareness and reading success in bilingual speakers (refer to Chapter 9 on bilingual literacy for additional discussion of bilingual phonemic awareness issues). As discussed in Swanson et al. (2005), phonological awareness has been found to be strongly related to reading development in English for child readers from a variety of language backgrounds. Phonological awareness in a child's native language has also been found to transfer to skills in a second language (Gottardo et al., as cited in Swanson et al., 2005). However, Swanson et al. (2005), who studied the effects of a reading intervention program designed to improve English phonological awareness skills in bilingual Spanish-English-speaking seventh-grade students, also observed that students who are still in the process of learning a second language can be at greater risk for reading failure when compared to their monolingual English-speaking peers. This is probably most likely to be the case with students who have not achieved a level of reading proficiency in their first and/or dominant language.

Writing

As students move into the school-age and adolescent years, written language becomes a very important part of the academic instructional and learning process (see Chapter 10 on writing and spelling development). However, as Nelson (1998) states, "learning to produce written language is a complex process involving the coordination of language formulation, phonological processing, graphomotor, and cognitive monitoring skills" (p. 380). Nelson goes on to say that "effective writers also use pragmatic knowledge to consider the needs of their listeners" (p. 380) and that written language, like spoken language, is used for many different purposes or functions.

Some of the different types of writing required by schools for adolescents, based on the work of Scott and Erwin (1982, as cited in Larson & McKinley, 2003), include personal experience narratives, book reports, written summaries of factual information, fictional stories, written expositions on how to do something, descriptive writing, reporting, persuasive writing, business correspondences (e.g., job interview applications), and personal correspondences (e.g., letters).

Research on the development of written language abilities in adolescence by Nippold (2000) revealed systematic and age-related changes that occur in the persuasive written discourse of adolescents. Specifically, Nippold (2000) found gradual age-related increases in the following in subjects aged 11 to 24 years: the use of relative clauses; mean length of utterances in terms of words per utterance; the use of literate words, including adverbial conjuncts such as *consequently,* abstract nouns such as *entertainment,* and metaverbs such as *acknowledge;* and the number of reasons used to support written arguments. In other research studies cited by Nippold (2000), adolescents have been found to produce more complex syntactic constructions in certain types of writing tasks (e.g., persuasive) than in others (e.g., narrative), suggesting that typically developing adolescents have the ability to recognize the need for and to change their style of writing depending on writing tasks demands.

Most of the cross-linguistic research that has been conducted on school-age and adolescent writers has focused on issues such as the potential impact of spoken dialect use patterns on written grammar. For example, Scott and Rogers (1996) cite several studies that demonstrate evidence of dialect-influenced patterns in the writing samples of elementary school-age students, as was found in the previously mentioned research of Thompson, Craig, and Washington (2004). Studies of older adolescent speakers have also revealed the impact of dialect background on writing style. For example, in a single-subject study that focused on the written essays produced by an African American college student, Garcia and Pearson (cited in Scott & Rogers, 1996) found that the ease and speed with which writing occurs can be affected by second-dialect proficiency issues. Specifically, these researchers provided evidence that when students have to pay close attention to the use of MAE dialect features in writing, fluidity of writing and clarity in the expression of ideas can be affected. There can also be a loss of voice. However, when students are given the opportunity to write without attention to dialect form, they can actively create written passages that are richer in content and flow. Scott and Rogers (1996) also report findings from research by Fowler that suggest that African American adolescents who are high dialect users sometimes need to take more time with academic writing tasks compared to those who are low or moderate dialect users. In addition, the robustness of the writing sample (number of words) can be affected.

Some studies have concentrated on culturally based differences in expository writing style that can occur in the writings of students from nonmainstream cultural backgrounds. Ball (1992), for example, studied the expository writing discourse styles of African American adolescents. Results from Ball's study revealed no differences between the preferred and most frequently used written expository organizational patterns produced by fifth- and sixth-grade African American students and those expected in mainstream American classroom settings. There were major differences, however, when comparing narratives produced by high school students from the two different cultural backgrounds. African American high school students tended to use more **narrative interspersion** (where the speaker or writer intersperses a narrative within expository text) and **circumlocution** (topic-associated style of writing) in written as well as oral communication tasks. This contrasted with the **topical nets** (topically organized or centered) and **matrices** (where attributes are organized according to discrete points among two or more dimensions) used most often by non–African American students at the same grade level.

Collectively, these studies suggest that both dialect and culture can influence the writing productions of students from diverse backgrounds. These differences have implications for the evaluation and instruction of writing for these students.

ADOLESCENT MOTIVATION AND BEHAVIOR

One last aspect of development that is key to understanding the maturation of language in adolescents is personal motivation. School professionals as well as parents often find it difficult to motivate their adolescent children and students during the teenage years, for numerous reasons. Two are the resistance to adult control and the need to have control of one's destiny. For many adolescents, regardless of cultural background, motivation generally comes from external versus internal motivators, such as their peer-group networks, parental or school professional expectations, and the need for social-group acceptance. As a result, teachers and other educational professionals may need to assist students in recognizing the positive aspects of school success.

CASE STUDY PERSPECTIVES

Case Study One Background: Trent

Trent is a 12-year-old African American student who is currently enrolled in a general education sixth-grade classroom. Outside the classroom, from the school's learning disabilities specialist, he receives resource support two times per week, 40 minutes each session. He also receives 30 minutes of speech and language consultation from the school speech-language pathologist, who works collaboratively with his classroom teachers to address some of his language-based learning weaknesses. His primary learning weaknesses are in the areas of auditory memory and attention, memory, and language processing.

Prior to the current year, Trent was being homeschooled by his mother, Mrs. Tate. However, after six years of homeschooling, Mrs. Tate was becoming increasingly frustrated with her son's lack of motivation to learn and his growing resistance to her teaching efforts. She was also becoming frustrated in getting him to "behave appropriately" in social situations and to interact socially with others in an appropriate and respectful manner.

Results from previous speech and language testing at a private clinic last year, using the *Clinical Evaluation of Language Fundamentals (CELF-4)* revealed below-age-level scores on the following subtests: "Word Definitions," "Understanding Spoken Paragraphs," and "Semantic Relationships." A review of Trent's performance on current classroom assignments revealed difficulties with assignments that involved new-word decoding, word definition, and reading comprehension. Trent also has difficulty answering questions about text reading passages and following verbal instructions from the teacher.

As part of last year's testing, Mrs. Tate was asked to rate her son's performance on several communication skills using the "Pragmatics Profile" of the CELF-4. She was asked to rate his skills using a four-point rating scale, with a rating of 1 given to social skills that are never displayed and a rating of 4 given to skills that are always demonstrated. Some of the items that were rated with a 1 included (1) asking for help from others appropriately, (2) reading social situations correctly and behaving/responding appropriately, (3) asking others for permission when required, and (4) using appropriate strategies for responding to interruptions and interrupting others. Follow-up observations of Trent's behavior and social interactions with others in the classroom by the speech-language pathologist confirmed these as continued areas of concern.

Two of the greatest concerns for Trent's teacher are understanding how to motivate Trent to complete difficult work assignments and getting him to be more compliant and attentive in the classroom. She also wants to engage Trent more in the learning process.

Case Study One Comments: Trent

The most appropriate approach for all professionals involved in working with Trent is a collaborative one, where they work with his teacher and parents to identify some of Trent's current interests, preferred learning style, and positive motivators. Vocabulary and reading comprehension activities that incorporate these interests should be identified and used when possible. Instruction should also be tailored toward providing Trent with active learning experiences where he has an opportunity to move around, touch, and talk about as well as listen to and read written information. For the present time, written text and verbally presented information should be brief, with frequent breaks. Reading and writing activities need to be at a level were Trent can be successful. In addition, the educational team needs to find ways to reward Trent for recognizing (e.g., stating) and also implementing good classroom listening and responding behaviors.

Academic motivation may be even more important when working with adolescents from culturally diverse communities where the pressures to conform to peer-group and social community standards are especially strong and where being academically successful is not necessarily always viewed as being "cool." For example, there are certain cultural communities where talking or acting in ways that are valued in the general education classroom setting is viewed negatively by peers within the student's home community. Examples include the use of MAE and certain mainstream cultural discourse styles; these examples have historically been equated with the African American community.

Students from such communities who wish to excel in the classroom setting may sometimes have to face conflicting community social perceptions. In order to succeed, they must have an unusually strong sense of self, the personal motivation to succeed, and their own sense of who they want to become in spite of what others may think. In some cases, students are able to meet this challenge by developing the ability to effectively switch between the code of the school and the code of the community, also known as **code switching** (e.g., switching between MAE and AAE). Switching between the school and community language standards in order to be accepted and survive within certain cultural community and peer networks is a strategy that has often been used by those facing this challenge.

In some cases, this issue has very strong implications for minority youth residing in communities where some teens also have to develop survival social communication skills that keep them out of potentially dangerous peer-group situations (e.g., gang affiliations). In these cases, students have the additional challenge of developing "street" verbal communication skills that are important for protecting their personal integrity and safety. This is the case for adolescents from a variety of cultural and language backgrounds who are living in communities where poverty and violence are a normal part of community life.

Teachers and speech-language pathologists can play a very important part in helping students to acquire the social communication skills that they need not only for the classroom and job settings, but also for the everyday social realities that adolescents face in their home communities after school. To do this, however, teachers and other professionals need to respect the fact that students have communication needs other than those in the normal classroom and to take the time to understand what those needs are and how they can best be addressed. Part of developing social communicative competence also involves helping students learn how to effectively code-switch between different styles of communication in a variety of simulated or role-play communication situations.

Finally, teachers and speech-language clinicians can be primary agents in helping students who may be shunned by their own cultural community to feel good about excelling with those styles of communication that they will need for other social settings. It is very important, however, that such approaches are done so that they do not denigrate but build acceptance for the legitimacy of other language uses and needs.

CASE STUDY PERSPECTIVES

Case Study Two Background: José

José is a 14-year-old high school student who is a bilingual Spanish-English speaker. Although English is currently his most dominant language, Spanish continues to be the primary language of the home. He continues to display the following language difficulties in both languages: (1) reduced sentence length and complexity; (2) difficulties generating and retelling stories using appropriate character referencing, temporal cohesion, and overall story grammar structure; (3) processing auditory commands in both languages; (4) reading comprehension; (5) writing; and (6) using age-appropriate social-negotiation and interpersonal communication skills with peers. He is currently enrolled in a high school classroom for students with special language needs, with additional speech and language support services provided in one session per week outside the classroom and 30 minutes of classroom consultation.

At a recent individual education plan (IEP) conference, José's parents expressed growing concerns about his social-communication skills because he is growing up in a community where gangs are becoming an issue. In the last two months, he has had difficulty defending himself after school with peers in his community who are beginning to pick on him. Weaknesses in social communication are supported by results from recent testing using the "Pragmatic Judgment" subtest of the *Comprehensive Assessment of Social Language (CASL)*, which was administered at the beginning of the current school year.

Case Study Two Comments: José

José is a perfect example of the types of challenges faced by adolescents with language learning difficulties and impairments who grow up in communities where pressure to conform to social peer groups such as gangs is a problem. José's parents, while recognizing the need for their son to develop his academic skills, also recognize the danger of him not being adequately prepared with the appropriate social-communication skills for survival in his community.

The most appropriate intervention plan for José is one where the speech-language pathologist (SLP) and teacher build his overall vocabulary and sentence production skills. They can expose him to various social-communication scenarios that model the most appropriate manner for responding to peers and communicating with them in difficult social situations. These scenarios can be presented via video, story reading tasks, and/or scripted role-plays. Using age-appropriate stories to demonstrate social-communication challenges will also improve his use and understanding of narrative structure (which is another weak area for him). In addition the teacher can incorporate story-writing tasks where José has an opportunity to practice various written expository tasks, such as (1) writing a paper on reasons for standing up to gangs, (2) writing a descriptive paper about actual situations he has had to face himself, and (3) writing a paper that outlines steps one can take to defend oneself against gangs. Active teaching and learning strategies should include approaches such as encouraging José to identify important questions that need to be asked in developing a well-written paper. Paper topics focusing on strategies for developing friendships with members of more positive group can also be useful. Collectively, these strategies also help to develop José's sense of personal self-worth, identity, self-esteem, autonomy, and independence.

SCHOOL DEMANDS AND CURRICULAR EXPECTATIONS FOR ADOLESCENT STUDENTS

In addition to the academic language issues previously addressed in this chapter, students will encounter other changes in expectations as they transition from elementary to middle school, and to high school. For example, while elementary classrooms tend to be more student-centered, secondary school classrooms are more subject-centered. Other changes that students encounter include having to enter classrooms where there is more emphasis on control and self-discipline, with less personal relationship between the teacher and students (Kimmel & Weiner, 1995).

Additional challenges discussed by Ehren (2002) include setting-specific differences, such as the fact that many high school campuses are fairly large and sprawling, with high levels of simultaneously occurring activities. Students must change classes frequently, and the time for transitioning between classes is fairly brief. Instruction tends to be departmentalized. In addition, students must adjust to several different teachers who use a variety of teaching methods. These environmental changes, as noted by Ehren (2002), can be very challenging to the adolescent with learning disabilities. High school is an environment where it is easy for students with disabilities to become confused and disorganized.

As students transition from middle school to high school, they are also faced with an increased amount of writing. They begin to encounter curricula that require increasingly complex types of written composition as well as a variety of writing tasks and assignments. These include note taking, taking exams, and completing lengthy term paper assignments (Sturm & Koppenhaver, 2000). As previously discussed, the types of written texts that they encounter also vary with respect to internal organization and structure. These differences change across grade levels, curriculum subject areas, and texts (Ehren, 2002).

CHARACTERISTICS OF LANGUAGE IMPAIRMENT IN ADOLESCENTS WITH EXCEPTIONALITIES

Spoken Language

Spoken language includes the following types of elements: phonological, morphological, semantic, syntactic, and pragmatics development. Each will be discussed below.

Phonological

Adolescent learners are not likely to display many of the phonological error patterns typically observed in a younger child's speech, such as persisting phonological processes that affect individual speech/sound and syllable structure. However, speech/sound sequencing difficulties can still be a problem for some older students. Other issues that affect speech intelligibility, such as inappropriate rate of speech and distorted productions of sounds due to resonance imbalance and/or oral-myofunctional disorders, can also be a problem, which can then translate to phonological awareness difficulties.

Morphological

As previously indicated, there are certain morphological markers that are still being acquired by adolescents. Therefore, it is possible for adolescents with language learning impairments to display continued difficulties with some of these forms long after they have been mastered by age-peers.

Semantic

This is probably one of the most likely areas of weakness for adolescent students with language learning difficulties. It is also an area of weakness that has a great potential for impact on academic success, with both written and spoken academic language requirements in the middle school and high school settings. Word difficulties can range from issues of word retrieval to receptive vocabulary and expressive vocabulary deficits. Weaknesses in receptive and/or expressive vocabulary are typically displayed as difficulties with word-association, word-categorization, word-definition, and word-use tasks. Difficulties with the comprehension of certain word meanings have important implications for the development of figurative language, and reading comprehension skills.

Syntactic

Two of the aspects of syntactic development that are likely to be most impaired with adolescents are the use of complex syntactic structures in both spoken and written language, and the production of sentences that are of appropriate length for a student's given age level. Students with syntactic language impairments may also struggle with correct use of later-developing conjunctions and adverbial conjuncts. In addition, they may display mazes that contain excessive numbers of words. The presence of mazes within their sentences may also be more frequent than for typically developing peers.

Pragmatics Development

Some of the aspects of conversational ability that can be impaired in adolescents with language weaknesses include (1) the ability to engage effectively in sustained conversation with others, (2) the ability to adapt conversation to the background of the listener, (3) the ability to make and respond to requests for conversational repair during breakdowns, (4) the ability to read the feelings and emotions of others, and (5) the ability to understand and take the perspective of others.

In the area of language function or use, adolescents may have difficulty using the most appropriate language strategies for engaging in specialized language uses such as persuasion and negotiation. They may miss the subtle figurative uses of language in humor, jokes, and everyday conversational exchanges with peers. They may also have difficulty acquiring the social communication registers needed for entry into certain social and job-related activities and groups.

The importance of developing effective social communication skills cannot be overstated. Results from studies reported by Whitmire (2000) reveal that adolescents with language disorders tend to be less liked by their peers; are attended to less by their peers; have poor social skills; adapt less well to the needs and feelings of their listener; have difficulty interpreting social cues; have difficulty understanding jokes, slang, and sarcasm; and have difficulty with social negotiation. These difficulties, according to Whitmire (2000), leave adolescents with language impairments without the emotional support from peers that allows them to build relationships with individuals outside their immediate family. There is also a vicious cycle where their inability to be accepted into peer networks deprives them of the opportunity to develop the types of interpersonal skills that they need for establishing intimate relationships with others. These social difficulties can lead to later social-emotional and psychological difficulties (Kimmel & Weiner, 1995, as cited in Whitmire, 2000).

In the narrative domain, adolescents may have difficulty constructing well-organized stories in spoken or written form that are cohesive and easy to understand, and that contain important information about character emotions, feelings, thoughts, and plans. They may produce stories that do not correspond to expected story grammar frameworks. They may also produce stories that are fairly simple in nature and more like the stories of younger students.

Reading and Writing

Many of the previously listed spoken language difficulties also affect student success with classroom reading and writing tasks. Adolescents who have difficulty using and understanding figurative language expressions such as metaphors, proverbs, idioms, and similes have difficulty comprehending literary texts that use these figurative language devices. Students with vocabulary difficulties have difficulties comprehending and producing written text that is meaningful.

Cognitive Processes

Some of the language difficulties experienced by adolescents are a direct by-product of underlying weaknesses or deficits in various cognitive and metacognitive processes, including attention, memory, and/or executive functioning and monitoring. Adolescents who have these additional cognitive limitations struggle with both social communication and academic tasks that rely on one or more of these abilities. Difficulties with planning or organization are also likely to affect writing skills because writing is a process that requires use of both of these cognitive processes. Students who have difficulties identifying patterns in text may have difficulty accessing the various forms of expository language found in their textbooks.

Teaching Strategies

There are a number of different roles that speech-language pathologists can play in promoting the language development of adolescents with language learning difficulties and impairments. These range from direct intervention to indirect intervention-consultation, including taking leadership by offering technical assistance to colleagues in developing and teaching a language-based curriculum for all students, not just those in the speech-language caseload; providing professional development workshops that expand teachers' understanding of effective language teaching strategies for youth with language difficulties; participating in the development of school policies that affect the type of curriculum offered; and participating in curriculum development to help develop curricula that are aligned with current state standards. Speech-language pathologists can play an important role in serving as advocates for adolescent students with specialized language needs.

There are also a number of teaching approaches that speech-language pathologists can use—and encourage their colleagues to use—in supporting the instruction of students with special language needs. Recommended instructional strategies include the use of **differentiated instruction** (instruction tailored to the unique needs of each student, Nelson, 2005) and scaffolding to support student learning (Ehren, 2006; Nelson, 2005). Therapy goals and approaches used by speech-language pathologists working with adolescents should be relevant to the curriculum and use materials that are actually used in the classroom setting (see Chapter 12 on consultation and collaboration issues) (Ehren, 2002, 2006). Students need to be taught to apply active reading comprehension and text analysis skills, which were discussed earlier in this chapter (Ehren, 2005). Especially with adolescents, it is important to involve them in ways that motivate them to learn (Ehren, 2002). Instruction should be geared toward the unique learning style preferences of students (Welsh, 2006). In addition, teachers and clinicians should attempt to use instructional strategies that address the unique socioemotional needs of adolescents. Useful strategies for doing the latter are provided by Winebrenner, 1998 (as cited in Hearne, 2000).

In addition to the above listed strategies, Hearne (2000) provides additional suggestions for working with second-language learners:

1. Using high-interest, low-vocabulary readers where the interest level is grade-appropriate but the actual vocabulary level is lower

2. Providing instruction at a level that is comprehensible to students given their levels of second-language proficiency

3. Using nonverbal input and instruction (e.g., through the use of accompanying gestures and visuals) to support verbal instruction

4. Creating a language-rich learning environment that contains L1 and L2 literature

5. Creating a classroom atmosphere that values differences and where all students feel welcome

6. Meeting with parents of every student to gain insight into the student's background, interests, ideas, and feelings, as well as insight into the student's home life

7. Encouraging students, whenever possible, to explore their own personal interests/talents and possible career options

8. Encouraging the development of bilingual skills and biliteracy as a method for enhancing a student's future career potential in American and international markets

9. Using bilingual teaching and analysis approaches to help build bridges between languages, such as using word cognate pairs (e.g., bebe-baby, differente-different, and estudiante-student) to help students learn how to spell words in their second language that look similar to words in their first language

---

INSTRUCTIONAL/CLINICAL STRATEGIES

Improving the Classroom Language and Learning Skills of Adolescents

Text-Processing Strategies
- Activate prior knowledge
- Analyze text
- Use visual imagery
- Use paraphrasing and summarizing
- Improve monitoring and repair during conversation

Reading Comprehension Strategies
- Interactive dialogue
- Content enhancement routines
- Choral reading
- Graphic organizers
- Texts that teach new or unfamiliar text structures using familiar words and vocabulary
- Training for students about how to negotiate texts
- Avoidance of "inconsiderate" texts (texts that lack organizational clarity and/or that emphasize trivial details verses fundamental principles)

Strategies for Encouraging Active Student Learning and Involvement
- Small groups with individual student feedback
- Groups that include students with varied learning styles (visual/spatial, kinesthetic, linguistic)
- Placing value on each learning style equally
- Teaching to student's learning strengths
- Teaching to each learning style equally

Strategies for Addressing Social-Emotional Behavioral Needs of Older Students
- Address needs for belonging and friendship (e.g., take time to chat with them about extracurricular interests)
- Address needs of self-worth (e.g., create a risk-free learning environment)
- Create the need for freedom, autonomy, and choice (e.g., encourage students to set their own short-term goals for behavior)
- Address the need for fun and enjoyment (e.g, incorporate fun into general education school tasks)

Sources: Ehren, 2002; Ehren, 2005; Welsh, 2006; Winebrenner, 1998, as cited in Hearne, 2000.

CONCLUDING REMARKS

Adolescent language development is just as crucial to school success as earlier preschool and school-age child development. Although most of the research to date on children's language development has focused on oral language development in younger children, there is a growing body of research on adolescents that provides evidence of continued growth in several different aspects of language and communication. Mastering the communicative expectations of adolescence is important not only to academic and school success but also to the development of social communication, personal identity, and self-esteem. The skills that develop and/or are refined during adolescence have important implications for later life. Adolescents who experience language impairments in one or more of these areas of communication are likely to be at risk for social as well as academic difficulties. When considering language development during the adolescent years, educators and speech-language pathologists need to remain cognizant of the cultural and linguistic differences that can exist within their student populations. These differences should never be viewed as deficits, even though they may have an impact on successful attainment of school-based standards. They are differences that should be addressed in a positive manner, as a means for improving the future educational and social opportunities for these and all children.

REFLECTION QUESTIONS

1. Refer to Case Study One. What types of language analyses would you conduct to assess José's current level of sentence length and complexity? Would you conduct the assessment in both Spanish and English, or just English? What strategies would you use for addressing his narrative difficulties?

2. Refer to Case Study Two. Design an instructional activity for Trent that you believe draws on his learning strengths. Give specific examples of how you would use some of the teaching strategies designed to address some of his most likely social-emotional behavioral needs.

3. Reflect on an adolescent student you know well personally or have taught or worked with in the school setting. How were some of the characteristics and descriptions of adolescence presented in this chapter exhibited by the student? Give specific examples of how these characteristics were displayed.

4. Imagine that you are a speech-language pathologist, general education teacher, or special education teacher who has been asked to be part of a school district task force focused on improving the language skills of high school minority students at risk for academic failure. What types of programs, support mechanisms, and strategies would you recommend for addressing this issue?

5. Assume that you are responsible for developing a thematic language unit for middle school or high school students in a community that is very diverse. You are interested in finding ways to build on the cultural knowledge and vocabulary that students already have as a way of enhancing their overall language and literacy skills. What strategies, methods, and materials would you use for accomplishing these tasks?

6. As previously stated, one important aspect of reading comprehension is the ability to use effective text analysis strategies, such as (1) activating prior knowledge, (2) predicting what will be addressed in a text, (3) asking important questions about the text, (4) using active self-questioning techniques, (5) using visual imagery, (6) paraphrasing and summarizing, and (7) monitoring and repairing breakdowns in communication. Provide specific examples of how you might apply each of these techniques in conducting a lesson from a middle school or

high school science or social studies text. Name the text and the chapter to be read, and state how you would use each of these strategies to help students in your class understand what they are reading in this text.

7. Social registers are an important part of social communication competence in adolescence and adulthood. Reflect on at least three different social registers that you have had to use in the past week. Where and with whom were they used, and how do these registers differ from each other in terms of vocabulary and style?

REFERENCES

Ball, A. F. (1992). Cultural preference and the expository writing of African-American adolescents. *Written Communication, 9*(4), 501–532.

Bedore, L. M., Peña, E. D., García, M., & Cortez, C. (2005). Conceptual versus monolingual scoring: When does it make a difference? *Language, Speech, and Hearing Services in Schools, 36*(3), 188–200.

Bradford, A. C., & Harris, J. L. (2003). Cultural knowledge in African American children. *Language, Speech, and Hearing Services in Schools, 34*(1), 56–68.

Champion, T. (2003). *Understanding storytelling among African American children: A journey from Africa to America*. Mahwah, NJ: Lawrence Erlbaum.

Edelman, M. W. (2006). Statement of purpose. In The Smiley Group, Inc. (Ed.), *The covenant with Black America* (pp. xiii–xiv). Chicago, IL: Third World Press.

Ehren, B. J. (2002). Speech-language pathologists contributing significantly to the academic success of high school students: A vision for professional growth. *Topics in Language Disorders, 22*(2), 60–80.

Ehren, B. J. (2005). Looking for evidence-based practice in reading comprehension instruction. *Topics in Language Disorders, 25*(4), 310–321.

Ehren, B. J. (2006, April). *Helping students with language impairment process text: An important literacy mission for SLPs*. Workshop presented at the annual meeting of the California Speech-Language-Hearing Association, San Francisco, CA.

Goldstein, B. A., Fabiano, L., & Washington, P. S. (2005). Phonological skills in predominantly English-speaking, predominantly Spanish-speaking, and Spanish-English bilingual children. *Language, Speech, and Hearing Services in the Schools, 36*(3), 201–218.

Gordon, E. W. (2006). Establishing a system of public education in which all children achieve at high levels and reach their full potential. In The Smiley Group, Inc. (Ed.), *The covenant with Black America* (pp. 23–45). Chicago, IL: Third World Press.

Green, L. J. (2002). *African American English: A linguistic introduction*. Cambridge, UK: Cambridge University Press.

Gutierrez-Clellen, V. F., & Quinn, R. (1993). Assessing narratives of children from diverse cultural/linguistic groups. *Language, Speech, and Hearing Services in Schools, 24*(1), 2–9.

Hearne, J. D. (2000). *Teaching second language learners with learning disabilities: Strategies for effective practice*. Oceanside, CA: Academic Communication Associates.

Helfand, D. (2005). Nearly half of blacks, Latinos drop out, school study shows. *Los Angeles Times*, pp. A1, A26.

Iglesias, S., & Goldstein, B. (1998). Language and dialect variation. In J. E. Bernthal & N. W. Bankson (Eds.), *Articulation and phonological disorders*, (4th ed, pp. 148–171). Boston, MA: Allyn & Bacon.

Kimmel, D. C., & Weiner, I. B. (1995). *Adolescence: A developmental transition*. New York: Wiley.

Kochman, T. (1981). *Black and White styles in conflict*. Chicago, IL: University of Chicago Press.

Lahey M. (1988). *Language disorders and language development*. New York: Macmillan.

Larson, V. L., & McKinley, N. L. (2003). *Communication solutions for older students: Assessment and intervention strategies*. Eau Claire, WI: Thinking Publications.

Loban, W. (1976). *Language development: Kindergarten through grade twelve*. Urbana, IL: National Council of Teachers of English.

McLaughlin, S. (1998). *Introduction to language development*. San Diego, CA: Singular Publishing Group.

Munro, P. (2002, April). *What slang can teach us about language*. Paper presented at the annual California State University, Fullerton, Linguistics Symposium, Fullerton, CA.

Nelson, N. W. (1998). *Childhood language disorders in context: Infancy through adolescence* (2nd ed.). Boston, MA: Allyn & Bacon.

Nelson, N. W. (2005). The context of discourse difficulty in classroom and clinic: An update. *Topics in Language Disorders, 25*(4), 322–331.

Nippold, M. A. (1998). *Later language development: The school-age and adolescent years* (2nd ed.). Austin, TX: Pro-Ed.

Nippold, M. A. (2000). Language development during the adolescent years: Aspects of pragmatics, syntax, and semantics. *Topics in Language Disorders, 20*(2), 15–28.

Owens, R. E. (2005). *Language development: An introduction* (6th ed.). Boston, MA: Pearson Education.

Paradis, J. (2005). Grammatical morphology in children learning English as a second language: Implications of similarities with specific language impairment. *Language, Speech, and Hearing Services in Schools, 36*(3), 172–187.

Qualls, C. D., & Harris, J. L. (1999). Effects of familiarity on idiom comprehension in African American and European American fifth graders. *Language, Speech, and Hearing Services in Schools, 30*(2), 141–151.

Qualls, C. D., O'Brien, R. M., Blood, G. W., & Hammer, C. S. (2003). Contextual variation, familiarity, academic literacy, and rural adolescents' idiom knowledge. *Language, Speech, and Hearing Services in Schools, 34*(1), 69–79.

Rickford, J. R. (1999). *African American vernacular english: Features, evolution, educational implications.* Malden, MA: Blackwell.

Scott, C. M., & Rogers, L. M. (1996). Written language abilities of African American children and youth. In A. G. Kamhi, K. E. Pollock, & J. L. Harris (Eds.), *Communication development and disorders in African American children: Research, assessment, and intervention.* Baltimore, MD: Paul H. Brookes.

Smitherman, G. (1977). *Talkin and testifyin: The language of black America.* Detroit, MI: Wayne State University Press.

Spears, A. K. (2001). Directness in the use of African American English. In S. L. Lanehart (Ed.), *Sociocultural and historical contexts of African American English* (pp. 239–259). Amsterdam: John Benjamins.

Stainburn, S. (2004a, March 22/March 29). Closing the gap. *U.S. News and World Report, 136*(10), 87.

Stainburn, S. (2004b, May). What's wrong with this picture? *Teacher Magazine, 15*(6), 70.

Sturm, J., & Koppenhaver, D. A. (2000). Supporting writing development in adolescents with developmental disabilities. *Topics in Language Disorders, 20*(2), 73–92.

Swanson, T. J., Hodson, B. W., & Schommer-Aikins, M. (2005). An examination of phonological awareness treatment outcomes for seventh-grade poor readers from a bilingual community. *Language, Speech, and Hearing Services in Schools, 36*(4), 336–345.

Thompson, C. A., Craig, H. K., & Washington, J. A. (2004). Variable production of African American English across oracy and literacy contexts. *Language, Speech, and Hearing Services in Schools, 35*(3), 269–282.

Vihman, M. M. (1998). Later phonological development. In J. E. Bernthal & N. W. Bankson (Eds.), *Articulation and phonological disorders* (4th ed., pp. 113–147). Boston, MA: Allyn & Bacon.

Welsh, R. (2006). *Engaging the non-traditional adolescent learner in the regular education and inclusion classroom.* Workshop presented at the annual meeting of the New Jersey Speech-Language-Hearing Association. Atlantic City, NJ.

Westby, C. E. (1994). The effects of culture on genre, structure, and style of oral and written texts. In G. Wallach & K. Butler (Eds.), *Language learning disabilities in school-age children and adolescents* (pp. 180–218). New York: Macmillan.

Whitmire, K. A. (2000). Adolescence as a developmental phase: A tutorial. *Topics in Language Disorders, 20*(2), 1–14.

Whitmire, K. A. (2005). Language and literacy in the age of federal initiatives. *Topics in Language Disorders, 25*(4), 302–309.

Wolfram, W., & Schilling-Estes, N. (2006). *American English: Dialects and variation* (2nd ed.). Malden, MA: Blackwell.

Wyatt, T. A. (1995). Language development in African American English child speech. *Linguistics and Education, 7*(1), 7–22.

Wyatt, T. A. (2002). Assessing the communicative abilities of clients from diverse cultural and language backgrounds. In D. E. Battle (Ed.), *Communication disorders in multicultural populations* (3rd ed., pp. 415–459). Boston, MA: Butterworth-Heinemann.

Part 2

Content Subject Development

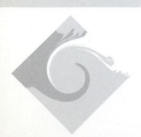

Chapter 7

Reading Development in the First Language

Vicky Zygouris-Coe

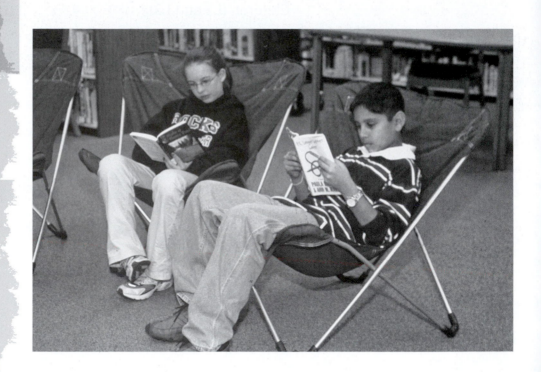

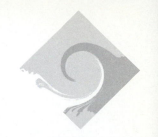

CHAPTER OUTLINE

Introduction

Reading and Policy Initiatives in the 21st Century

Theoretical Perspectives
   The Reading Process

Theories of Reading Development
   Reading from a Language Perspective
   Psycholinguistics and Reading
   Sociolinguistics and Reading
   Transactional Perspective of Reading

Reading Development
   Emergent Literacy
   Acquiring Concepts About Print
   Alphabetics
   Phonological Awareness
   Phonemic Awareness
   Phonics
   Fluency
   Vocabulary
   Comprehension
   Language-Rich, Print-Rich Environments and Reading

Case Study Perspectives
   Case Study One Background: Rebecca
   Case Study One Comments: Rebecca
   Case Study Two Background: Thomas
   Case Study Two Comments: Thomas
   Case Study Three Background: Tyler
   Case Study Three Comments: Tyler

Instructional Suggestions and Strategies
   Suggestions for Collaboration Among Educators
   Suggestions for Collaboration with Families

Concluding Remarks

INTRODUCTION

The ability to read is a complex phenomenon. It is the major avenue to learning, and it must be mastered in school. Students must acquire the knowledge, skills, and strategies that will allow them to read, write, and think critically. As a consequence, difficulty in learning to read influences a child's motivation and ability to learn.

   Reading refers to the process of constructing meaning from text, whereupon readers decipher symbols to create meaning. Reading is complex because it requires applying knowledge of print and other symbols, knowledge of possible meanings of these symbols, and knowledge of the world to the reading task. All school professionals need to understand the current nature of reading problems in schools. Students face greater demands in schools today with high-stakes testing and performance requirements exacted by federal- and state-mandated tests. Reading is so critical to our society that it has risen to the level of a major health problem (National Institute of Child Health and Human Development [NICHHD], 2001). Early identification of young children with reading difficulties and timely intervention are extremely critical in helping children learn to read.

Children vary in their experiences of oral language, in their preparation for learning to read words accurately and fluently, in their experiences with written language, and in their motivation to read. Most children who struggle in learning to read words fluently exhibit weaknesses in their phonological/phonemic areas of language competence. These weaknesses can be inherent or can be attributed to a lack of opportunities to learn at an early age. Such weaknesses are usually expressed by delays in phonological/phonemic awareness and phonics skills development.

Unfortunately, not all children experience the benefits of effective reading instruction in school. About 40% of all children read below basic levels on national reading assessments. The cost of reading failure to our society and to individuals is rather high. The National Institute of Child Health and Human Development (NICHHD, 2001) considers reading failure a national public health problem. Researchers have found a high correlation between poor early reading and subsequent school failure (Juel, 1988; Torgesen, Wagner, Rashotte, Alexander, & Conroy, 1997). Reading failure is linked to adolescent substance abuse as well as to criminal behavior (National Institute of Child Health and Human Development, 2000). For example, there is a relationship between poor reading performance in the early years and later incarceration.

Parents need to support their children's literacy development. In addition, school professionals need to teach reading effectively. Speech-language pathologist and teacher knowledge about the reading process, how children learn to read, and effective reading instruction provides the foundation for reading success. Young children learn to read from experts who know and use effective reading instructional practices.

In 2005, the National Center for Educational Statistics released its report "NAEP 2004: Trends in Academic Progress: Three Decades of Student Performance in Reading and Mathematics." This report documents trends in student reading performance from 1971 through 2004. Overall, the national trend in reading shows the average reading score at age 9 was higher in 2004 than in any previous assessment year. The data indicates that there is no statistically significant difference in 13- and 17-year-olds' average reading scores from 1999 to 2004.

For children to read well by the end of third grade, their progress needs to be closely monitored by school professionals and parents during the preceding years (Hiebert, Pearson, Taylor, Richardson, & Paris, 1998). The National Research Council (NRC) report "Starting Out Right: A Guide to Promoting Children's Reading Success (1998b)" suggested that the more children know about literacy before they enter school, the better they are equipped to succeed in reading. The main accomplishments include (1) oral language skills, (2) print awareness, (3) phonological and phonemic awareness, (4) letter knowledge, (5) appreciation for literate forms, and (6) motivation to learn.

According to Snow, Burns, and Griffin (1998a) and the National Reading Panel (2000a), school professionals must employ scientifically based reading strategies to enable reading success. The term **scientifically based reading research** refers to research that applies rigorous, systematic, and objective procedures to obtain valid knowledge relevant to reading development, reading instruction, and reading difficulties and empirical (valid and reliable) methods of data collections and analysis. Scientifically based reading research (SBRR) has identified five essential components of effective reading instruction:

1. **Phonemic awareness:** The ability to hear, identify, and manipulate individual sounds—or phonemes—in spoken words.

2. **Phonics:** The relationship between the letters of written language and the sounds of spoken language.

3. **Fluency:** The capacity to read text accurately and quickly, silently and aloud.

4. **Vocabulary:** The words students must know to understand oral and written communication effectively.

5. **Comprehension:** The ability to understand and gain meaning from what has been read (Armbruster, Lehr, & Osborn, 2001).

READING AND POLICY INITIATIVES IN THE 21ST CENTURY

In April 1997, the National Institute of Child Health and Human Development (NICHHD), in consultation with the Secretary of Education, was charged with convening a National Reading Panel (NRP) that would assess the status of research-based knowledge, including the effectiveness of various approaches to teaching children to read. The NRP built on the previous work of the National Reading Council (NRC), which was published in *Preventing Reading Difficulties in Young Children* (Snow, Burns, & Griffin, 1998b). The National Reading Panel released its findings in 2000 and made recommendations about teaching methods that have been shown to increase student reading, learning, and achievement. In January 2002, President George W. Bush signed the **No Child Left Behind (NCLB)** Act. This act was a major reform of the Elementary and Secondary Education Act (ESEA) (originally passed in 1965). According to the NCLB legislation, all children must meet basic standards set by states' core curricula in reading and mathematics. In particular, the legislation requires states to guarantee that all children read proficiently by third grade, and that all states must meet this goal within 12 years.

The NICHHD studies (in Snow, Burns, & Griffin, 1998b) reported that for 85 to 90 percent of poor readers, prevention and early intervention strategies can increase reading skills to average reading levels. These strategies combine instruction in phoneme awareness, phonics, vocabulary and spelling, reading fluency, and reading comprehension. This research also indicates that if early intervention is delayed until 9 years of age (i.e., the time that most children with reading difficulties first receive assistance), approximately 75 percent of these students will continue to have difficulties learning to read throughout high school and their adult years. Because of the convergence of research and best practice, it is now clearer what it will take to enable children to become skilled readers. Undoubtedly, speech-language pathologists and teachers play a crucial role in developing and supporting children's reading development in the classroom. Scientifically based reading research has created many discussions about reading, reading instruction, and school professionals using scientific, evidence-based, and empirically proven practices.

In addition, all states are required to report student data by school and to disaggregate the data for students by poverty level, special education status, first language, and race/ethnicity. Several recent reports have identified dramatic demographic changes in the United States, with special emphasis on shifts in the cultural and linguistic composition of school students (U.S. Census Bureau, 2003). One out of every five American students entering school knows a language other than English. It is estimated that by 2030, language minority students will account for about 40% of the school-age population. This data calls for well-prepared speech-language pathologists and teachers, school professionals who will be able to meet students' diverse needs and help them become successful readers and writers. Programs such as **Reading First** clearly define the parameters and expected reading outcomes in grades K–3 for all children.

According to the Reading First model, to prevent reading failure in grades K–3, speech-language pathologists and teachers will need (1) an increase in the quality, consistency, and reach of scientifically based reading instruction in every K–3 classroom; (2) timely and valid assessments of reading progress to identify struggling readers; and (3) immediate, intensive, skillful, and appropriate interventions to prevent students from falling behind.

THEORETICAL PERSPECTIVES

The Reading Process

Reading is a language process. Language enables communication. Language is used to describe, inquire, share, encourage, and persuade others. Children's oral language reflects the experiences they have had with people, objects, print, and the world. Oral language is the cornerstone on which reading is built. Because reading is a language process, speech-language pathologists and teachers need to utilize children's language experiences and connect oral to written language. Anderson, Hiebert, Scott, and Wilkinson (1985) discuss the relationship between oral language and the reading process as such:

> Reading instruction builds especially on oral language. If this foundation is weak, progress in reading will be slow and uncertain. Children must have at least a basic vocabulary, a reasonable range of knowledge about the world around them and the ability to talk about their knowledge. These abilities form the basis for comprehending text (p. 30).

Children typically come to school with knowledge about their oral language. They use oral language to communicate with parents, siblings, peers, and teachers. Children's oral language should be viewed as the foundation for reading and writing before children enter school. It also reflects what children understand when they read.

Reading is a cognitive process. **Cognition** refers to the active process of organizing and understanding experiences. Each person has a system (i.e., a schema) for organizing knowledge about people, events, objects, and experiences. The more experiences children have with the environment, the more that the **schemata** or organizational systems develop. Active involvement with the environment helps form and evolve concepts. Because reading is a cognitive process, speech-language pathologists and teachers should provide many opportunities for students to interact with text, with others in class, and with learning in general.

Reading is an affective process. Positive experiences with print and reading help develop a positive self-concept. The successes or difficulties children experience with reading affect their motivation. Children's self-concept, interests, motivations, and attitudes toward reading are closely connected with their home, school, and community backgrounds. Creating positive experiences and helping children develop positive attitudes toward reading is an important part of any reading program. Because reading is an affective process, speech-language pathologists and teachers should create supportive and motivating learning environments and provide diverse materials to meet all students' interests and needs.

Reading is a social process. Social culture plays an important role in a child's experiences and attitudes toward reading. If reading is valued at home or at school, it's likely that the child will also value reading. How often adults discuss various issues with children or read and talk about books with children reinforces the reader's background knowledge and comprehension. Societal changes, school and curricula changes, increasing student and family diversity, and the challenges of a technological society emphasize improving children's reading skills. Because reading is a social process, speech-language pathologists and teachers should provide many opportunities for students to interact, cooperate, and collaborate with others in class.

Reading is a physiological process. Auditory and visual acuity, auditory and visual perception, and consequently neurological functioning also affect the reading process. Parents' socioeconomic status, poverty, and negative home environments play a crucial role in children's overall health, growth, and ability to read.

Reading is a developmental process. Literacy development begins at birth. Children's ability to communicate, use language, and later read and write is related to their developmental growth. Children who become successful readers possess appropriate sensory, perceptual, cognitive, and social skills as they progress through the school years. Children's concepts about literacy develop from the earlier years by observing and interacting with their significant others. Children move through various stages of reading development at different rates. Some children may require more time to learn how to decode than others. Chall (1996) viewed reading development as a series of five stages ranging from preschool through college levels (see Table 7–1). Although the stages are not entirely separate from each other, they do provide an overall framework for reading development.

THEORIES OF READING DEVELOPMENT

Reading from a Language Perspective

The bond between language development and reading is very strong. Without language, there would be no reading. Reading is very much a language process; therefore, the ability to read is affected by language skills (Catts, 1989, 1993; Catts & Kahmi, 1999; Snow, Tabors, Nicholson, & Kurland, 1995). Reading is the process of constructing meaning from text.

TABLE 7–1
Stages of Reading Development

Stage	Description
Stage 0	**Prereading:** This stage ranges from age 0 to 6, before reading instruction takes place. Children begin to associate sounds and words; identify rhymes and alliteration; and develop phonological awareness and print, alphabet, and language knowledge. Reading to children and playing games with sounds in words helps to develop their phonological awareness. Parents can help develop a child's phonological awareness through rhyming, playing with sounds, music, and reading aloud to children.
Stage 1	**Initial reading or decoding:** This stage takes place during the beginning of grade 1. In this stage, the student learns about sound/symbol correspondences. Readers also learn about what it means to read something, what letters are for, and the subtle differences between similar-sounding words. Teach frequent, highly regular sound/spelling relationships systematically; break words into their sounds; show children how to sound out words; use interesting stories to develop language comprehension; and read aloud to children.
Stage 2	**Confirmation and fluency:** This stage ranges from the end of grade 1 to the end of grade 3. Students learn to decode words fluently and accurately. They develop their fluency through rereading familiar text and through exposure to familiar words. Provide students with continued explicit instruction in advanced structural analysis skills; teach them to identify syllable patterns in words to enhance their recognition skills; practice reading familiar text and quality literature; and help them improve their vocabularies through a study of word parts: prefixes, suffixes, and roots.
Stage 3	**Learning the new (single) viewpoint:** This stage ranges from grades 4–8. Children learn to use their reading skills to construct meaning from text. Readers gain more independence and read from content area textbooks and other texts. This stage is characterized by learning and exploration.
Stage 3a	In this first part (grades 4–6), students read new information for assigned purposes, and they learn to enjoy acquiring conventional knowledge through reading.
Stage 3b	In the second part of the stage (middle school grades), students read to acquire and synthesize information from varied sources and begin to develop their personal preferences and interests.
Stage 4	**Multiple viewpoints:** This stage ranges from high school to early college. In this stage, readers critically analyze texts, synthesize information from different texts, acknowledge multiple viewpoints, and continue to expand their interests.
Stage 5	**A world view:** This is the most mature level of reading, and it usually ranges from late college to graduate school. In this stage, adults weigh information from multiple perspectives and selectively add new information to their world view. Adults are motivated by their own purposes and tastes, and they increase their efficiency of reading for career purposes as well as for cultivating their reading interests.

Psycholinguistics and Reading

A psycholinguistic view of reading combines psychological understanding of the reading process with an understanding of how language works. According to this

FIGURE 7–1
The Three Cueing Systems

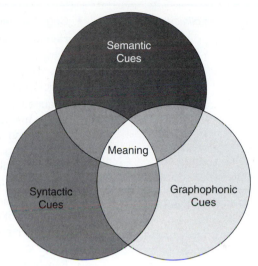

view of reading, readers actively interact with written language in an effort to make sense of text. Reading is viewed as an active and interactive process. Readers search for and coordinate cues from three distinct systems in written language (Figure 7–1): the phonological (or graphophonemic), the semantic, and the syntactic (Melvin, 1979; Rosenblatt, 1994).

The phonological system refers to the sounds of the language. **Phonological awareness** refers to the ability to identify, think about, and manipulate phonological processes. **Phonemic awareness** is the ability to manipulate sounds. Children learn to talk without being consciously aware of individual phonemes. Terms associated with phonology include the following:

1. **Phoneme** is the smallest unit of sound within a language (e.g., when the word *bat* is pronounced, three phonemes are utilized: /b/, /a/, /t/).

2. **Grapheme** is a written symbol (letter or letter combination) used to represent a phoneme.

3. The English **graphophonic system** is composed of 26 graphemes and approximately 44 phonemes.

4. **Grapheme-phoneme relationship** refers to the letter-sound correspondence.

5. **Phonics** refers to different approaches designed to teach the letter-sound relationships.

Research has shown that children need to learn about the relationships between word spellings and pronunciations in order to become successful readers (Adams, 1990; Chall, 1996; Stahl, 1999). Understanding the importance of language in literacy development and instruction is necessary for a quality instructional program (see Table 7–2).

TABLE 7–2
Predictors of Reading Success and Failure

Physical and clinical factors	• Cognitive deficiencies • Hearing problems • Early language impairment • Attention deficit/hyperactivity disorders • Vision problems
Predictors of school entry	• Acquired proficiency in language • Verbal memory • Lexical and syntactic skills • Overall language • Phonological and phonemic awareness • Oral vocabulary
Acquired knowledge of literacy	• Reading readiness • Concepts of print • Phonemic awareness • Letter identification
Family-based risk factors	• Family history of reading difficulties • Home literacy environment • Opportunities for verbal interaction • Home language other than English • Use of a nonstandard dialect of English in the home • Socioeconomic status
Neighborhood, community, and school-based factors	• Environmental risks • Low-performing schools • Low expectations • Lack of resources • Conflicting community values • Negative peer pressure

Sociolinguistics and Reading

Halliday (1975) viewed language as a tool that children use to understand their interactions with others in their environment. They also learn that language is purposeful and intentional. According to Halliday (1975), if children have difficulty learning to read, it is due to beginning instruction not making connections to oral language.

According to Halliday (1978), language is a complex system for creating meaning through socially shared conventions. Before beginning school, children learn the language of their home and community. In this setting, children make gains in language development from experience with having books read aloud and from book discussions. According to Cambourne and Turbill (1987), the optimal conditions for literacy learning in the classroom are as follows:

1. *Immersion*—Students are surrounded by literacy experiences and examples of written text in their environment.

2. *Demonstration*—Students participate as people use language to work and play; students are involved with prediction, questioning in reading, and other language arts activities.

3. *Authenticity*—Students are involved with real-life activities that have purpose and meaning.

4. *Responsibility*—Students take responsibility for their own learning by working cooperatively and independently to be productive.

5. *Expectations*—Parents, teachers, and students have a positive attitude that they will learn and be successful.

6. *Approximation*—Students are expected to try to accomplish tasks that are challenging while receiving encouragement. Student attempts at the application of new learnings are recognized and accepted, then bridged through instruction to conventional applications.

7. *Feedback*—Students are given much feedback on the progress they are making as literacy learners by teachers, parents, and peers.

Because reading is uniquely human, learning to read requires sharing, interacting, and collaborating with significant others in the child's environment. Because a large part of learning to read depends on the social and cultural context of the classroom, opportunities must abound for discussions and conversations between teacher and child and also among children.

Transactional Perspective of Reading

Transactional theory suggests a "reciprocal, mutually defining relationship" (Rosenblatt, 1986) between the reader and the literary text. Transactional theory proposes a great deal of emphasis on the role of the reader as he or she interacts with and constructs meaning from text.

Such a conception affirms the significance of the unique reader and suggests that reading cannot be independent of the reader's individuality, background knowledge, and experiences. Transactional theory stipulates that the reader's characteristics and knowledge must be respected and considered and that readers initially understand any text only on the basis of prior experience. They cannot make sense of a text except through personal experiences or experiences with other texts. Transactional theory invites the reader to reflect on what she or he brings to any reading, and to acknowledge and examine the responses possibly evoked.

READING DEVELOPMENT

Emergent Literacy

Children begin developing literacy long before they enter school. By the time they enter school, children have acquired a fairly extensive oral language vocabulary and a fairly complex syntactic system (except for those children with disabilities). By the age of 2 or 3, children can identify signs (e.g., Taco Bell, Wendy's), labels (e.g., favorite toys, cereals, foods), and logos (e.g., Disney). Because children bring with them much emergent literacy knowledge, speech-language pathologists and teachers must build on what they already know. As children observe and interact with parents' and peers' reading and writing, they experiment and develop their own theories about reading and writing. **Emergent literacy** refers to knowledge about print and unconventional literacy behaviors. This begins before school and leads into conventional reading and writing (Zygouris-Coe, 2002).

Emergent literacy is a fairly new term used to conceptualize early reading and writing development. Teale and Sulzby (1986) in their influential volume *Emergent Literacy: Writing and Reading* introduced this term, which assumes that the child acquires some knowledge about language, reading, and writing before formally entering school. Currently, this term has been expanded to include listening, viewing, thinking, speaking, reading, and writing (Cooper, 1997).

Literacy activities occur and are embedded within content areas such as art, play, social studies, and science (Morrow, 1997). Studies as early as 1966 have shaped the current outlook on emergent literacy (Clay, 1967; Durkin, 1966; Holdaway, 1979; Taylor, 1983; Teale, 1982; Teale & Sulzby, 1989). Teale and Sulzby (1989) view emergent literacy as the reading and writing behaviors that precede and develop into conventional literacy. These behaviors are developed through meaningful experiences and daily interactions with peers and adults (Heath, 1983; Sulzby, 1985). Children's concepts about literacy are molded from the earliest experiences and interactions children have with readers and writers as well as through their own attempts to read, write, and construct meaning (Sulzby & Teale, 1991).

Early experiences with written language provide children with a solid foundation for school literacy learning (Sulzby & Teale, 1991; Teale & Sulzby, 1986, 1996). Before they enter kindergarten, many children have devoted countless hours to storybook reading and programs such as *Sesame Street* (Adams, 1990). From these experiences, especially those with storybooks, children gain an interest in books, the capacity to understand and talk about stories, and the ability to connect the information in stories to their background knowledge (Purcell-Gates, McIntyre, & Freppon, 1995). Children also learn that print is read in stories. In addition, children who have had many experiences with storybook reading are able to identify many of the alphabet letters and have acquired some beginnings of phonemic awareness.

Acquiring Concepts About Print

Understanding how print works and the roles it plays in people's lives is otherwise known as the big picture of literacy (Purcell-Gates, 1997). This big picture is the blueprint for the development of reading and writing. Children will need to develop **concepts of print** to indicate that they can:

1. Write and read what is said.
2. Read words, not pictures.
3. Know that what is said is divided into words.

4. Understand that words are made up of letters.

5. Understand that sentences are made up of words.

6. Understand that space separates written words.

7. Understand that sentences begin with capital letters and end with a period, an exclamation mark, or a question mark.

8. Read from left to right and from top to bottom.

9. Read a book from front to back.

Children must also develop phonological awareness and arrive at an understanding of the **alphabetic principle.** The alphabetic principle refers to the ability to associate sounds with letters and use these sounds to form words. The alphabetic principle is composed of two parts: (1) alphabetic understanding (i.e., words are made up of letters that represent sounds), and (2) phonological recoding or beginning decoding (i.e., sounds and letters correspond to the pronunciation and spelling of words). Because English is alphabetic, decoding is a fundamental means of recognizing words.

According to Juel (1991), a major difference between good and poor readers is the ability to use letter-sound correspondence to identify words. Also, students who acquire and apply the alphabetic principle early in their reading experience long-term reading benefits (Stanovich, 1986). The combination of instruction in phonological awareness and letter-sound correspondence appears to be productive for successful early reading (Haskell, Foorman, & Swank, 1992).

Alphabetics

Research on early reading suggests that children move through phases in word identification (Ehri, 1994; Snow, Burns, & Griffin, 1998a). During the earliest phase, the **logographic phase,** they "read" a word based on visual cues (e.g., MacDonald's golden arches logo). Although they may have little knowledge of how to process print out of context (Ehri, 1994, p. 328), they may possess a great deal of information regarding print.

According to Ehri (1994), children may know that print:

1. Has to do with the real world.

2. Is different than drawing.

3. Can stand for spoken language.

4. Occurs in different places.

5. Is made up of letters.

Gradually, young readers begin to link letters with sounds in the reading and **spelling-alphabetic phase.** Invented spelling can support their developing phonemic awareness and understanding about sound-letter correspondences. Over time, with exposure, practice, and knowledge, they enter the **orthographic phase,** and they are able to use spelling patterns or letter sequences that support word identification. With practice, and meaningful experiences, fluency and automaticity are developed through wide reading.

Phonological Awareness

Phonological and phonemic awareness are important elements of emergent literacy. Phonological awareness refers to an awareness of syllables and sounds apart from whole words. Torgesen and Mathes (1998) stated that "phonological awareness is most commonly defined as one's sensitivity to, or explicit awareness of, the phonological structure of words in one's language. In short, it involves the ability to notice, think about, or manipulate the individual sounds in words" (p. 2). **Phonemic awareness** is an understanding that words can be divided into a sequence of phonemes (Chard & Dickson, 1999).

Becoming phonologically and phonemically aware prepares children for later reading instruction (Adams, Foorman, Lundberg, & Beeler, 1997, 1998; Chard, Simmons, & Kameenui, 1998). Rhyming and rhyming games help young children to develop an awareness of the phonological structure of words. Acquiring phonological awareness involves two tasks: learning that words can be divided into segments of sound smaller than a syllable, and learning about individual phonemes themselves (Torgesen, 1998). As children acquire more knowledge about the distinctive features of phonemes, they become more skilled at identifying the different sounds in words.

Phonological awareness assists children's reading and construction of meaning. Research indicates that children who understand the relationships between phonemes and letters and who use this knowledge for word identification become better readers than children who have difficulty acquiring these skills (Beck & Juel, 1995; Share & Stanovich, 1995).

Phonological awareness is important in learning beginning word-reading skills because it helps children:

1. Understand the alphabetic principle.

2. Notice the regular ways sounds and letters are represented in words.

3. Generate possibilities for words in context that are only partially sounded out.

Smith, Simmons, and Kameenui (1998) concluded that, although phonological awareness training is beneficial for most students, the degree and nature of instruction may vary according to the child's unique reading needs. They stated that phonological awareness can be developed before reading, and it assists in the development of reading skills. Instruction in phonological awareness should be fun, interactive, and developmentally appropriate. Early instruction in rhyming and onset-rime relationships, and integrated instruction in segmenting and blending can be beneficial to reading development (Gough, 1995; Snider, 1995).

Phonological awareness involves the auditory and oral manipulation of sounds. As children grow older, however, their basic phonological awareness does not necessarily develop into the more sophisticated phonemic awareness. Most early phonological awareness activities are taught in the absence of print, but there is increasing evidence that early writing activities, including spelling words as they sound (i.e., invented or temporary spelling), appear to promote more sophisticated phonemic awareness (Ehri, 1998; Treiman, 1993).

It is possible that during spelling and writing activities, children begin to combine their phonological sensitivity and print knowledge and apply them to building words. Even if children are unable to hold and use a pen or pencil, they can use letter tiles or word-processing programs to practice their spelling. Torgesen, Wagner, and Rashotte (1994) concluded that training for at-risk children must be more explicit or more intense than what is typically prescribed for children with severe reading disabilities. Therefore, instruction must target phonological awareness. The second tier of instruction includes more work in segmenting and blending phonemes (e.g., Snider, 1995).

In the design of phonological awareness instruction, the following general principles increase students' success (Chard & Osborn, 1999):

1. Start with continuous sounds, such as /s/, /m/, and /f/, that are easier to pronounce than stop sounds, such as /p/, /t/, and /k/.

2. Model each activity as it is first introduced.

3. Move from larger units (words, onset-rime) to smaller units (individual phonemes).

4. Move from easier tasks (e.g., rhyming) to more complex tasks (e.g., blending and segmenting).

5. Use additional strategies to help struggling early readers manipulate sounds. These strategies may include using concrete objects (e.g., blocks, bingo chips) to represent sounds.

Research suggests that by the end of kindergarten, children should be able to demonstrate phonemic blending and segmentation and to use sounds to spell simple words. Speech-language pathologists and teachers need to be aware that through appropriate assessments, students can be identified as having or lacking these abilities. Achieving these abilities requires that speech-language pathologists and teachers be knowledgeable about effective instructional approaches to teaching phonological and phonemic awareness at all ages and aware of the ongoing progress for each of their students through effective assessment.

Phonemic Awareness

Phonemic awareness is a powerful predictor of reading success (Adams, 1990; Juel, 1994, 1998; Snow, Burns, & Griffin, 1998). Phonemic awareness refers to a child's understanding and awareness that speech is composed of a series of individual sounds or phonemes (Yopp, 1992). Stanovich (1994) concluded that phonemic awareness tasks "are the best predictors of the ease of early reading acquisition— better than anything else that we know of, including IQ" (p. 284). Phonemic awareness helps children understand how spoken language relates to written language. Torgesen, Wagner, and Rashotte (1994) concluded that at-risk children can truly benefit from intense, explicit instruction. They also suggested that phonemic awareness instruction needs to be fun, interactive, and developmentally appropriate.

Yopp (1992) suggested various strategies that help develop children's phonemic awareness. The following is a summary of her recommendations:

1. Incorporate activities that are fun and playful, and natural ways of teaching that avoid rote memorization and drill.

2. Use activities that help reinforce and extend children's awareness of sounds in words (e.g., sound matching, sound isolation, sound segmentation, sound addition, sound deletion, and sound substitution).

3. Practice activities that encourage interaction among children.

4. Incorporate activities that allow children to experiment with language.

5. Practice activities that help meet students' individual differences.

6. Use sharing books that capitalize on word play.

7. Make words.

8. Read and recite nursery rhymes.

9. Share riddles and rhymes that focus on songs.

10. Sing songs that include word play.

11. Play games that encourage word play.

Research has shown that a young child's sound-letter knowledge is the single best predictor of first-year reading achievement (Adams, 1990, 1996). Adams (1996), Honig (1996), and Riley (1996) agree that the most powerful predictor of later reading success is the child's knowledge of the alphabet. A child who can easily and accurately recognize letters will be better prepared to meet the school literacy requirements. Phonological and phonemic awareness greatly contribute to this skill.

Phonemic awareness is critically important as children move into the later stages of literacy development. Current research indicates that phonemic awareness is the best predictor of a child's ability in learning to read.

It is important to remember that phonemic awareness is not phonics; however, research (e.g., the *National Reading Panel* [2000]) suggests the following:

1. Phonemic awareness is absolutely important in reading acquisition.

2. Phonemic awareness is best taught in kindergarten and first grade.

3. Average students need only 20 hours of phonemic awareness instruction in a year.

4. Children need to be taught to listen to the sounds of language because what we say is not what children see in print.

5. Teaching children to manipulate phonemes in words is highly effective under many different kinds of teaching conditions and with a variety of learners across age and grade levels.

Yopp (1992) suggested that students who have developed phonemic awareness can manipulate the spoken language in isolating a sound in a word, blending individual sounds to form a word, substituting sounds in a word, and segmenting a word into its constituent sounds. The types of activities a student must experience in order to be phonemically aware (Armbruster, Lehr, & Osborn, 2001) include identifying phonemes, categorizing phonemes, blending phonemes to form words, segmenting words into phonemes, deleting or adding phonemes to form new words, and substituting phonemes to make new words.

Critical skills in phonemic awareness involve the following:

1. **Sound isolation** (i.e., identifying sounds). Example: The first sound in *mat* is *mmmm.*

2. **Blending** (i.e., putting sounds together). Example: *mmm + aaa + ttt* is *mat*.

3. **Segmenting** (i.e., breaking words down into sounds). Example: The sounds in *mat* are /m/ + /a/ + /t/.

Blending and segmentation of words at the phoneme level are the two most critical skills that must be taught. Speech-language pathologists and teachers can achieve better results when they teach phonemic awareness explicitly (through modeling) to small groups of children rather than to the entire class. Because phonemic awareness is an auditory skill, the manipulation of sounds combined with letters (e.g., letter tiles, magnetic letters, letter squares) helps children's phonemic awareness skills. As children develop their phonemic awareness, they ready themselves for literacy development in connecting sounds to written symbols (graphemes).

Phonics

Phonics is the association of sounds and letters to written symbols (Snider, 1995); it is a system of teaching reading that builds on the alphabetic principle, in which a central component is the teaching of correspondences between sound pronunciations and letters or groups of letters (Adams, 1990). The goal of phonics instruction is to help readers identify unknown words on their own. Phonics is best learned in the context of reading and writing.

Children who are adept at using phonics are able to decipher words that are not readily recognizable. Best practices establish the need to embed the teaching of phonics into the reading program through child-appropriate activities, shared reading, and read-aloud activities. Because poor readers do not analyze each letter in a word (Stanovich, 1992; Velluntino & Scanlon, 1987), phonics instruction should help children focus their attention on all the letters by emphasizing the full analysis of words. Research indicates there are many methods of teaching phonics, but for the most part, instruction can be classified as either analytic or synthetic (Heilman, Blair, & Rupley, 2002).

Analytic phonics involves teaching words by the whole-word method. This involves teaching a skill lesson by using either an inductive or deductive approach.

1. When using the inductive approach, the speech-language pathologist or teacher gives generalizations and encourages the students to come up with a conclusion. For example, a number of words beginning with a certain letter are presented (*bell*, *bat*, and *bag*). The children are expected to find out what is the same in all the words and then give other examples.

2. When using the deductive method, words in the children's oral vocabulary are listed on the board (*cup*, *candy*, and *cap*). The children are told that all the words begin with *c* and are then asked to provide other examples.

One feature of **synthetic phonics** is the direct instruction of basic phonic elements. Instruction begins by teaching the sounds of letters, and then syllables, progressing to monosyllabic words, then phrases, and eventually sentences. After the letter sounds are learned, children form words by blending all the letters together.

Word families or **phonograms** are another approach used for identifying words. Other components include rhyming parts, or onset and rimes. The onset is the consonant that precedes the vowel, while the rime is the part of the word that follows containing the vowel (b *ake*, c *ane*, b *at*). When this approach is used, direct instruction is typically not given because the children can figure out the word by using the phonograms or rimes.

Analogy phonics is teaching students unfamiliar words by comparing them to similar known words. For example, -*ame* is in *game*, and when the phoneme /f/ is substituted, it becomes *fame*. The **embedded phonics** approach involves teaching students phonics by embedding the words in text, which is a more implicit approach to teaching reading. In this approach, a student uses sound-letter correspondences and context clues to identify a new word. **Phonics through spelling** is teaching students to segment words into chunks to assist in spelling new similar words. For example, if the student knows how to spell *day*, then with help, she or he can spell *today*.

Word identification and decoding are broader than phonics. Phonics is only one of several important approaches to identifying words. Other decoding clues include (1) word parts (prefixes, suffixes, base words) and familiarity with similar words (analogy), (2) meaning (semantic) clues, and (3) the grammar and syntax of a sentence (Adams, 1990). For young learners, acquisition of the word identification skills describes their ability to understand the alphabetic principle of the language they are learning.

The goal of every reading program is for students to develop **automaticity** in word identification. Automaticity refers to the ability to quickly identify and recognize the word. This essential behavior has been found to be a strong predictor of successful reading (Snow, Burns, & Griffin, 1998). The learner's needs for word identification changes as children come in contact with more multisyllabic words. Developmentally speaking, as children's linguistic abilities increase, they become more sophisticated in their word identification strategies. At grade 3 and beyond, children's use of prefixes, suffixes, and affixes provide additional clues for the identification of new words.

To become capable readers, children must be able to use a number of identification strategies, some of which include building sight vocabulary and using the whole-word approach, the phonics approach, structural analysis, and contextual analysis. **Sight words** are words children recognize instantly. Many of these are structure words and words with irregular patterns that must be learned visually so that they are recognized automatically. These words have to be learned by the whole-word approach.

The **whole-word approach,** traditionally called the look and say method, concentrates on learning words as wholes, not through analysis. This is usually accomplished through the use of shared reading with predictable books, guided reading, big books, the language experience approach (LEA), and direct instruction, especially by building background knowledge prior to reading content area material. Because of the repetitive patterns in predictable books, words are visually recognized and easily memorized. Selection of stories related to the child's familiar experiences facilitates memorization and subsequent learning of the words.

Structural analysis is utilized by older students and readers who are able to identify letter clusters such as prefixes, suffixes, and affixes. Readers who use the cluster technique must be able to recognize the root word. The ability to recognize and associate sounds with these clusters provides more effective word identification. It also enhances the ability to recognize words.

A third strategy for the teaching of whole words is the use of **contextual analysis.** While this is a helpful strategy, it does not always allow for accurately predicting the correct word. Contextual clues are helpful only when a child recognizes most of the words in the sentence. Three different types of context clues are frequently used: semantic or word meaning, syntactic or word order, and picture clues.

1. *Semantic (or meaning) clues.* For example, when reading a story about cats, good readers develop the expectation that the story will contain words associated with cats, such as *tail, purr,* and *whiskers.* Sentence context clues are more specific. In the sentence "My cat likes to_____," words such as *play, jump,* and *scratch* make sense.

2. *Syntactic (or word order) clues.* In the previous example, the order of the words in the sentence indicates that the missing word must be a verb. Other parts of speech, such as adjectives *(nice, brown)* or nouns *(man, fence),* do not make sense.

3. *Picture clues.* Illustrations can often help with the identification of a word. In the example, if a picture of a cat leaping through the air accompanies the text, the word *jump* seems like a very good possibility.

Context clues are often helpful, but they are not specific enough to predict the exact word. Often several choices are possible. However, when context clues are combined with other clues, such as phonics, accurate word identification is usually possible. Ehri (1995) suggests that words become sight words after a thorough analysis of their orthographic structure. Ehri (1995) proposed that this process takes place in four phases: pre-alphabetic, partial alphabetic, full alphabetic, and consolidated alphabetic.

The **pre-alphabetic phase** corresponds to Chall's (1996) early reading stage. During this phase, beginning readers remember sight words by making connections between certain visual attributes of a word and either its pronunciation or its meaning (e.g., the tail at the end of the word *dog,* or the two eyes in the middle of the word *look*). Letter-sound relationships are not involved in the recognition process. This can be an effective strategy as long as the number of words encountered remains low; however, it becomes increasingly ineffective as a child's repertoire of sight words increases.

At the **partial alphabetic recognition phase,** students begin to read sight words by making the connections between some of the letters in written words (usually the initial and/or final letters because of their salience) and their corresponding sounds. The advantage here is that the alphabetic system is available to aid in word recognition. Children are helped in this phase by both knowledge of letter names and a certain amount of phonological awareness (Stahl & Murray, 1998).

As learners continue to develop an understanding of the alphabetic system, they move toward the **full alphabetic coding phase.** This parallels the initial stage of conventional literacy outlined in Chall's model. At this point, readers recognize how most graphemes represent phonemes in conventional spelling. This allows readers to easily recognize different words with similar spellings (e.g., *bat, bait,* and *brat*) because each word's representation is sufficiently complete. It also enables them to read new words by determining how the unfamiliar spellings are pronounced.

However, while learners at the full alphabetic phase can decode words, words that are encountered sufficiently often become sight words and recognition is immediate. This immediate recognition also occurs for words that are phonetically irregular and therefore not decodable using sound-symbol correspondence rules.

During the final phase, the **consolidated alphabetic phase,** learners come to recognize letter patterns that occur across different words as units; this becomes part of their generalized knowledge of the orthographic system. This final stage reduces the memory load for the reader, making it easier to learn new words and speeding up the process of word recognition, by increasing children's awareness of the ways letters co-occur in the spelling system. This final phase ensures that the learner establishes automaticity and accurate word recognition, which are fundamental to the reading process.

Fluency

To gain meaning from text, students must be able to read fluently. Fluent readers are automatic with phonological awareness and decoding; they focus their attention on constructing meaning from text (Kuhn & Stahl, 2000). However, many students with reading problems have difficulty reading fluently (Rasinski & Padak, 1998). They often do not have an adequate sight vocabulary, and they must work hard to decode many words in the text. Usually, their oral reading is filled with long pauses, ongoing repetitions, and monotonous expressions. Because they labor so hard on decoding, usually little comprehension occurs. Children who experience reading difficulties are often caught in a vicious circle (Stanovich, 1986): their lack of interest in reading leads to less reading; as a result, they read less, they do not have a developed vocabulary, and reading becomes more difficult.

Fluency is the effortless, automatic ability to read words with appropriate prosody and accuracy in connected text with no noticeable cognitive or mental effort. Fundamental skills are so automatic that they do not require conscious attention. LaBerge and Samuels (1974) described the fluent reader as someone whose decoding processes have become automatic, that is, requiring no conscious processing.

Such capacity then enables readers to allocate their attention to comprehending text. Effective fluency-building instruction rests on selecting appropriate instructional tasks (e.g., letter sounds students can produce accurately but not fluently), scheduling sufficient practice (multiple opportunities per day), and systematically increasing correct response rates.

For a child to become a fluent reader, he or she must possess a number of skills (Juel, 1991; National Reading Panel, 2000; Johns & Berglund, 2002), such as automaticity (accuracy), quality (the reader's ability to use proper prosodic features such as pitch, juncture, and stress in one's voice), rate (attaining appropriate speed according to the reader's purpose or type of passage), and comprehension. Readers who can identify words instantly have sufficient attention to focus on the text's meaning (Samuels, 2002). To ensure adequate comprehension, automatic word recognition must be developed. Students must develop automatic word recognition through

TABLE 7–3
Fluency Benchmark Standards for Grades K–3

Grade Level	Benchmark Standards
Kindergarten	"Reads" familiar texts emergently, i.e., not necessarily verbatim from the print alone.
Grade 1	Reads aloud with accuracy any text that is appropriately designed for the first half of grade 1.
Grade 2	Accurately decodes orthographically regular multisyllable words and nonsense words. Accurately reads many irregularly spelled words and spelling patterns such as diphthongs, special vowel spellings, and common word endings.
Grade 3	Reads aloud with fluency any text that is appropriately designed for grade level.

extensive reading of connected text rather than through recognizing words in isolation (Kuhn, 2004).

Snow, Burns, and Griffin (1998) reported desired reading fluency standards for kindergarten through third grade. These standards are listed in Table 7–3.

Fluency instruction must be well organized and delivered consistently. According to the National Reading Panel (2000), students benefit from direct instruction using guided, oral, repeated reading procedures that include support from teacher, peers, and parents. Such instruction has a positive impact on word recognition, fluency, and comprehension. Repeated readings, choral reading, and partner reading can be effective as part of a well-designed reading fluency program.

Children's reading and fluency also develop when they are exposed to varied models of fluent reading. Observing, listening to, and imitating fluent reading models help students learn how to become fluent readers themselves. They need access to quality reading books and materials, and they also need time to read at home and in school.

Additional strategies for improving students' ability to read passages fluently include reading familiar texts to build students' reading confidence and also success, using patterned books to provide support for word recognition, assisted reading (reading with a fluent reader), **echo reading** (student imitates the teacher's performance or echoes the text), and **neurological impress method (NIM)** (teacher begins by reading at a fast and loud pace; as student gains confidence, the teacher starts to read more softly). Last, **reader's theater** is an involving way for students to develop fluency (National Reading Panel, 2000; Partnership for Reading, 2001). Reader's theater involves rehearsing and performing a script with dialogue before an audience. The script may be one from a book or from a literature response activity. This activity allows students to participate in reading along with other, perhaps more skilled readers. This allows all readers to feel part of a group. In addition, it may provide good models of reading and accomplishment.

A speech-language pathologist or teacher can determine whether a student is a fluent reader simply by listening to his or her oral reading. Wilson (1988) identified three problems with fluency.

1. In choppy reading, students repeat words, stumble, and treat the text as a continuous list of words.

2. In monotonous reading, readers have little expression in the rise and fall of their voices. Their reading reflects their perception that reading is a task of pronouncing words.

3. In hasty reading, students race through the text, ignoring punctuation and sentence breaks. In their haste to get through the text, they even make errors on familiar words.

To determine a student's fluency, simply listen to the student read a text at an instructional or independent level. Reading rate in passages is a good indication of fluency. As the student reads orally or silently, the reading should be timed. Calculate words per minute (WPM). Multiply the number of words in the passage by 60 and then divide by the number of seconds it took to read the passage. Table 7–4 provides a list of fluency rates. Another way to assess students' fluency is by timed administration of word lists.

Vocabulary

Vocabulary refers to the ability to understand and use words to acquire and convey meaning. The four types of vocabulary involved in language include listening, speaking, reading, and writing vocabulary. Vocabulary is very important to reading comprehension. "Readers cannot understand what they are reading without knowing what most of the words mean. As children learn to read more advanced texts, they must learn the meaning of new words that are not part of their oral vocabulary" (National Institute for Literacy, 2001, p. 34).

Research demonstrates that children learn most words indirectly, that is, through everyday experiences with oral and written language (National Reading Panel, 2000; Stahl, 1986). By age 6, most children have an oral vocabulary of up to 14,000 words (Clark, 1993). However, children do need to learn words directly through explicit instruction in order to comprehend oral and written text. The National Reading Panel (2000) has given specific teaching recommendations and has emphasized that teachers need to use varied methods to teach vocabulary.

TABLE 7–4
Fluency Rates

Grade Level	Minimum Words Per Minute (wpm)	Fluent Oral Reading (wpm)
Grade 1	60 wpm	80 wpm
Grade 2	70 wpm	100 wpm
Grade 3	80 wpm	126 wpm
Grade 4	90 wpm	162 wpm
Grade 5	100 wpm	180 wpm

There are three ways that children learn vocabulary indirectly. First, they participate in oral language daily. The more conversations with other people children have, the more words they learn. Second, they learn words by being read to. Reading aloud to children helps them learn new words and engages them in conversations about books. Third, children learn new words through their own reading. This is one of the reasons for daily reading time.

Students learn vocabulary when they are taught individual words and word-learning strategies directly. Vocabulary learning is supported by developing word consciousness. **Word consciousness** is a disposition toward words that is both cognitive and affective (Anderson & Nagy, 1992; Graves & Watts-Taffe, 2002). The student who is word conscious knows many words well, is interested in words, enjoys using words well, enjoys seeing or hearing others use words well, looks for new words, is aware of the power of words, uses words skillfully, and realizes that words can be used to foster clarity and understanding or to confuse matters.

When a child has minimal vocabulary, then it affects reading progress in school (e.g., National Reading Panel, 2000; RAND Reading Study Group, 2002). Vocabulary learning is a tremendous task. However, knowing which words to teach and how to foster students' vocabulary development is important for strengthening all students' vocabularies, especially those who enter school with limited vocabularies (National Reading Panel, 2000; RAND Reading Group, 2002). Children from disadvantaged backgrounds where books and language-oriented experiences are not often part of their daily lives are at greater risk for reading failure.

As beginning readers, children use the words they have heard to make sense of the words they see in print. They have a much more difficult time reading words that are not already part of their oral vocabulary. Not all children come to school with the same experiences or vocabulary knowledge. Although a great deal of vocabulary is learned indirectly, some vocabulary should be taught directly. This can be done through specific vocabulary instruction (teaching specific words, engagement with words, and repeated exposure to words in many contexts) and word learning strategies (using dictionaries and other reference aids, using word parts, and using context clues). Recent research shows that speech-language pathologists and teachers can narrow the gap through explicit, **robust vocabulary instruction.** A robust approach to vocabulary instruction involves directly explaining the meanings of words. Beck, McKeown, and Kucan (2002) found that words are learned best when learned in context with thought-provoking and interactive follow-up activities in the classroom. They identified the following tiers of words for vocabulary instruction.

1. Tier I (high-frequency words) includes high-frequency, basic sight words that rarely require instruction in school (e.g., *the, play,* and *come*).

2. Tier II (rich words) includes high-frequency words for mature language users (e.g., *coincidence, disposition,* and *industrious*). Instruction in these words can add to a student's general ability. This includes words students encounter through listening or reading experiences in a wide variety of situations and texts. Speech-language pathologists and teachers should focus on vocabulary instruction.

3. Tier III (low-frequency words) includes words whose frequency use is quite low and limited to specific domains. These words are usually found within a content area such as math or science (e.g., *isotope, galaxy,* and *eclipse*). Such words are often important for understanding a particular text but do not usually appear across the content areas in many types of texts.

Vocabulary is learned best through direct, hands-on experiences. Children need to read meaningful words in meaningful contexts (Stahl, 1986; Rasinski, 1998). Speech-language pathologists and teachers should offer both definitions and context during vocabulary instruction. Effective vocabulary instruction connects new vocabulary to students' background knowledge and also expands their understanding (Stahl, 1986). Students need to have multiple exposures to new reading vocabulary words. Common strategies used in vocabulary instruction include word banks, specific word identification, problem solving with words, teaching of synonyms and antonyms, euphemisms, **onomatopoeia** (creating words that imitate sounds, e.g., buzz, vrrrroom), semantic maps, and word maps.

Associate words with definitions but move beyond by having students manipulate words in rich and varied ways. The following is a list of key suggestions for robust vocabulary instruction: (1) describe how words relate to other words; (2) relate words to children's familiar experiences; (3) apply words to unusual contexts; (4) associate new words with consequences; (5) use semantic groups, webs, and visual organizers; (6) teach context clues; (7) problem-solve with words; and (8) focus on conceptual understanding.

Comprehension

The National Reading Panel (NRP, 2000) defined comprehension as the intentional thinking during which meaning is constructed between the reader and text, and concluded that comprehension is enhanced when readers relate what they are reading to their own experiences and knowledge. Comprehension can be improved by teaching students cognitive strategies when they have difficulties understanding what they are reading (NRP, 2000). The NRP identified seven types of instruction that improve comprehension of non-impaired readers: (1) comprehension monitoring, (2) cooperative learning, (3) graphic organizers, (4) question answering, (5) question generating, (6) story structure, and (8) summarization.

According to the National Reading Panel (2000), teaching a combination of these methods is more likely to improve results on standardized comprehension reading tests. Furthermore, their research shows that comprehension is improved when trained speech-language pathologists and teachers use a combination of these strategies in natural settings. Later in this chapter, these strategies and approaches will be described in further detail.

Comprehension is an active and accurate process. It is the main purpose for reading. Many low-achieving students are unable to read effectively because they lack comprehension skills. Good readers know that the purpose of reading is understanding the text, that is, comprehension. They activate and use their background knowledge to comprehend, read with purpose, utilize many strategies to construct meaning, have metacognitive awareness, and read critically. Proficient reading comprehension is influenced by:

1. Accurate and fluent word recognition skills.
2. Oral language skills (vocabulary).
3. Fix-up strategies (knowledge in use of cognitive strategies to repair meaning when it breaks down).
4. Reasoning and inferential skills.
5. Motivation.

According to the National Research Council report (1998), there are three core obstacles to becoming a good reader: (1) difficulty learning to read words accurately and fluently; (2) insufficient vocabulary, poor general knowledge, and lack of reasoning skills to support comprehension of written language; and (3) poor motivation to read and/or develop an appreciation of reading.

One way the reader constructs meaning from text is by using **strategies**: planned procedures designed to help the reader meet a goal. Comprehension strategies include preparing, organizing, expanding, and monitoring. Readers can use several effective strategies before, during, and after reading to help them develop comprehension from text.

Before-reading strategies are designed to help the reader relate new information to what she or he already knows about a topic. Some key before-reading strategies include previewing, activating background knowledge, setting purpose and goals, and making predictions. **During-reading strategies,** or organizational strategies, are at the heart of constructing meaning because they involve selecting important details and building connections among them. Some of these strategies include comprehending the main idea, determining important details, organizing details (many times through graphic organizers), sequencing, and summarizing. **After-reading strategies** help the reader construct connections between information from text and prior knowledge. The reader generates inferences, images, questions, judgments (i.e., evaluating information), and elaborations.

Reciprocal teaching is an effective way to build students' comprehension. It is built on four strategies that good readers use to comprehend text: (1) predicting, (2) questioning, (3) clarifying, and (4) summarizing (Palinscar & Brown, 1984). For reciprocal teaching to be effective, certain instructional prerequisites must be in place. Speech-language pathologist or teacher scaffolding provides readers the support they need to become successful at using all four strategies. Students view the modeling of each strategy, try the strategies for themselves in a supported environment, and work independently using the strategies to comprehend text.

Teaching **question-and-answer relationships (QAR)** facilitates students' comprehension by providing them with a strategy for reading and answering questions (Raphael, 1986). QAR identifies two sources of information for answering questions, that is, in the book and in the reader's head.

In-the-book questions are classified as either right-there questions or think-and-search questions. The answer to right-there questions can be found in one or more sentences in the text. Students can point to these answers (e.g., definitions). The answers to think-and-search questions are pieced together using information from different parts of the text.

In-my-head questions are classified as either author-and-you questions or on-my-own questions. The answers to author-and-you questions are not found in the text. Instead, they require students to activate their background knowledge, make connections, and think inferentially. Students must think about what they already know and what the author is telling them, and synthesize how both pieces of information fit together.

Duke and Pearson (2002) summarized the research on teachers who are effective at developing children's comprehension. They recommended nine teaching principles:

1. Carefully choose texts matched to specific strategies, purposes, and readers.

2. Provide explicit comprehension instruction.

3. Create authentic situations and reasons for children to read real texts.

4. Ensure that children are reading the different kinds of text to aid comprehension.

5. Provide many text and hands-on opportunities to build vocabulary and word knowledge.

6. Focus on developing decoding skills and reading fluency.

7. Make sure children regularly engage in writing texts for others. This will demonstrate the text features that aid and hinder understanding.

8. Foster an environment in which children and school professionals engage in high-quality talk to revise or confirm meanings about text.

9. Conduct ongoing assessment to determine children's application of strategies and knowledge.

Effective comprehension instruction requires purposeful and explicit teaching. Scaffolded step-by-step instruction includes explicit explanations and modeling of strategies. Effective speech-language pathologists and teachers have a repertoire of strategies for developing students' text comprehension (e.g., writing, discussions, and many opportunities to interact with texts). School professionals should remember that effective comprehension instruction begins before children can read independently. Speech-language pathologists and teachers need to carefully select appropriate texts and materials (Center for the Improvement of Early Reading Achievement, 2002).

Students need experiences with varied texts and genres. Good comprehension instruction focuses on teaching students how to make connections between what they know and what they read. Effective comprehension instruction requires ongoing assessment to inform instruction and monitor students' progress (Center for the Improvement of Early Reading Achievement, 2002).

Language-Rich, Print-Rich Environments and Reading

A print-rich environment is one in where children interact with many forms of print, including signs, centers, word displays, labeled murals, charts, poems, and other printed material. It is important for children to recognize print in their surroundings, understand that print carries meaning, know that print is used for many purposes, and experience print through writing. According to the National Council of Teachers of English (1997) resolution, children need many opportunities to read and write from an early age and they need experiences with different types of text and other print/nonprint materials (e.g., literature, information books, nursery rhymes, songs, poems, predictable books). School professionals also need to allocate sufficient (and consistent) time daily to engage children in varied reading and writing experiences.

Environmental print, that is, print in the everyday environment at home and school, helps surround children with written language. **Family literacy** refers to the ways in which children learn to read, write, think, behave, and communicate within the context of everyday family experiences (Auerbach, 1990, 1995a, 1995b, 1997; Neuman, Caperelli, & Kee, 1998; Weinstein-Shr & Quintero, 1995). Studies of early readers indicate that learning to read is strongly associated with positive home environments (Neuman & Roskos, 1993; Strickland & Morrow, 1990a). Through quality interactions with adults, access to a variety of reading materials at home, observation of family members reading, and being read to by adults, children understand the many purposes of reading. Consequently, they may become involved in different kinds of reading activities. Literate environments provide children with access to print and books, include supportive adults who demonstrate literacy behaviors and involve children with storybook reading and writing.

Hart and Risley (1995) spent 2 and a half years studying the spoken interactions between parents and children in 42 families. They wanted to find why, despite best efforts in preschool programs to equalize opportunity, children from low-income homes remained well behind their more economically advantaged peers years later in school. They found that language development in young children was overwhelmingly correlated with socioeconomic status. By age 3, the recorded spoken vocabularies of the children from the professional families were larger than those of the parents in the welfare families. Between professional and welfare parents, there was a difference of almost 300 words spoken per hour. Thus, children in professional families would hear 11 million words, while children in welfare families would hear just 3 million before they began school. Positive interactions and vocabulary experiences, oral language concepts, and emergent literacy concepts improve the potential for school success for the at-risk children.

Duke (2000) also studied the differences in print environments and experiences offered to children in different socioeconomic-status (SES) school settings. The results of her study indicated differences between the low- and high-SES classrooms in terms of (1) the amount, (2) the types, and (3) the nature of print experiences. She reported that a child in a low-SES first-grade classroom experienced distinctively different print environments and experiences than those of his or her high-SES counterpart.

According to Duke (2000), a child in a low-SES classroom:

1. Encountered less print on the walls and other surfaces of the classroom.
2. Had fewer books and magazines in the classroom library.
3. Received fewer references to classroom environmental print.
4. Had fewer opportunities to use the classroom library.
5. Received a smaller proportion of exposure to extended forms of text.
6. Experienced print integrated across the curriculum less often.
7. Had fewer opportunities to choose what he or she read.
8. Had fewer opportunities to write for audiences beyond the teacher.

9. Engaged in activities in which she or he had a high degree of authorship less often.

10. Engaged in activities such as copying, taking dictation, and completing worksheets more often.

Duke (2000) concluded that schools themselves may contribute to the relatively lower levels of literacy achievement among low-SES children. Speech-language pathologists and teachers can enhance students' word learning by introducing words in context, covering illustrations in predictable text, examining words in isolation and in context, working with sentence strips, and reviewing words over time. Word study should be meaningful and engaging. It should incorporate the text, the reader, and the task (Johnson, 1998).

Morrow (1993) suggested that school professionals can learn from parents who create a language-rich literate environment at home. She recommended that school professionals stop looking at families as deficient and begin examining the positive contributions that families make in interactions or storybook reading. Strickland and Morrow (1989) proposed that school professionals should concentrate on developing and improving the existing family skills. They suggested that school professionals need to create safe classroom environments and child-centered environments, and have materials available for all children to use. Stories should be part of daily reading routines, especially during the early emergent literacy years and the beginning primary school years. Last, because of the importance of reading to children at home, home-school partnerships should be created.

CASE STUDY PERSPECTIVES

Three case studies are presented to illustrate how best practices and strategies may be implemented with speech-language pathologists, classroom teachers, parents, and other school professionals.

Case Study One Background: Rebecca

Rebecca is a monolingual fifth-grade student who is experiencing difficulties in reading and writing. Rebecca is currently reading at fourth-grade level. She perceives herself to be a very good reader because she practices reading every night. The materials she enjoys reading the most include her science and social studies books, informational books, humorous books, and comic strips. She enjoys reading. She says that reading makes her feel happy, relaxed, good, and comfortable.

Based on assessment data, Rebecca's reading strengths include her reading rate, reading accuracy, fluency, and ability to retell the story in her own words using details. She also shows strength in using decoding strategies as she focuses on onset-rime relationships and the initial letter of new words. Rebecca can decode but has difficulty with comprehension. Other phonics weaknesses shown from assessments include her difficulty in blending letter sounds when three sounds are said to her, as well as manipulating sounds into words.

Furthermore, Rebecca shows reading weaknesses using self-correcting strategies when reading long passages. Miscues are made throughout the leveled passages without being self-corrected. She also shows a weakness in reading effectively with punctuation. Her reading expression does not reflect question marks, exclamation points, and commas. Rebecca has difficulties with consonant digraphs and structural analysis.

Case Study One Comments: Rebecca

Rebecca would benefit from explicit comprehension instruction during reading. As Rebecca reads a text, the speech-language pathologist (SLP) or teacher can check for comprehension by asking questions, help her notice errors so she can learn to self-check her reading, and connect text to background knowledge. Strategies that would help this student improve her reading include the speech-language pathologist or teacher making inferences, which will enable her to judge, conclude, question, or reason about what she has read. Rebecca should learn to self-monitor for meaning. The speech-language pathologist or teacher should help Rebecca visualize the events of the story by asking questions and making predictions. In addition, the speech-language pathologist or teacher should connect the text with Rebecca's background knowledge of literature and of outside experiences.

One recommendation is for the teacher to introduce new vocabulary words that will be in an upcoming reading passage. Before introducing a new text, the teacher should write the new words and explain to the class the meaning of each. This would benefit Rebecca because she would be prepared to effectively read and comprehend the new words in the text. The strategy for this instruction includes the speech-language pathologist or teacher writing the new words on the board or chart paper, reading one word at a time. Rebecca repeats. The SLP or teacher explains what the word means, writes the meaning next to the word, and checks for Rebecca's understanding.

In addition, Rebecca's fluency would benefit from listening to fluent reading, choral reading, and guided reading. During guided reading, the speech-language pathologist or teacher should teach reading strategies and skills that model how Rebecca can use these strategies as she reads independently.

Rebecca would also benefit from the use of graphic organizers after reading, which would help her organize her thoughts and allow her to visualize the text. It would also help her develop her comprehension by mapping out the story's setting, characters, problem, main events, resolution, etc. One example is the use of story maps. Story maps allow the student to determine the setting, characters, problem, and outcome. Story webs, which show the beginning, middle, and end of a story, would also be an appropriate aid.

Case Study Two Background: Thomas

Thomas is a monolingual third-grade student who is experiencing reading difficulties. Thomas has a tendency to read fast, and he repeats sentences that he has read because he loses track of the passage. During his reading, he also repeats words. When the speech-language pathologist or teacher gives a reading assignment, Thomas seems less than thrilled to complete the assignment. Thomas usually tries to find something else to do rather than read. Thomas's retelling skills are adequate as long as he does not have to read the story himself.

Case Study Two Comments: Thomas

Thomas would benefit from guided reading. He needs to hear fluent reading, that is, when the speech-language pathologist or teacher has the student follow along while reading the passage. This would help Thomas learn to read fluently. Thomas should be taught to use a pointer or pencil while learning a pacing technique.

Echo reading is another strategy to consider. This involves the speech-language pathologist or teacher reading a short phrase or sentence and the student echoing the phrase back, using the same rate and intonation that the SLP or teacher used. This strategy may assist Thomas recognize his reading rate and the intonation he uses while reading.

Reader's theater is an activity that provides purpose for reading. This strategy involves students reading a script aloud. Students practice their vocal expressions, which assists with reading fluently. It is a cooperative setting where students learn fluency from one another. The script has short assigned segments instead of long passages. Therefore, passage length rarely discourages them. This strategy may help to build up Thomas's confidence when reading with his fellow classmates.

Case Study Three Background: Tyler

Tyler is a monolingual first-grade student. Tyler has a specific learning disability (SLD) and receives additional special instruction in reading and mathematics from the special-education resource teacher during two periods of the day. Tyler has a limited vocabulary and a poor attitude toward reading. His alphabetic principle is underdeveloped; as a result, Tyler struggles with basic sight-word vocabulary.

Tyler's instructional reading level is at the primer level, and his independent reading level is at the preprimer level. Assessment results show that Tyler is far below grade level on his comprehension and below basic in the performance standard. Tyler has difficulties in (1) blending and segmenting, (2) manipulating sounds in words, (3) syllabication, and (4) distinguishing oddity in words.

Case Study Three Comments: Tyler

Tyler would benefit from phonemic awareness and phonics instruction to help build (1) phonemic awareness, (2) letter knowledge, (3) word identification skills, (4) fluency, and (5) comprehension. Tyler would initially benefit from explicit instruction in phonemic awareness and phonics. Games, practice, and sustained reading would help Tyler build his basic vocabulary, confidence in reading, and eventual fluency. Tyler needs to develop his reading automaticity. He would benefit from reading connected texts, reading and rereading familiar texts, and also being read to by fluent readers (e.g., teacher, parents, peers).

INSTRUCTIONAL SUGGESTIONS AND STRATEGIES

Research indicates that effective primary reading teachers have a sophisticated understanding of literacy instruction (Chi, Glaser, & Farr, 1988; Erickson & Smith, 1991; Hoffman, 1992; Pressley, Rankin, & Yokoi, 1996). Morrow, Tracey, Woo, and Pressley (1999) examined the nature of exemplary early literacy instruction and concluded that school professionals who were identified as exemplary had a balanced perspective for literacy instruction. Students of exemplary teachers were exposed both to the direct, explicit instruction for skill development in the context of authentic literature and to integrated instruction that emphasized writing and content area connections.

In studying over 10,000 children for 15 years, the National Institute of Child Health and Human Development (NICHHD) and the United States Department of Education have documented the following necessary components of effective beginning reading instruction:

1. Create appreciation for the written word.
2. Develop awareness of printed language and the written system.
3. Teach the alphabet.
4. Develop students' phonological awareness.
5. Teach the relationship between sounds and letters.
6. Teach children how to sound out words.
7. Teach children how to spell words.
8. Help children develop fluent, reflective reading.

According to this recent research, all successful early reading programs must do the following:

1. Base instruction on accurate diagnostic information.
2. Develop print concepts.
3. Develop knowledge of letter names and letter shapes.
4. Convey the understanding that spoken words are composed of sounds (phonemic awareness) and that letters correspond to these sounds.
5. Provide systematic and explicit instruction in sound/symbol relationships (phonics).
6. Connect instruction to practice in highly decodable text that contains the sounds and symbols taught.
7. Make use of rich and varied literature by reading to children regularly.

Snow, Burns, and Griffin (1998) shared various conclusions and recommendations about literacy development during the early years. Table 7–5 summarizes their conclusions and recommendations.

Suggestions for Collaboration Among Educators

Research by Snow, Burns, and Griffin (1998) shows that children who have early experiences with reading before they enter school are more likely to succeed in learning how to read. Educators can help their young children become readers by selecting activities and experiences that promote reading success. Collaboration between the general education classroom teacher and the speech-language pathologist or special education classroom teacher should promote reading (refer also to Chapter 12 on school professional collaboration models). Braaten and Mennes (1992) defined collaboration as school professionals working together while attempting to solve a mutually defined problem. They share the problem, have similar perspectives of the situation, and view each other as equal partners.

TABLE 7–5
Early Reading Development

Conclusions	Recommendations
Important experiences related to reading begin early in life. Prevention steps designed to reduce the number of children with inadequate literacy-related knowledge (e.g., concepts of print, phonemic awareness, receptive vocabulary) at the onset of formal schooling would reduce the number of children with reading difficulties.	Organizations and governing bodies concerned with the education of young children should promote public understanding of early literacy development.
Children who are at-risk for reading difficulties should be identified as early as possible. Speech-language pathologists, teachers, pediatricians, social workers, preschool practitioners, and parents play significant roles in identifying children who need assistance.	Public authorities and education professionals should provide research-derived guidelines for parents, pediatricians, and preschool professionals so that children who need intervention are identified as early as possible and are given the necessary support for language and literacy development.
Providing preschool opportunities to lower-income families in ways that fully support language and literacy development is possibly one of the more important public policy issues raised by welfare reform.	All children, especially those at risk for reading difficulties, should have access to early childhood environments that promote language and literacy factors in an integrated fashion. The following should be included in home and preschool activities: • Adult-child shared book reading that stimulates verbal interaction to enhance language development and knowledge about print concepts. • Activities that direct young children's attention to the phonological structure of spoken words (e.g., games, songs, and poems that emphasize rhyming or manipulation of sounds). • Activities that highlight the relations between print and speech.
Central to the goal of primary prevention of reading difficulties is the teacher's knowledge base, experience, and support provided to the teacher.	School professionals at all levels need to understand the course of literacy development and the role of instruction in optimizing literacy development.
Preschool teachers' role is a very important one in promoting literacy through acquisition of rich language and emergent literacy skills.	Programs that educate early childhood professionals should require mastery of information about the many kinds of knowledge and skills that need to be acquired in the preschool years. Their knowledge base should include at least the following: • How to provide rich conceptual experiences that promote growth in vocabulary and reasoning skills. • Knowledge about lexical development.

Conclusions	Recommendations
	• Knowledge about the early development of listening skills.
	• Information on young children's sense of story.
	• Information on young children's sensitivity to the sounds of language.
	• Information on young children's understanding of print, and the developmental patterns of emergent reading and writing.
	• Information on young children's development of concepts of space, including directionality.
	• Knowledge of fine motor development.
	• Knowledge about how to motivate children to read.

Book and Print Awareness

To help children understand how books and print communicate information, the speech-language pathologist or teacher should take time to explain how a book is held, the direction in which text is read, and when to turn a page. Create a book with the child by having him or her dictate a story. Let the child illustrate the pages and share the new creation with others. Provide different types of books, such as fiction, poetry, and nonfiction books. Discuss the differences among the types of print genres available.

Phonological and Phonemic Awareness

Learning about syllables is important to understanding the structure of language. Have children begin by breaking their own names into syllables. Organize the children into groups and think of other names that share the same number of syllables as their own name. For phonemic awareness, play a game to hear all the sounds in a word. Tell the children to break a word into parts and put it back together again. Say the sound /r/ and then the rime -*an*. Have them put the word together to make the word *ran*. Practice this with other words, keeping the initial sound (onset) the same and changing the end sounds from the syllable (rime). Afterward, switch and keep the rime and change the onset. Give the child a picture of a simple word such as a dog barking. Have the child spell the word *bark* and then make each individual sound for that word.

Language and Comprehension

To help children bridge prior knowledge with new information understanding, allow time for children to discuss ideas that interest them. Allow other children to add information to the first child's ideas. Guide children in dramatic retellings of favorite stories. Let them enhance the stories with their own prior knowledge. When reading to children, ask for summaries of parts of the book. Allow them to discuss their feelings about why certain characters acted as they did in the story.

Try to activate prior knowledge when dealing with new subjects. Bring in other books or objects to help the children grasp new ideas. Review new vocabulary and have them use it in meaningful sentences. Use story books to develop strategies such as finding the main idea, predicting, determining cause and effect, sequencing, and comparing and contrasting.

Letter Recognition, Decoding, and Word Recognition

Children should practice writing letters and words and then keep them in a file folder for later review. Make each day a letter day. Have each child participate when it is his or her special day for writing initials on the blackboard. Whenever anyone sees or hears a word that starts with such letters, he or she can write them down in their alphabet folder and share it with others at the appropriate time. Have children work on sight words (e.g., *the, have, said, one*) with games such as Concentration. This can be accomplished by having 10 to 12 sight words printed twice on different rectangle squares. Lay the words face down. Have the children match simple sight words and say the word when they make an appropriate match. Make a word wall in the children's room. Put up 5 to 6 new words a week. Some words can be brought to the attention of the class by the student who uses a new word or brings something new to class.

Spelling and Writing

Allow children to make their own letter and word dictionaries. This is a great way to enhance their confidence as emergent writers. Have students add pictures and illustrations to help their understanding of words. Begin their writing on something familiar to them, for example, their families. As children progress into the second and third grades, their writing themes become broader. Create a special chair in the room where an author sits. Have children sit in the author's chair when they read a story that they wrote. Children often hear many nursery rhymes when they are young; have them write their own poems or nursery rhymes and share them with the class.

Comprehension and Making Connections

When sharing books, choose examples that can make connections to the child's life. For example, when reading a book about how plants grow, have the child describe all the different kinds of plants that are in his or her yard. Have children give presentations on the books that they have heard or on experiences that are similar to those in the book.

Wordless Picture Books. Provide children with wordless picture books, such as *Good Dog* or *Carl* by Alexandra Day and *Tuesday* by David Wiesner. Give them the opportunity to create their own language and vocabulary for the story. During writing time, allow them to write their own dialogue and interpretations of the story.

Rhyming Books. Rhyming books help develop children's phonological awareness skills. Children need practice in manipulating sounds within words they know. See Figure 7–2 for a representative list of quality rhyming books.

Predictable and Patterned Books. **Predictable and patterned books** (i.e., books with recurring word or sentence themes, such as *Brown Bear, Brown Bear, What Do You See* by Bill Martin, Jr.) help young readers learn the concept of a story. They also help children join in the reading of a story, even though they may not know all of the words. See Figure 7–3 for a representative list of quality predictable and patterned books.

FIGURE 7–2
Rhyming Books That Promote Emergent Literacy

- *The Big Bug Dug* by M. Serfozo
- *Chimps Don't Wear Glasses* by L. Numeroff
- *Commotion in the Ocean* by G. S. Andreae and D. Wojtowycz
- *Dinosaur Chase* by C. Otto
- *Five Little Monkeys Jumping on the Bed* by E. Christelow
- *The Foot Book* by Dr. Seuss
- *A Giraffe and a Half* by S. Silverstein
- *The Grumpy Morning* by P. Edwards
- *Is Your Mama a Llama?* by D. Guarino and S. Kellog
- *Miss Mary Mack* by M. A. Hoberman
- *Moose on the Loose* by C. P. Ochs
- *Moses Supposes His Toeses Are Roses* by N. Patz
- *One Fish Two Fish Red Fish Blue Fish* by Dr. Seuss
- *Peanut Butter and Jelly: A Play Rhyme* by N. Westcott
- *Sheep in a Jeep* by N. Shaw
- *Sometimes I Wonder If Poodles Like Noodles* by L. Numeroff
- *Zoom! Zoom! Zoom! I'm Off to the Moon!* by D. Yaccarino

FIGURE 7–3
Predictable and Patterned Books That Promote Emergent Literacy

Repetitive Words and Phrases

- *Brown Bear, Brown Bear, What Do You See?* by B. Martin, Jr.
- *Chicken Soup With Rice* by M. Sendak
- *Dear Zoo* by R. Campbell
- *Do You Want to Be My Friend?* by E. Carle
- *Goodnight Moon* by M. Brown
- *The Very Busy Spider* by E. Carle
- *The Very Lonely Firefly* by E. Carle

Repetitive and Cumulative Patterns

- *Are You There Bear?* by R. Maris
- *Buzz Buzz Buzz* by B. Barton
- *Hippity Hop, Frog on Top* by N. Wing
- *"I Don't Care!" Said the Bear* by C. West
- *Little Pink Pig* by P. Hutchins
- *A Most Unusual Lunch* by R. Bender
- *Runaway Bunny* by M. Brown

Suggestions for Collaboration with Families

Parents are the child's first teachers. There are many activities that parents can do with their young emergent readers to promote literacy. The most important activities include daily and varied oral interactions, reading aloud to children, and exposing children to print and varied texts.

There are many ways to read to children. **Read-alouds** involve reading a book or part of a book out loud to a child. **Shared reading** involves an adult reading aloud as well as showing the child the text and pictures. The child follows along and is invited to read along with the adult.

Follow Directions

One way to help a child learn about the importance of reading is have him or her help you follow directions, such as when baking a cake. All emergent readers benefit from watching others and following directions needed to complete a task. As the directions are given, read them to the child and then discuss what they mean.

Environmental Print

Environmental print is print used and seen in everyday life, such as signs, newspapers, letters, and lists. Environmental print is important for a child's literacy development because it brings the importance of reading into perspective for emergent readers.

Play Reading Games

Learning to read should not be rote and disengaging. Games that contain needed skills help emergent readers get excited about reading. Games like Concentration (matching) and bingo can be designed to promote recognition of alphabet letters and sight words.

Create a Reading Environment

Provide a comfortable place to read, with plenty of light and places to sit. Have books readily available. Decorate the area with creative posters about reading. Provide materials that show children different kinds of printed materials and discuss what the materials are used for and what they mean. Books, newspapers, magazines, letters, and lists are suggestions.

Print Functions and Print Awareness

Discuss the differences among the types of print genres. Have the children decide why someone might want a book of poetry versus a dictionary or a menu versus a recipe book. Use authentic print; for example, read menus and signs to the child that are encountered in everyday life. Discuss their meaning and how they differ from books. When reading books, remember to mention the title, author, and illustrator of the book. Touch the title and author's name with a finger as they are named.

Discuss what an author and illustrator did as it pertains to the book. Have children identify a letter, a word, a sentence, and different punctuation marks on a page of a book. Give the child a book and ask him or her, "Which way do you open the book?" "Where do you begin reading?" "Where is the end of the book?" Have them point and show the correct parts. Demonstrate with a pointing finger, for example, the direction in which text is read on a page. Have the child run his or her fingers under the sentence as you read them the information on that page.

Practice Readiness Skills

When working with younger emergent readers (birth to age 3), practice readiness skills needed for reading. **Readiness skills** include listening, sequencing, and the knowledge and manipulation of sounds in words (phonemic awareness). For example, cook a new recipe with the child and say the directions out loud.

Sing Songs

All emergent readers benefit from singing and listening. Sing songs with rhyme and rhythm; this will help children become aware of the different sounds in words. Teach emergent readers the alphabet song and nursery rhymes. Make up songs and make sure the children are adding appropriate rhyming words.

CONCLUDING REMARKS

Reading is a complex and multilayered process. The demands for literacy are always increasing in school and society. Reading problems have become a national dilemma. Speech-language pathologists, teachers, general-education teachers, preschool teachers, parents, caregivers, and the community at large play critical roles in preparing a child to be a successful reader. There are no simple answers for developing early literacy behaviors. There is a need for all individuals to understand the complex cognitive, social, and cultural influences of emergent literacy. There is also a need to understand the unique characteristics of children and families, discover their strengths, and capitalize on ways to help all students succeed in school (Yaden, Rowe, & MacGillivray, 1999).

Speech-language pathologists and teachers bear the primary responsibility for instructing students who have reading problems. Reading problems are associated with difficulties in life, including poverty, unemployment, and even problems with the law. Effective educators understand that the development of literacy skills is not automatic but unique for every child. Effective school professionals make instructional decisions based on their knowledge of reading and writing, research, and children's unique strengths and needs. SLPs and teachers need to respect children's home language and culture, and use it as a base to build and expand children's language and literacy experiences. "If we start early and finish strong, we can help every child become a good reader" (United States Department of Education, America Reads Challenge, 1998, p. 15). (Refer again to Table 7–5.)

REFLECTION QUESTIONS

1. When you place a book upside down in front of Michelle, a kindergarten student, she turns it over, looks at the front cover, and attempts to read the title of the book. She then turns to the first page of the book, studies the pictures, reads as many words as she can recognize, and makes up the ones she cannot. What inferences

can you make about Michelle's alphabetic principle? What experiences would help Michelle develop her reading skills?

2. Explain to a teacher the need for explicit instruction in phonemic awareness. Describe three key phonemic awareness activities that would help all children develop their reading skills.

3. Explain to a parent the role of oral language in reading development. Advise the parent to involve themselves and their child in three fundamental oral language activities. Name those activities.

4. What are the four characteristics of reading fluency development? Describe three core ways for speech-language pathologists and teachers to build the fluency development of all children in the classroom.

5. What is the role of explicit instruction in phonics, vocabulary, and comprehension? Discuss what speech-language pathologists and/or teachers need to do to develop students' phonemic awareness, vocabulary, and comprehension skills.

6. What is the role of assessment in planning for instruction? Discuss how speech-language pathologists and/or teachers should use assessment data to plan for instruction that will meet the diverse reading needs of students.

7. Why is there so much variation in students' reading skills? Using research and personal experiences, discuss ways speech-language pathologists and/or teachers can balance the wide range of reading skills and experiences students bring with them to the classroom.

REFERENCES

Adams, M. (1990). *Beginning to read: Thinking and learning about print.* Cambridge, MA: MIT Press.

Adams, M. J. (1996). *Beginning to read.* Cambridge, MA: MIT Press.

Adams, M. J., Foorman, B. R., Lundberg, I., & Beeler, T. (1997). *Phonemic awareness in young children: A classroom curriculum.* Baltimore, MD: Brookes.

Adams, M., Foorman, B., Lundberg, I., & Beeler, T (1998). *Phonemic awareness in young children.* Baltimore, MD: Brookes.

Anderson, R. C., Hiebert, E. H., Scott, J. A., & Wilkinson, I. A. G. (1985). *Becoming a nation of readers.* Washington, DC: National Institute of Education.

Anderson, R. C., & Negy, W. E. (1992). The vocabulary conundrum. *American Educator, 16*(4), 14–18, 44–47.

Armbruster, B. B., Lehr, F., & Osborn, J. (2001). *Put reading first: The research blocks for teaching children to read.* Washington, DC: U.S. Department of Education.

Auerbach, E. (1990). *Making meaning, making change.* Boston, MA: University of Massachusetts.

Auerbach, E. R. (1995a). From deficit to strength: Changing perspectives on family literacy. In G. Weinstein-Shr & E. Quintero (Eds.), *Immigrant learners and their families* (pp. 63–76). McHenry, IL: Center for Applied Linguistics and Delta Systems.

Auerbach, E. R. (1995b). Which way for family literacy: Intervention or empowerment? In L. M. Morrow (Ed.), *Family literacy: Connections in schools and communities* (pp. 11–27). New Brunswick, NJ: International Reading Association.

Auerbach, E. R. (1997). Reading between the lines. In D. Taylor (Ed.), *Many families, many literacies: An international declaration of principles* (pp. 71–81). Portsmouth, NH: Heinemann.

Beck, I. L., and Juel, C. (1995). The role of decoding in learning to read. *American Educator, 19*(2), 21–25.

Beck, I., McKeown, M. G., & Kucan, L. (2002, March). *Bringing words to life: Robust vocabulary development.* New York: Guilford.

Braaten, B., & Mennes, D. (1992). A model of collaborative service for middle school students. *Preventing School Failure, 36*(3), 10–15.

Cambourne, B., & Turbill, J. (1987). *Coping with chaos.* Rozelle, Australia: Primary English Teaching Association.

Catts, H. W. (1989). Defining dyslexia as a developmental language disorder. *Annals of Dyslexia, 39,* 50–64.

Catts, H. (1993). The relationship between speech-language impairments and reading disabilities. *Journal of Speech and Hearing Research, 36,* 948–958.

Catts, H., & Kamhi, A. (1999). *Language and reading disabilities.* Needham Heights, MA: Allyn & Bacon.

Center for the Improvement of Early Reading Achievement (2002). Improving the reading comprehension of America's children: 10 research-based principles. Ann Arbor, MI: University of Michigan. Available online at http://www.ciera.org/library/instresrc/compprinciples/.

Chall, J. S. (1996). *Stages of reading development,* (2nd ed.). New York: Harcourt Brace.

Chard, D. J., & Dickson, S. V. (1999). Phonological awareness instructional and assessment guidelines. *Intervention in School and Clinic, 34,* 261–270.

Chard, D. J., Simmons, D. C., & Kameenui, E. J. (1998). Word recognition: Research bases. In D. C. Simmons & E. J. Kameenui (Eds.), *What reading research tells us about children with diverse learning needs: Bases and basics* (pp. 141–168). Mahwah, NJ: Erlbaum.

Chi, M. T. H., Glaser, R., & Farr, M. J. (1988). *The nature of expertise.* Hillsdale, NJ: Erlbaum.

Clark, A. (1993). *Associative engines: Connectionism, concepts, and representational change.* Cambridge, UK: Cambridge University Press.

Clay, M. (1967). The reading behavior of five year old children: A research report. *New Zealand Journal of Educational Studies, 2*(1), 11–31.

Cooper, J. D. (1997). *Literacy: Helping children construct meaning* (3rd ed.). Boston, MA: Houghton Mifflin.

Duke, N. K. (2000). 3.6 minutes per day: The scarcity of informational texts in first grade. *Reading Research Quarterly, 35,* 202–224.

Duke, N., & Pearson, D. (2002). Effective practices for developing reading comprehension. In A. Farstrup & S. Samuels (Eds.), *What research has to say about reading instruction* (pp. 205–242). Newark, DE: International Reading Association.

Durkin, D. (1966). *Children who read early.* New York: Teachers College Press.

Ehri, L. C. (1994). Development of the ability to read words: Update. In R. Ruddell and H. Singer (Eds.), *Theoretical models and processes of reading* (4th ed., pp. 323–358). Newark, DE: International Reading Association.

Ehri, L. C. (1995). Phases of development in learning to read words by sight. *Journal of Research in Reading, 18*(2), 116–125.

Ehri, L. C. (1998a). Grapheme-phoneme knowledge is essential for learning to read words in English. In J. Metsala & L. Ehri (Eds.), *Word recognition in beginning literacy* (pp. 3–40). Mahwah, NJ: Erlbaum.

Ehri, L. C. (1998b). Research on learning to read and spell: A personal historical perspective. *Scientific Studies of Reading, 2*(1), 97–114.

Erickson, K. A., & Smith, J. (Eds.). (1991). *Toward a theory of expertise.* Cambridge, UK: Cambridge Press.

Gough, P. B. (1995). The new literacy: Caveat emptor. *Journal of Research in Reading, 18*(2),79–86.

Graves, M. F., & Watts-Taffe, S. M. (2002). The place of word consciousness in a research-based vocabulary program. In A. E. Farstrup & S. J. Samuels (Eds.), *What research has to say about reading instruction* (3rd ed., pp. 140–165). Newark, DE: International Reading Association.

Halliday, M. (1975). *Learning how to mean.* London: Edward Arnold.

Halliday, M. (1978). *Language as social semiotic.* Baltimore, MD: Edward Arnold.

Hart, B., & Risley, T. (1995). *Meaningful differences.* Baltimore, MD: Paul H. Brookes.

Haskell, D. W., Foorman, B. R., & Swank, P. R. (1992). Effects of three orthographic/phonological units on first-grade reading. *Remedial and Special Education, 13,* 40–49.

Heath, S. B. (1983). Research currents: A lot of talk about nothing. *Language Arts, 60*(8), 999–1007.

Heilman, A. W., Blair, T. R., & Rupley, W. H. (2002). *Principles and practices of teaching reading.* Upper Saddle River, NJ: Prentice-Hall.

Hiebert, E. H., Pearson, P. D., Taylor, B. M., Richardson, V., & Paris, S. G. (1998). *Every child a reader: Applying reading research in the classroom.* Ann Arbor: CIERA/University of Michigan.

Hoffman, R. R. (1992). *The psychology of expertise: Cognitive research and empirical.* Albany, NY: Springer-Verlag.

Holdaway, D. (1979). *The foundations of literacy.* Sydney, Australia: Ashton Scholastic (distributed by Heinemann, Portsmouth, NH).

Honig, B. (1996). *Teaching our children to read: The role of skills in a comprehensive reading program.* Thousand Oaks, CA: Corwin Press.

Johns, J. & Berglund, R. (2002). *Fluency: Question, answers, evidence-based strategies.* Dubuque, IA: Kendall/Hunt.

Johnson, A. P. (1998). Classifying and super word web: Two strategies to improve productive vocabulary. *Journal of Adolescent and Adult Literacy, 42,* 204–208.

Juel, C. (1988). Learning to read and write: A longitudinal study of 54 children from first through fourth grades. *Journal of Educational Psychology, 80,* 437–447.

Juel, C. (1991). *Beginning reading.* In R. Barr, M. L. Kamil, P. B. Mosenthal, & P. D. Pearson (Eds.), *Handbook of reading research* (Vol. II, pp. 759–788). New York: Longman.

Juel, C. (1994). *Learning to read and write in one elementary school.* New York: Springer-Verlag.

Juel, C. (1998). What kind of one-on-one tutoring helps a poor reader? In C. Hulme and R. M. Joshi (Eds.) *Reading and spelling: Development and disorders* (pp. 449–471). Mahwah, NJ: Lawrence Erlbaum.

Kuhn, M. (2004). Helping students become accurate, expressive readers: Fluency instruction for small groups. *The Reading Teacher, 58*(4), 338–344.

Kuhn, M. R., & Stahl, S. A. (2000, March). *Fluency: A review of developmental and remedial practices* (Rep. No. 2-008). Ann Arbor, MI: Center for the Improvement of Early Reading Achievement. Available at www.ciera.org/library/reports/inquiry-2/2-008/2-008.pdf

LaBerge, D., & Samuels, S. J. (1974). Toward a theory of automatic information processing in reading. *Cognitive Psychology, 6,* 293–323.

Melvin, M. P. (1979). Psycholinguistics and the teaching of reading. *The Elementary School Journal, 79,* 276–328.

Morrow, L. M. (1993). *Literacy development in the early years: Helping children read and write* (2nd ed.). Boston, MA: Allyn & Bacon.

Morrow, L. M. (1997). *Literacy development in the early years: Helping children read and write.* Boston, MA: Allyn & Bacon.

Morrow, L. M., Tracey, D. H., Woo, D., & Pressley, M. (1999). Characteristics of exemplary first-grade literacy instruction. *The Reading Teacher, 52*(5), 462–476.

National Council of Teachers of English. (1997). *On reading, learning to read, and effective reading instruction: An overview of what we know and how we know it.* Urbana, IL: The National Council of Teachers of English.

National Institute for Literacy. (2001). *Put reading first: The research building blocks for teaching children to read.* Washington, DC: The Partnership for Reading: National Institute for Literacy; National Institute of Child Health and Human Development; and U.S. Department of Education.

National Institute of Child Health and Human Development. (2000). Report of the National Reading Panel. *Teaching children to read: An evidence-based assessment of the scientific research literature on reading and its implications for reading instruction: Reports of the subgroups* (No. 00-4754). Washington, DC: U.S. Government Printing Office.

National Institute of Child Health and Human Development (2001). Report of the National Reading Panel. *Teaching children to read: An evidence-based assessment of the scientific research literature on reading and its implications for reading instruction* (NIH Publication No. 00-4769). Washington, DC: U.S. Government Printing Office.

National Reading Panel. (2000a). *Teaching children to read: An evidence-based assessment of the scientific research literature on reading and its implications for reading instruction* (National Institute of Health Pub. No. 00-4769). Washington, DC: National Institute of Child Health and Human Development.

National Reading Panel. (2000b). *Teaching children to read: An evidence-based assessment of the scientific research literature on reading and its implications for reading instruction: Reports of the subgroups.* Bethesda, MD: National Institute of Child Health and Human Development.

National Research Council. (1998). *Preventing reading difficulties in young children.* Washington, DC: National Academy Press.

National Research Council. (1999). *Starting out right: A guide to promoting children's reading success.* Washington, DC: National Academy Press.

Neuman, S. B., Caperelli, B. J., & Kee, C. (1998). Literacy learning, a family matter. *The Reading Teacher, 52,* 244–252.

Neuman, S. B., & Roskos, K. A. (Eds.). (1998). *Children achieving: Best practices in early literacy.* Newark, DE: International Reading Association.

Palinscar, A., & Brown, A. (1984). Reciprocal teaching of comprehension-fostering and comprehension-monitoring activities. *Cognition and Instruction 1,* (2), 117–175.

Partnership for Reading. (2001). *Put reading first: The research building blocks for teaching children to read.* Washington, DC: The Partnership for Reading.

Report available online at www.nifl.gov/partner shipforreading.

Pressley, M., Rankin, J., & Yokoi, L. (1996). A survey of the instructional practices of outstanding primary-level literacy teachers. *Elementary School Journal, 96*, 363–384.

RAND Reading Study Group. (2002). *Reading for understanding: Towards an R&D program in reading comprehension.* Available online at http://www.rand.org/multi/achievementforall/reading/readreport.html.

Raphael, T. (1986). Teaching question answer relationships, revisited. *The Reading Teacher, 6*(39), 516–522.

Rasinski, T. V. (1998). How elementary students referred for compensatory reading instruction perform on school-based measures of word recognition, fluency, and comprehension. *Reading Psychology: An International Quarterly, 19*, 185–216.

Riley, R. (1996). Improving the reading and writing skills of America's students. *Learning Disability Quarterly, 19*, 67–69.

Rosenblatt, L. (1986). The aesthetic transaction. *Journal of Aesthetic Education, 20*(4), 122–128.

Rosenblatt, L. (1994), The transactional theory of reading and writing. In R. B. Ruddell, M. R. Ruddell, & H. Singer (Eds.), *Theoretical models and processes of reading* (4th ed.). Newark, DE: International Reading Association.

Samuels, S. J. (2002). Reading fluency: Its development and assessment. In A. E. Farstrup & S. J. Samuels (Eds.), *What research has to say about reading instruction* (3rd ed., pp. 166–183). Newark, DE: International Reading Association.

Share, D. L., & Stanovich, K. E. (1995). Cognitive processes in early reading development: A model of acquisition and individual differences. *Issues in Education: Contributions from Educational Psychology, 1*, 1–57.

Smith, S. B., Simmons, D. C., & Kameenui, E. J. (1998). Phonological awareness: Synthesis of the research. In D. C. Simmons (Ed.), *What reading research tells us about children with diverse learning needs: The bases and basics* (pp. 61–127). Mahwah, NJ: Lawrence Erlbaum.

Snider, V. E. (1995). A primer on phonemic awareness: What it is, why it's important, and how to teach it. *School Psychology Review, 24*, 443–455.

Snow, C., Burns, M., & Griffin, P. (1998a). *A guide to promoting children's reading success.* Washington, DC: National Research Council; National Academy Press.

Snow, C., Burns, M., & Griffin, P. (1998b). *Preventing reading difficulties in young children.* Washington, DC: National Research Council; National Academy Press.

Snow, C., Tabors, P., Nicholson, P., & Kurland, B. (1995). SHELL: Oral language and early literacy skills in kindergarten and first grade children. *Journal of Research in Childhood Education, 10*, 37–48.

Stahl, S. A. (1986). Three principles of effective vocabulary instruction. *Journal of Reading, 29*(7), 662–668.

Stahl, S. A. (1999). In J. S. Chall (Series Ed.), *From reading research to practice: Vol. 2. Vocabulary development.* Cambridge, MA: Brookline Books.

Stahl, S. A., and Murray, B. A. (1998). Issues involved in defining phonological awareness and its relation to early reading. In J. Metsala and L. C. Ehri (Eds.), *Word recognition in beginning literacy* (pp. 65–87). Mahwah, NJ: Erlbaum.

Stanovich, K. E. (1986). Matthew effects in reading: Some consequences of individual differences in the acquisition of literacy. *Reading Research Quarterly, 21*, 360–406.

Stanovich, K. E. (1992). Speculations on the causes and consequences of individual differences in early reading acquisition. In P. Gough, L. Ehri, and R. Treiman (Eds.), *Reading acquisition* (pp. 307–342). Hillsdale, NJ: Lawrence Erlbaum.

Stanovich, K. E. (1994). Constructivism in reading education. Special issue: Implications of constructivism for students with disabilities and students at risk: Issues and directions. *Journal of Special Education, 28*(3), 259–274.

Strickland, D. S., & Morrow, L. M. (1989). Assessment and early literacy (emergent readers and writers). *The Reading Teacher, 42*(8), 634–635.

Sulzby, E. (1985). Children's emergent reading of favorite storybooks: A developmental study. *Reading Research Quarterly, 20*(4), 458–481.

Sulzby, E., & Teale, W. (1991). Emergent literacy. In R. Barr, M. Kamil, P. Mosenthal, & P. D. Pearson (Eds.), *Handbook of reading research* (Vol. II, pp. 727–757). New York: Longman.

Taylor, D. (1983). *Family literacy: The social context of learning to read and write.* Exeter, NH: Heinemann.

Teale, W. H. (1982). Toward a theory of how children learn to read and write naturally. *Language Arts, 59*, 555–570.

Teale, W. H., & Sulzby, E. (Eds.). (1986). *Emergent literacy: Writing and reading.* Norwood, NJ: Ablex.

Teale, W. H., & Sulzby, E. (1989). Emergent literacy: New perspectives. In D. S. Strickland and L. M. Morrow

(Eds.), *Emerging literacy: Young children learn to read and write.* Newark, DE: International Reading Association.

Torgesen, J. K. (1998). Instructional interventions for children with reading disabilities. In B. K. Shapiro, P. J. Accardo, & A. J. Capute (Eds.), *Specific reading disability* (pp. 197–220). Timonium, MD: York Press.

Torgesen, J. K., & Mathes, P. G. (1998). *What every teacher should know about phonological awareness.* Tallahassee, FL: Florida State University, Florida Department of Education.

Torgesen, J. K., Wagner, R. K., & Rashotte, C. A. (1994). Longitudinal studies of phonological processing and reading. *Journal of Learning Disabilities, 27*(5), 276–286.

Torgesen, J. K., Wagner, R. K., Rashotte, C. A., Alexander, A. W., & Conway, T. (1997). Preventive and remedial interventions for children with severe reading disabilities. *Learning Disabilities: A Multidisciplinary Journal, 8*(1), 51–61.

Treiman, R. (1993). *Beginning to spell.* New York: Oxford University Press.

U.S. Census Bureau. (2003). *The Hispanic population in the United States: Population characteristics.* Washington, DC: Author.

United States Department of Education, America Reads Challenge (1999). *Start early, finish strong: How to help every child become a reader.* Washington, DC: Author.

Velluntino, F. R., & Scanlon, D. M. (1987). Phonological coding, phonological awareness, and reading ability: Evidence from a longitudinal and experimental study. *Merril-Palmer Quarterly, 33*(3), 321–363.

Weinstein-Shr, G., & Quintero, E. (Eds.). (1995). *Immigrant learners and their families.* McHenry, IL: Center for Applied Linguistics and Delta Systems.

Wilson, M. (1988). Critical thinking: Repackaging or revolution? *Language Arts, 65*(6), 543–551.

Yaden, D. B., Rowe, D. W., & MacGillivray, L. (1999). Emergent literacy: A matter (polyphony) of perspectives. In M. Kamil, P. B. Mosenthal, P. D. Pearson, & R. Barr (Eds.), *Handbook of reading research* (Vol. III). Mahwah, NJ: Lawrence Erlbaum. Also available as CIERA Report 1-005.

Yopp, H. K. (1992). Developing phonemic awareness in young children. *The Reading Teacher, 45,* 696–703.

Zygouris-Coe, V. (2002). The media specialist: The catalyst in school literacy plans. *Florida Media Quarterly, 28*(1), 28–30.

Reading and Writing Development for Bilingual Children (L1 and L2)

Alejandro Brice and Roanne G. Brice

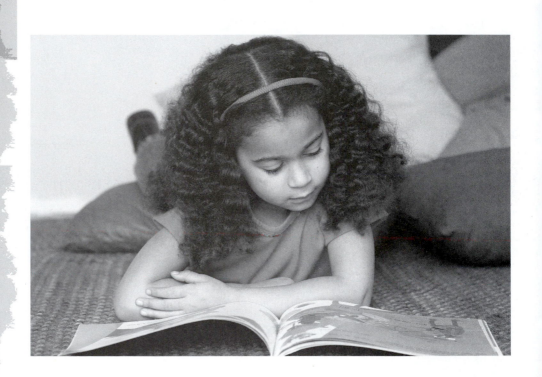

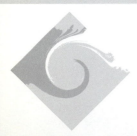

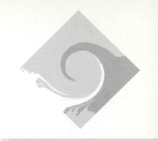

CHAPTER OUTLINE

INTRODUCTION

The ability to read is the most fundamental skill for children's success in school. Most children achieve this goal without any difficulty, while other children find it extremely difficult learning to read at even a basic level. It has been estimated that 95% of all school-age students can be taught to read (Spafford & Gosser, 1996). However, the issue of reading is more difficult for younger students; that is, 20 to 30% of elementary students have significant problems learning to read (Lyon, 1998; McEwan, 2002; Moats, 1999; Shaywitz, 1996). In addition, the U.S. Department of Education estimates that up to 38% of all fourth-grade students read below the most basic reading level (U.S. Department of Education, 2003b). Among all students, African American, Hispanic, English-language learners (ELLs), and students with disabilities are among the groups noted for reading failure (U.S. Department of Education, 2002).

Focus on Hispanic Students

Recent U.S. Census Bureau (2003) data indicates that the Hispanic population in the United States has reached a total of 35.3 million. In addition, the U.S. Census Bureau (2001) found that 35.7% of all U.S. Hispanics were less that 18 years of age (i.e., preschool or school age) compared with 23.5% of non-Hispanic Whites. It is safe to assume that a large percentage of these young Hispanic children are students who do not have a strong command of English. In addition, within the past decade, the English-language-learner student enrollment has increased at nearly eight times the rate of all student enrollment (Padolsky, 2002).

Since implementation of No Child Left Behind in 2002, the identification of children in need of reading remediation has significantly increased. Many students in schools come from diverse backgrounds, particularly homes where Spanish is the primary language. Less than one-third of all fourth-graders performed at the expected grade level, according to the National Assessment of Educational Progress Report (U.S. Department of Education, 2003a). Only 13% of Hispanic students performed at the expected fourth-grade level. These results indicate that Hispanic students are at risk for reading failure and as a group, they will need to close the educational gap with the other students (Brice, 2004).

Current research indicates that a large portion of Hispanic students with limited English skills are at risk for educational failure (England, Collins, & Algozzine, 2002) and are more than likely to be referred and placed in exceptional education programs (Brice, 2002; Ortiz, 1992; Wilkinson & Ortiz, 2003; Winzer & Mazuek, 1998). If referred, these students are most likely to be placed in exceptional-education services due to reading difficulties (Burnette, 1998; Donovan & Cross, 2002; International Reading Association, 2003). In sum, there is a high academic and reading failure rate of Hispanic/ELL students (U.S. Department of Education, 2003b). The International Reading Association (2003) is "particularly concerned that lack of appropriate reading instruction and early reading interventions among low-performing minority children is contributing to the overrepresentation of these children in . . . disability categories" (p. 2). Several researchers have noted that first- and second-language issues are associated with Hispanic students learning to read (Carlisle & Beeman, 2000; Ciscero & Royer, 1995; Durgunoglu, 2002; Durgunoglu & Öney, 2000). These studies will be discussed in further detail later in the chapter. However, a preliminary discussion of general bilingual issues is warranted.

Bilingual Issues

Speech-language pathology program placement, assessment, and instruction are often based on research and practices from monolingual students with disabilities. Vaughn, Mathes, Linan-Thompson, and Francis (2005) stated, "Special education identification, placement, and instruction decisions for students who are English-language learners

(ELLs) have been largely based on research and practices used with monolingual students with disabilities (Artiles & Ortiz)" (p. 58). Generalizing from monolingual students who may be at risk for reading difficulties to bilingual students who may be at risk for reading difficulties is problematic.

Most school professionals are English speaking and view learning from a monolingual perspective, although many preparation programs and school districts are now addressing the learning needs of ELL students. In addition, school professionals charged with teaching reading and writing have never taken formal Spanish coursework (Escamilla, 2000). Escamilla (2000) stated, "In fact, most teachers who are charged with teaching children to read and write in Spanish have never taken formal coursework in methods of teaching reading in Spanish (Guerrero, 1997)" (p. 102).

It should be noted that use of two languages does not create confusion, but rather upholds learning. Escamilla (2000) stated that her work demonstrated that children who are beginning Spanish-English bilinguals regularly use their two languages concurrently in reading and in classroom situations. Furthermore, these bilingual students use both languages (i.e., English and Spanish) even when they have had access only to formal instruction in Spanish. Escamilla's (2000) research indicates that use of both Spanish and English in literacy events "is not a source of confusion, but one of support" (p. 105). Consequently, it is apparent that Spanish reading skills are transferring to English reading. This seems to be true in Spanish as well as with other languages.

Ramírez (2000) stated that certain gaps of knowledge remain on how "the development of primary language listening skills influence[s] the development of second language listening skills and reading acquisition" (p. 28). He also noted that the synthesis of the current and future reading research with ELL students will "help contextualize biliteracy development within the current national literacy initiatives" (p. 30). Therefore, a greater understanding and discussion on the development of bilingualism and reading is warranted.

Gaps in the Bilingual Reading Research Database

In addressing issues relevant to the development of reading for English-language learners, the U.S. Department of Education commissioned the Office of Bilingual Education and Minority Language Affairs (OBEMLA) to gather reading information. As a consequence, a sponsored research symposium "High Standards in Reading for Students from Diverse Language Groups: Research, Practice, and Policy" resulted. This symposium presented the most current research on issues related to the teaching of reading skills to bilingual, English-language-learner students. In summary, the Office of Bilingual Education and Minority Language Affairs (2000) noted several gaps in reading research for the English-language-learner students. These gaps for future reading research are listed here:

1. Research gaps exist in how literacy in one's first language influences the acquisition of literacy in the second language (i.e., English). OBEMLA stated, "[W]hile there are similarities between different languages in how reading skills develop, there are also marked differences. These language differences impact the development of literacy skills in the second language" (p. 2). It was noted that not all studies incorporated comparisons of two languages into the respective reading

research designs. Therefore, OBEMLA concluded that more research with regard to how learning to read English is different for ELL students versus native English speakers was needed.

2. Research gaps exist regarding the use of English reading curricula with Spanish-speaking students. Increasing evidence indicates that the use of English pedagogy in Spanish curricula is not developmentally and/or culturally appropriate. Therefore, this area warrants further research.

3. Research gaps also exist on what speech-language pathologists and teachers need to know in order to provide effective literacy instruction to English-language-learner students. Future research is needed in defining best practices for teaching reading to ELL students who may or may not have literacy skills in their own language.

HOW LITERACY IN THE FIRST LANGUAGE AFFECTS LITERACY IN THE SECOND LANGUAGE

Cummins (1984) stated that a **common underlying proficiency (CUP) model** exists in the bilingual brain. According to this model, learned aspects of one language are transferable to the learning of a second language. This suggests that a positive transfer between the two language exists; that is, the two languages are interdependent (Cummins, 1984). Cummins (1984) stated that "a theoretical model of bilingual proficiency is proposed in which a 'common underlying' proficiency is hypothesized to underlie the surface manifestations of both L1 [first language] and L2 [second language] making possible the transfer of cognitive/academic skills across languages" (p. 6).

On the other hand, the **script-dependent hypothesis** asserts that skills in one language are influenced by its orthography and phoneme-grapheme correspondence. That is, language-specific rules influence the ability or inability of languages to transfer information. Lipka, Siegel, and Vukovic (2005) suggest that language-specific circuits regarding reading exist. Therefore, the script-dependent hypothesis would suggest that a child whose first language is Spanish would not experience difficulties in reading Spanish but might experience considerable difficulty in reading English due to some features of reading not transferring because first-language features interfere with the process. What is most likely is that some features of literacy transfer (common underlying proficiencies model), while some language-specific features may not transfer (script-dependent hypothesis).

Three known features seem to have a pronounced effect on second-language literacy acquisition: (1) age of second-language acquisition, (2) first-language proficiency levels, and (3) second-language acquisition proficiency levels (Illes, Francis, Desmond, Gabrieli, Glover, Poldrack, Lee, & Wagner, 1999). Hakuta (1986) stated, "The real question is the identification of the conditions under which the two languages maintain separation and those under which they are apparently merged" (pp. 94–95). Moats (1999) stated:

> The language skills that most reliably distinguish good and poor readers are specific to the phonological or speech-sound processing system . . . [other] skills include awareness of linguistic units that lie within a word (consonants, vowels) . . . and fluency in recognition and recall of letters (p. 16).

Therefore, it is not surprising that a number of studies in literacy research have focused on phonological or phonemic awareness. Research with monolingual children has indicated substantial evidence that learning to read is dependent upon a child's phonological and phonemic skills (Adams, 1990; Carlisle, Beeman, Davis, Spharim, 1999; Hulme, Hatcher, Nation, Brown, Adams, & Stuart, 2002; National Reading Panel, 2000; Snow, Burns, & Griffin, 1998; Wagner & Torgesen, 1987). Research on bilingual literacy is relatively sparse (Denton, Anthony, Parker, & Hasbrouck, 2004), and research on the cross-linguistic transfer (e.g., Spanish to English) on literacy development is even more limited (Durgunoglu & Öney, 2000).

This chapter will address the following bilingual literacy issues: (1) cross-linguistic transfer (Spanish to English) of phonological/phonemic awareness, (2) cross-linguistic transfer of Spanish to English phonics, (3) cross-linguistic transfer of Spanish to English vocabulary, (4) cross-linguistic transfer of reading fluency, (5) cross-linguistic transfer of comprehension, (6) language of instruction affecting transfer of attained reading skills in Spanish to English reading, (7) reading development in other languages, (8) writing and bilingual strategies, and (9) brain regions involved in bilingual reading. In our review of the literature, we found that the majority of studies investigating bilingual literacy issues focused on phonological/phonemic awareness issues versus phonics, vocabulary, fluency, or comprehension.

Phonological and Phonemic Awareness

Phonological awareness is the ability to manipulate syllables and sounds within words. Phonemic awareness is a subcategory of phonological awareness, which refers to awareness and sensitivity to phonemes. Examples of phonemic awareness include (1) identifying and making oral rhymes, (2) identifying syllables in spoken words, (3) identifying and working with onsets (initial consonant-vowel or consonant-consonant of words) and rimes (the syllable that follows the onset) in spoken syllables, (4) identifying and working with individual phonemes in spoken words, (5) deleting sounds or syllables from words, and (6) grouping words that begin with the same sounds.

As previously stated, phonological and phonemic awareness studies in Spanish have been limited. A number of studies have included only Spanish speakers (Chiappe, Siegel, & Gottardo, 2002; Cisero & Royer, 1995), while other studies have included bilingual speakers (e.g., Spanish-English bilinguals or Spanish-Catalan bilinguals) (Brice, 2004; Brice, Castellon-Perez, & Ryalls, 2004; Navarra, Sebastián-Galles, & Soto-Franco, 2005). Only a small number of studies have addressed phonemic awareness skills solely in Spanish (Adrian, Alegria, & Morais, 1995; Dickinson, McCabe, Clark-Chiarelli, & Wolf, 2004). As with English phonemic awareness studies, a variety of procedures to elicit phonemic and/or phonological awareness have been used: (1) phoneme discrimination (Brice et al., 2004; Navarra et al., 2005), (2) rhyming (Cisero & Royer, 1995), (3) phoneme deletion (Dickinson, et al., 2004), and (4) rapid automatized naming (Chiappe, et al., 2002).

There exists a great need for specific research in how Spanish phonemic awareness affects English phonemic awareness and beginning reading (i.e., cross-linguistic transfer). Grandmaison, Cormier, Comeau, and Lacroix (1996) stated that few studies provide data that "support the expectation that phonological processing skills play a role in the prediction of reading achievement in a second language" (p. 5).

Spanish Phonological and Phonemic Awareness

Rhyming seems to develop prior to literacy acquisition among Spanish speakers (Adrian, Alegria, & Morais, 1995). However, conscious manipulation of syllables appears to be difficult for Spanish-speaking nonreaders. Spanish-speaking students tend to develop prereading skills in a particular order. They gain sensitivity to (a) syllables, (b) onsets, (c) rimes, and finally (d) individual phonemes (Denton, Hashbrouck, Weaver, & Riccio, 2000). Spanish-speaking children from Argentina who were either prereaders or beginning readers could identify the number of syllables in words about 50% of the time, but could only identify sounds (phonemes) from 5% (preschoolers) to 35% (first graders) of the time (Manrique & Gramigna, 1984). Spanish-speaking prereaders showed sensitivity to rhyme (words ending the same way) and alliteration (words beginning the same way) (Carillo, 1994). Hence, syllable identification seems easier for some Spanish-speaking children. A student's ability to segment Spanish words into syllables may be more important than his or her ability to segment words into phonemes. In Spanish, there is a continued emphasis on the letter-sound and syllable correspondence, up to third grade, more so than in English (Signorini, 1997). Spanish is more phonetically based than English; thus, the letter-sound correspondence plays a less significant role in decoding words than it does in English. Children who received instruction in Spanish letter-sound correspondence were able to isolate onset from rime in simple words (Carillo, 1994). According to Adrian et al. (1995), tasks that separated prereaders from early readers included (1) **phoneme segmentation** (pronouncing separate sounds in words) and (2) segmenting tasks. These phonemic awareness tasks also separated average from poor first-grade readers. According to Adrian et al. (1995), rhyme detection is a skill that no longer needs instruction by first grade.

Some of the more difficult phonemic awareness tasks for Spanish speakers include **phoneme deletion** (repeating the word without a sound), **syllable deletion** (repeating the word without a syllable), word reversal, and phoneme reversal. For Spanish-speaking prekindergarten and kindergarten children, continuants (e.g., /m/ or /s/) were easier to identify on phoneme isolation tasks than were stops (e.g., /p/ or /t/). Initial consonants in a blend (CC) were more difficult to identify than were initial single consonants (CV) (González & Garcia, 1995).

Spanish-English Phonological and Phonemic Awareness

Currently, there is a need for research in how Spanish phonemic awareness affects English phonemic awareness and consequently beginning reading. Lindsey, Manis, and Bailey (2003) found that Spanish phonological awareness has a relationship to word reading, as it does in English. In their study, they found that phonological awareness skills transferred from Spanish to English and were also predictive of word identification skills, i.e., letter knowledge and word knowledge. They found that Spanish phonological awareness to Spanish word identification was no greater than Spanish phonological awareness to English word identification. Spanish phonological awareness was equally successful in producing word identification in either language. Consequentially, phonological awareness appeared to be a general, not a specific, cognitive reading process.

Brice (2004) investigated English phonemic awareness and phonic skills in four groups of kindergarten students with and without disabilities. The groups consisted of 20 high-reading-level English monolinguals, 20 low-reading-level English monolinguals, 20 high-reading-level English-Spanish-speaking bilinguals, and 20 low-reading-level English-Spanish-speaking bilinguals. Brice (2004) found an existing achievement gap between monolingual and bilingual students with and without disabilities, even at the kindergarten level, on a phoneme and letter identification task. All students (high monolingual readers, high bilingual readers, low monolingual readers, and low bilingual readers) in her study consistently identified words with voiced phonemes more often than words with voiceless phonemes. Therefore, the issue of voicing seems to have an important role in helping young emerging readers differentiate among the different phonemes. These results support the earlier findings of Ricio, Amado, Jiménez, Hasbrouck, Imhoff, & Denton (2001), who found that identifying initial sounds, final sounds, and rime seems to relate to reading fluency in Spanish and transfer to reading fluency in English. Hence, some phonemic awareness tasks can transfer between Spanish and English.

Phonics

Phonics is the sound-to-letter (graphophonemic) connection between spoken sounds and written letters (Armbuster, Lehr, & Osborn, 2001). Some English-language-learner students may be at risk for reading difficulties because they face the simultaneous and dual language challenges of learning to speak and read English simultaneously (Brisk & Harrington, 2000). These students will most likely struggle to acquire basic phonemic awareness and phonics skills. Ramírez (2000) clarified this point when he stated:

> [L]anguage development emerges as a unique issue for English-language learners, specifically, the importance of oral receptive language and production skills. Knowing the sounds of [a] language is a precondition for being able to match it to print. Learning the actual patterns of a language requires extensive experiences with the words of that language through reading and writing (pp. 15–16).

Durgunoglu (as reported in Carlisle & Beeman, 2000) stated that English spelling is influenced by good skills in phonological awareness and letter knowledge in the native language. In addition, Lindsey et al. (2003) found that letter knowledge, print concepts, sentence memory, and rapid automatic naming speed all showed correlations with English word identification and reading comprehension.

Other factors such as short-term, immediate, and working memory have also influenced phonics abilities in transference from the native language to English. Lindsey et al. (2003) found that Spanish-English-speaking children were able to transfer word decoding skills (including phonics abilities) from Spanish to English. English vocabulary development and English memory for sentences, however, developed more slowly. Spanish measures in kindergarten (print knowledge, phonological awareness, rapid auditory naming [RAN], and expressive language) correlated with English reading measures (English print knowledge, phonological awareness, RAN,

TABLE 8–1
Teaching English Phonics Skills

Phonics Skill	Strategy
Analogy phonics	Teach students new words to known words by means of analogy (e.g., recognizing that the rime segment [syllable that follows the initial CC or CV of a word] of an unfamiliar word is identical to a known or familiar word. For example, recognizing in the word *br-ick* that the *ick* is the same as in the word *s-ick*.
Analytic phonics	Teach students to analyze letter-sound relations in previously rehearsed and learned words to avoid incorrect pronunciation sounds in isolation. For example, the "at" sound appears in the words *pat* and *cat*.
Embedded phonics	Embed phonics instruction in text reading, and use a more implicit approach that relies on incidental teaching.
Phonics through spelling	Teach students to segment words into phonemes and to select letters for those phonemes (i.e., teach students to spell words phonemically).
Synthetic phonics	Teach students to convert letters into sounds (phonemes) and then to blend these sounds to form identifiable words.

Source: National Reading Panel, 2000.

expressive language, letter-word identification, and passage comprehension) in second grade. In addition, phonological awareness and rapid auditory naming were unique predictors of English word identification. In sum, print knowledge in Spanish was found to be the strongest predictor of English letter-word identification and English passage comprehension. The strongest English language predictors for reading were phonological awareness and RAN.

Children learning English as a second language may need specific English reading instruction in (1) learning a core set of frequently used English consonants and short vowel sounds, (2) blending and segmenting sounds to read and spell in decodable text, (3) separating sounds with similar visual and auditory features, (4) learning that some letters represent more than one sound, (5) learning that letters in English can make more than one sound, and (6) learning that English sounds can be represented by a single letter or combination of letters. See Table 8–1.

Vocabulary

Two basic types of vocabulary exist, that is, oral and print (National Reading Panel, 2000). A connection between vocabulary and reading has long been established (National Reading Panel, 2000). Carlisle, Beeman, Davis, and Spharim (1999) stated that bilingual children might experience difficulties in reading English because of their limited English vocabulary. In their study, they found that performance on definitions in English and Spanish was affected by word knowledge in the language of the task (e.g., Spanish word knowledge) and performance of definitions in the other language (e.g., English). Overall, the child's level of bilingualism did not affect his or her word definitions. Native- and second-language vocabulary and phonological awareness each contributed independently to English reading

TABLE 8–2
Teaching Vocabulary

1. Vocabulary should be taught through both direct and indirect means.
2. Vocabulary should incorporate repetition and multiple exposure to vocabulary items.
3. Learning vocabulary in stimulating contexts is valuable.
4. Vocabulary tasks should be restructured when necessary.
5. Vocabulary learning should involve active student involvement.
6. Computers and Internet sites can be used to assist teaching vocabulary.
7. Vocabulary can be learned incidentally.
8. How vocabulary is assessed can have different effects on how it is taught.
9. Reliance on a single vocabulary method of instruction does not result in the best learning situations for the students.

comprehension. For young bilinguals with limited native-language development, vocabulary development in both languages was important for English reading comprehension. Carlisle et al.'s (1999) results provide support that first- and second-language vocabulary contributed to both formal and informal definitions in the same language. The child's degree of bilingualism contributed to the child's ability to give informal definitions in Spanish but not in English. The child's degree of bilingualism also contributed to giving formal definitions in both languages. Therefore, some transfer in informal definitions was found (from L1 to L2 only), while cross-transfer of formal definitions between L1 and L2 was found. However, a significant factor in reading comprehension was the extensiveness of the child's vocabulary in the first language and the second language, and also his or her phonological awareness. Therefore, phonological awareness skills also affect vocabulary development in both languages.

Proctor, Carlo, August, and Snow (2005) stated that English vocabulary knowledge appears to be significant for English-language learners reading English. Carlisle et al. (1999) found that with beginning-level Spanish-English readers, English vocabulary and phonological awareness each made independent contributions to English reading comprehension. Depth of vocabulary and word comprehension are factors in word knowledge and reading comprehension.

Vocabulary can be taught directly by (1) teaching specific words before a reading activity, (2) teaching word learning strategies, (3) providing instruction for specific words, and (4) teaching specific words before reading activities. See Table 8–2.

Reading Fluency

Fluency is the ability to read text quickly and accurately. Fluent readers group words together. Fluency is important because it provides a bridge between word recognition and comprehension. Lindsey, Manis, and Bailey (2003) stated that accurate word recognition is vital for fluent reading and reading comprehension. Oral reading practice and feedback given by speech-language pathologists and teachers can influence a child's abilities in word knowledge, reading speed, and oral accuracy. Strategies for teaching fluency in Spanish reading should be similar to general reading fluency strategies, which include (1) student-adult reading, (2) choral reading, (3) reader's theater, (4) use of explicit instruction and modeling, (5) tape-assisted reading, and (6) partner reading (see Chapter 7).

Reading Comprehension

Comprehension involves both literal comprehension and inferential comprehension. **Literal comprehension** is the ability to understand the factual meaning of the text, while **inferential comprehension** allows the reader to make conjectures, assumptions, deductions, and conclusions from the reading.

Carlisle and Beeman (2000) found that successful Latino bilingual readers were able to apply their knowledge of Spanish to their English reading comprehension. Unsuccessful bilingual readers treated their two languages as unrelated and did not employ strategies for using their first language. Miller, Heilmann, Nockerts, Iglesias, Fabiano, and Francis (2006) found that cross-language comparisons revealed that English oral language skills (narrative skills, number of different words measured as lexemes, number of words read per minute) predicted Spanish reading comprehension and word reading efficiency. In addition, Spanish oral language skills predicted English reading skills. Therefore, reading abilities in the native language seem to aid comprehension abilities in the second language. This supports building strong reading skills in the native language and then building on these skills for English reading.

Durgunoglu and Öney (2000) stated that an important aspect of listening comprehension for bilingual children is vocabulary and background knowledge. Background knowledge is also related to experiences with one's language and culture. In addition, cognate knowledge between Spanish and English should assist English reading comprehension. **Cognates** are similar-sounding and -meaning words in two languages, for example, *exitar* (Spanish) and *to excite* (English).

Comprehension improvement occurs when school professionals demonstrate, explain, model, and implement reading interaction with students in teaching them how to comprehend a text. In studies where even a few hours of preparation were given, school professionals taught students who were poor readers, but adequate decoders, to apply various strategies to texts. These skills were taught in reading groups, with the school professional demonstrating, guiding, or modeling the strategies, and with directed scaffolding.

Language of Instruction

The question of which language to use for providing therapy and instruction has long been debated. Brice and Roseberry-McKibbin (2001) reported, "The current literature supports the notion that the native or home language is the best medium for working with children and adds to the child's ability to communicate in the second language (i.e., English)" (p. 10). This is supported by the research from Thomas and Collier (2002). They reported that children who had a minimum of two to three years of instruction in their native language had superior school achievement when compared to children whose experiences were in English only. Hence, the language of instruction interacts with the child's level of language proficiency.

Carlisle and Beeman (2000) investigated the relationship between instruction in Spanish and English and related literacy proficiency levels in both languages. They performed an exploratory study of teaching literacy skills to first-grade Hispanic students. At the beginning of the fall, Spanish-English-speaking first- and second-grade students were administered language and reading tests. During the spring semester (for the first-grade students), the students were given listening and reading comprehension tests and writing tests in both Spanish and English. Students taught in Spanish did not differ from those taught in English on English reading and writing; they were significantly stronger on Spanish reading and writing. Therefore, instruction in Spanish was beneficial to reading and writing in Spanish and English. For the second-grade students, Spanish and English vocabulary gains were significant. Spanish literacy instruction resulted in Spanish reading comprehension gains. English literacy instruction did not result in English reading comprehension gains. Carlise and Beeman (2000) stated, "Three factors emerge from various studies of biliteracy. These are proficiency in the native language, proficiency in the second language, and the extent to which students have opportunities in school to develop their native- and second-language abilities" (p. 333).

READING DEVELOPMENT IN OTHER LANGUAGES

Vandergrift (2006) investigated the influence of the first-language (English) listening comprehension and proficiency in the second language (French) to second-language listening comprehension (French). The study was conducted in an urban school in Canada. The students completed tests in both languages, listened to conversation in French, and later completed multiple-choice listening comprehension questions. Vandergrift found that first-language listening comprehension and second-language proficiency contributed to French (L2) comprehension. Second-language proficiency was a better predictor of L2 listening comprehension than L1 comprehension. Therefore, listening comprehension appears to be a general skill affected by language proficiency and abilities.

Palmer, Chen, Chang, and Leclare (2006) reported that Chinese students read classroom assigned texts for memorization and spelling. Chinese students may not be as prepared for English syntax because Chinese grammar tends to be simple compared to English. In addition, Palmer reports, "[T]here are also obvious differences in semantics and word choices between the Chinese and English languages" (p. 250). An example is the absence of articles in Chinese; therefore, Chinese language interference may impede a Chinese-English-speaking student using articles in written English.

Gottardo, Chiappe, Yan, Siegel, and Gu (2006) investigated the relationship between first- and second-language phonological awareness (i.e., processing) and also reading skills in Chinese-English-speaking students. They studied 40 students who spoke Cantonese as their first language and were enrolled in an English-speaking school in Canada. The students' ages ranged from 6 to 13 years. Measures of word reading, pseudoword reading, and character reading, were administered. Their findings indicated that phonological awareness and rapid naming were related to English reading. For Chinese reading measures that required phonological strategies, however, pseudocharacter reading was related to phonological processing. The authors concluded, "[P]honological processing is most strongly related to reading tasks that require the use of phonological information in non-alphabetic languages" (p. 389).

Verhoeven (2000) studied the reading and spelling development of Dutch-speaking children and non-native-Dutch-speaking children from various countries. A total of 2,143 children from 118 elementary schools participated. Tests for word decoding, word spelling, grapheme knowledge, word blending, and phoneme segmentation in Dutch were administered. The students were enrolled in first and second grades. The linguistically diverse group of students was able to keep up with their Dutch peers when compared on word decoding (word blending) in their first year of school. They did exhibit difficulties with Dutch alphabet knowledge. The author believes that this finding was attributable to their less than full Dutch auditory discrimination abilities, which in turn impeded their ability to quickly map correct Dutch pronunciation to letters. After two years of school instruction, the linguistically diverse students were "as efficient as . . . their native-Dutch speaking peers" (p. 326). All children made the most progress with consonant-vowel-consonant (CVC) words, followed by consonant-consonant (CC) blends, and then by multisyllabic words. This finding seems to indicate a developmental progression of reading that is universal across orthographic languages.

The linguistically diverse students fell behind their Dutch-speaking peers in spelling and phoneme segmentation. They also lagged behind their Dutch-speaking peers in terms of Dutch vocabulary. Their lesser vocabulary skills put them at risk for reading at both the word and sentence levels. The linguistically diverse group of children also showed lags in terms of their Dutch reading comprehension. Apparently, the linguistically diverse group of children was able to acquire some emerging reading skills in a period of two years, but they still lagged behind in other areas. This is not surprising because it may take five to seven years to fully acquire academic skills such as reading (Cummins, 1984). The author recommended strengthening their native language skills and vocabulary skills in Dutch prior to formal L2 reading.

WRITING AND BILINGUAL STRATEGIES

As with oral language, children progress through various writing stages; however, the fundamental difference is that spoken language is acquired, while writing needs to be taught. Children in kindergarten begin to (1) use letters, (2) phonetically spell words, and (3) write words and brief sentences. Children in kindergarten also begin to write stories about people and events in their lives, and to use lower- and uppercase letters. Students begin with short CVC words and then progress to more complex words (Duran & Shefelbine, 2003).

Children whose first language is Spanish have an advantage because Spanish is more of a phonetic language than English. Therefore, Spanish orthography is easier for bilingual Spanish-speaking students to acquire. These students may not go through the same stages of **invented spelling** (spelling words as they may sound or as children believe they should be spelled) as English-speaking children because of the closer sound-to-letter correspondence in Spanish than in English. In addition, the reading research generally suggests that reading skills transfer from the native language to English; therefore, it would seem apparent that most writing skills would also transfer from one orthographic language to another.

Students in kindergarten and first grade use their phonics skills (sound-to-letter correspondence skills) to write unknown words. Students at this stage begin to recognize that writing is communication and also a process; for example, they give descriptions of events (Duran & Shefelbine, 2003).

Typically, second-grade students begin to write complete sentences that are coherent. They write using the process of prewriting, drafting, revising, and editing their work. Children should be encouraged to use their native-language skills in thinking through these cognitive writing stages.

Interactive writing occurs when the speech-language pathologist (SLP) or teacher and the student co-write collaborative stories. SLPs and teachers model, demonstrate, and provide feedback through this interactive stage. Students can then chorally read with the SLP and/or school professional on their jointly created story (Duran & Shefelbine, 2003).

Writing is a process that occurs in stages: prewriting, drafting, editing and revising, and publishing (Graves, 1985). In the prewriting stage, the students and school professional talk freely about what they know and what the story should involve. This language experience approach enables students to express themselves on topics that they know and feel comfortable about. Encouraging students to talk and think creatively should be done in the language children feel most comfortable in expressing themselves. In the drafting stage, students write their initial story. The focus is not on spelling, punctuation, or grammar. In the editing and revising stages, the focus turns to correct grammar and/or spelling. Students can then publish their written work. This final step allows students to share their work and to feel proud of their written accomplishments.

BRAIN REGIONS FOR BILINGUAL READERS

Bilingual Brain Activation

Current trends in neuroimaging have allowed researchers to investigate which areas of the brain are activated (i.e., involved) during reading for bilingual individuals. (See also Chapter 1 for a discussion of the neurological correlates of language.) Results from a study by Kim, Relkin, Lee, and Hirsch (cited in Simos, Billingsley-Marshall, Sarkari, Pataraia, & Papanicolaou, 2005) using functional magnetic resonance imaging (fMRI) to compare early versus late bilinguals found that late bilinguals exhibited proximally close brain activation areas for the bilinguals' two languages in the inferior frontal lobe regions (areas for the generation of utterances and language). No separation was found for the two languages in the posterior temporal lobes (the areas necessary for perception, analysis, and comprehension of spoken language). For the early bilinguals, no significant separation of the two languages in any of the brain areas was noted. Simos et al. (2005) stated that for Indo-European languages (e.g., French, Italian, Spanish, German, Portuguese, Dutch, and English), cortical regions of activation are not expected to be language-specific, but instead to depend on variables such as the age when the second language was acquired and the language proficiency levels for each language. In sum, Simos et al. (2005) found activated regions of the brain common to both languages, and one or two activation regions that were language-specific.

Do two languages demonstrate language invariance versus language-specific circuits, that is, overlapping versus distinct language systems for literacy? Pugh, Sandak, Frost, Moore, and Menel (2005) stated, "There is some evidence suggesting that fluent bilingual readers tend to engage primarily overlapping circuits for both L1 and L2" (p. 24). They also stated, "Whereas most studies have reported largely overlapping systems for the spoken forms of L1 and L2 in fluent bilinguals, the degree of overlap appears to depend heavily upon factors such as age of acquisition and perhaps most importantly, degree of proficiency" (p. 25). Lexical retrieval does not appear to differ in transparent (e.g., Spanish) versus opaque (e.g., English) orthographies.

Word Recognition

Nueroimaging studies for alphabetic languages (e.g., Italian and English) indicate that left hemisphere cortical regions involved in word recognition and sentence processing include occipitotemporal, tempoparietal, and inferior frontal networks. Pugh et al. (2005) stated, "Language-specific differences appear to be mostly a matter of degree, and not of kind" (p. 26). The dorsal system includes the angular gyrus, the supramarginal gyrus, the inferior parietal lobe, and the posterior portion of the superior temporal gyrus (also known as Wernicke's area). The dorsal region seems to involve mapping letters onto their respective phonemic and semantic language aspects; correspondingly, it decodes print in beginning readers (Pugh et al., 2005). The inferior frontal gyrus (Broca's area) is associated with phonological recoding for reading (phonological memory, syntactic processing). The tempoparietal lobe is more affected by low-frequency words. The ventral system (forward portion of the brain) is late developing and supports fluent reading after initial reading instruction. See Figure 8–1.

Children with Reading Disabilities

Pugh et al. (2005) found that children with reading disabilities underuse the left hemisphere posterior dorsal areas and ventral areas (e.g., superior temporal area, supramarginal gyrus, and the angular gyrus) in word and pseudoword reading. Reduced connectivity between these areas for reading-disabled children has been noted. Therefore, children with reading disabilities compensate with reduced left hemisphere functions and include increased right hemisphere posterior sites and increased dual hemisphere activation in the inferior frontal gyrus. The higher the reading rate among children, the greater the response of the left hemisphere ventral cortex. In sum, the left hemisphere ventral system appears to be critical for fluent word recognition (Pugh et al., 2005).

FIGURE 8–1
Broca's Area, Inferior Parietal Lobe, Supramarginal Gyrus, Angular Gyrus, and Wernicke's Area

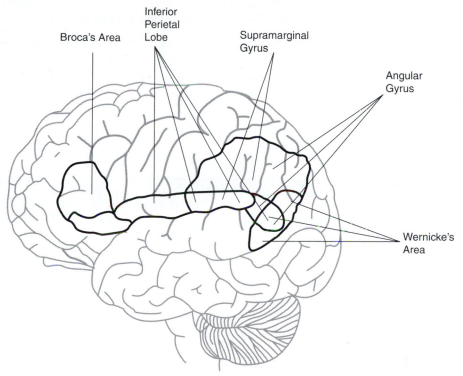

Research by Fletcher, Simos, Shaywitz, Shaywitz, Pugh, and Papanicolaou (2000) indicates that anterior regions of the brain in the left hemisphere involving the frontal lobes have to do with production, while posterior brain regions (temporal and parietal lobes) involve comprehension. Activation patterns are different according to whether translation or alternating languages is required. Translation leads to activation in the prefrontal and subcortical areas, whereas alternating languages activate areas of the frontal lobes (Broca's area) associated with phonological coding. Activation profiles of poor readers compared to adults who read well have found reduced blood flow in the left temporoparietal area when reading and processing phonological tasks. Normal activation in the left inferior frontal areas for the poor readers was noted. Left angular gyrus activity was observed during a phonological task with proficient readers, but it was noted to be absent in poor readers. According to Fletcher et al. (2000), listening to words involved the angular gyrus, Wernicke's area, and the superior temporal gyrus. Children with reading problems activated the temporoparietal areas of the right hemisphere.

Summary of Findings

With regard to how the brain organization is different in monolingual versus bilingual individuals, findings across studies (Fletcher et al., 2000; Pugh et al., 2005; Simos et al., 2005) indicate that the organization of language is likely to vary according to:

1. The age at which the person became bilingual: early bilinguals show less separation between areas of the brain than late bilinguals.

2. The level of proficiency: Individuals who are more proficient show less separation than those who are less fluent.

3. The area of the brain and the task involved: there is more separation in anterior areas of the brain (production) than in posterior areas (perception and comprehension).

CASE STUDY PERSPECTIVES

Case Study One Background: Robert

Robert is a high-reading-level English monolingual student of kindergarten age. He has taken the Dynamic Indicators of Basic Early Literacy Skills (DIBELS), which are standardized, individually administered tests of early literacy development. For kindergarten, the DIBELS measures initial sounds fluency, letter naming fluency, phoneme segmentation fluency, and nonsense word fluency. All of Robert's DIBELS scores were in the low-risk range. In addition, his kindergarten teacher reported near the end of the school year that he was very low risk for literacy difficulties based on his classroom performance.

Case Study One Comments: Robert

Robert is developing normally with his phonemic awareness, letter, and fluency skills. The classroom kindergarten teacher has expressed no concerns, so it appears that no special intervention is needed. Robert should be able to blend and segment sounds, and read and spell decodable real words.

Case Study Two Background: Carol

Carol is a low-reading-level English monolingual student. She is receiving speech and language therapy twice weekly for articulation errors. Her DIBELS scores varied and she was judged to be at risk and moderate risk for reading difficulties. In addition, the kindergarten teacher reported near the end of the school year that she was at moderate to high risk for reading difficulties based on classroom performance. Carol has difficulties with beginning sounds, rhyming, blending, and segmenting. In addition, it has been noted that she has difficulty staying on task and completing assignments without the school professional redirecting her back to the task.

Case Study Two Comments: Carol

Carol should continue with her speech therapy for her articulation errors because these production mistakes may influence her ability to correctly perceive and identify speech sounds. The speech-language pathologist (SLP) and classroom teacher should also provide direct therapy and instruction in identifying beginning sounds, rhyming patterns, blending sounds in single consonant-vowel-consonant (CVC) syllables, and decoding simple CVC syllables. The lessons should be short to maintain her attention. However, the SLP and teacher should model, demonstrate, provide opportunities for practice, and provide immediate feedback.

Case Study Three Background: Stella

Stella is a high-reading-level Spanish-English bilingual kindergarten student. Stella has had very limited exposure to English (less than one year, i.e., while in kindergarten). On four of the six DIBELS tests she scored low risk. Her kindergarten teacher reported that Stella's low risk is also based on her classroom performance. Stella speaks mostly English and some Spanish at school.

Her parents reported that both of them speak Spanish in the home. Stella speaks English and Spanish equally at home. The school professional has noted that Stella has good listening skills, can complete initial and final phoneme identification tasks, and can identify initial and final letters, yet she displays some difficulty switching classroom tasks.

Case Study Three Comments: Stella

It would be expected that Stella is still acquiring oral English. Cummins (1984) refers to this as basic interpersonal communication skills (see Chapter 4). In fact, this stage of acquisition can take from two to three years of speaking the second language. In addition, Stella is still acquiring her cognitive academic language skills, which can take up to seven years of speaking English. Therefore, Stella's ability to complete cognitively challenging tasks of initial and final phoneme identification and initial and final letters is a testament to her high abilities. It would be natural to need more time to process a second language; thus, her difficulty switching classroom tasks may be attributed to her learning English as a second language. Stella should receive additional classroom support from the teacher to assist her with English-processing abilities.

Case Study Four Background: Javier

Javier is a Spanish-English-bilingual kindergarten student with low reading abilities. All of his DIBELS scores placed him at risk for reading difficulties. His kindergarten classroom teacher reported him to be at very high risk for reading difficulties based on his classroom performance. His performance is lower than that of other bilingual students in the classroom. Javier has difficulty in initial phoneme and letter identification and in segmenting beginning sounds. He is unable to identify final sounds or letters. He speaks mostly English with some Spanish at school. His parents reported that they both speak only Spanish at home, while he speaks mostly Spanish and some English.

Case Study Four Comments: Javier

It appears that Javier may have reading difficulties and also may have difficulties associated with his learning English as a second language. Javier's difficulties may not be solely due to his speaking a second language. He should be monitored through a response-to-intervention assessment. If he continues to demonstrate difficulties, he should then be referred for a bilingual speech-language evaluation by a professional trained in assessing bilingual children, and optimally a diagnostician who is Spanish-English-speaking. In addition, Javier should receive assistance from the classroom teacher and SLP in identifying English sounds and English letters, letter naming fluency, and CVC word identification. He should also be provided therapy to segment CVC words. As they did for Carol in Case Study Two, the SLP and teacher should model, demonstrate, provide opportunities for practice, and provide immediate feedback.

INSTRUCTIONAL STRATEGIES

Types of collaboration with general-education classroom teachers, exceptional-education teachers, and/or other school professionals vary from consultation to collaboration, to co-teaching lessons (refer to Chapter 12 for further discussion). It is recommended that speech-language pathologists (SLPs) and classroom teachers make appropriate accommodations and provide strategies to enhance reading instruction. Additional strategies may be needed to enhance reading and writing instruction. Therefore, it is suggested that speech-language pathologists, classroom teachers, and exceptional-education teachers work together to implement the following practices:

1. Specific instruction for students should be provided for place of articulation of sounds, manner of articulation, and aspects of voicing (i.e., if sounds are voiced or voiceless). This should assist phonemic awareness instruction. Direct instruction in place, manner, and voicing may reduce the number of phonemic interference errors between the native language and English for those bilingual students.

2. It is suggested that the general-education classroom teacher have the student say words aloud during initial and final phoneme identification tasks. The student receives auditory feedback as he or she says the words. In addition, the SLP and/or teacher should pay attention to errors and provide immediate corrective feedback by giving a correct model.

3. It is recommended that SLPs and other school professionals (1) teach a core set of frequently used consonants and short vowel sounds, (2) begin to blend and segment sounds to read and spell in decodable text, (3) separate the sounds with similar visual and auditory features, (4) teach that some letters represent more than one sound, (5) teach that different letters can make the same sound, and (6) teach that sounds can be represented by a single letter or a combination. In addition, the SLP and school professional may add a kinesthetic component to the teaching of letters (e.g., manually tracing letters) or color-code consonants and vowels to aid discrimination and differentiation between consonants and vowels.

4. It is recommended that segmentation skills, specifically syllable and phoneme segmentation, be taught and reinforced. The SLP and teacher may segment longer words into syllables for easier phoneme and grapheme identification. Phoneme segmentation should begin with one-syllable words. As the students become more proficient at this task, then words of multiple syllables may be taught. This will help bilingual students and students with disabilities process sufficient chunks of information according to their auditory memory capabilities.

5. Allow students to draw from their personal experiences, using a language experiences approach (LEA), in creating personal stories. When writing, it is helpful for students to draw pictures to add their personal contextualization to the story (Figueroa & Ruiz, 1997). Figueroa and Ruiz stated that when children bring their own experiences to literacy, then they are more likely to be engaged and active participants in their learning.

CONCLUDING REMARKS

The abilities to read and write are the most basic skills necessary for all children, including bilingual children, to achieve success in school. Speech-language pathologists, general-education classroom teachers, and exceptional-education teachers all play a key role in teaching bilingual students to read and write. Speech-language pathologists, educators, and students can benefit from the latest research. This chapter has attempted to provide information regarding reading and writing skills in students from bilingual-speaking backgrounds. The aim is that *all* children will learn to read and write, have access to the general-education curriculum, and ultimately succeed in school and life. Therefore, as SLPs, teachers, and school professionals, our job is to give all students the means to succeed. Success for bilingual students means that they must learn to read and write early, become academically successful, graduate from high school, and become productive members of our diverse society.

REFLECTION QUESTIONS

1. Robert in Case Study One is developing normally with his English phonemic awareness and phonics skills. However, Carol from Case Study Two is having difficulties with beginning sounds, rhyming, blending, and segmenting. How can Robert and Carol be paired together in reading lessons for the general-education classroom?
2. Refer to Case Study Two. Carol is experiencing frustration with reading. She has verbally expressed that she does not like reading and does not wish to participate in any reading activities. How can reading be fun and also instructional for her?
3. How can Carol (see Case Study Two) and Javier (see Case Study Four) receive reading assistance from the SLP in the classroom?
4. Refer to Case Study Three. How is bilingualism an asset for Stella in reading instruction?
5. Refer to Case Study Three. Stella is developing her English skills and is having success in the classroom. However, she still needs additional practice, particularly with a proficient reader demonstrating, modeling, and providing feedback. How can Stella receive this extra time in reading?
6. How can Stella's knowledge of Spanish orthography assist her with English spelling?
7. Refer to Case Study Four. Javier is an English-language-learning student with reading difficulties. How can a monolingual English-speaking SLP provide some Spanish reading instruction?

REFERENCES

Adams, M. J. (1990). *Beginning to read: Thinking and learning about print.* Cambridge, MA: MIT Press.

Adrian, J., Alegria, J., & Morais, J. (1995). Metaphonological abilities of Spanish illiterate adults. *International Journal of Psychology, 30*(3), 329–353.

Armbuster, B. B., Lehr, F., & Osborn, J. (2001). *Put reading first: Kindergarten through grade 3.* Jessup, MD: The Center for the Improvement of Early Reading Achievement.

Brice, A. (2002). *The Hispanic child: Speech, language, culture and education.* Boston, MA: Allyn & Bacon.

Brice, A., Castellon-Perez, Y., & Ryalls, J. (2004). Speech recognition of code switched words by proficient Spanish-English bilinguals. *Journal of Distinguished Language Studies, 2*, 13–22.

Brice, A., & Roseberry-McKibbin, C. (2001). Choice of languages in instruction: One language or two? *Teaching Exceptional Children, 33*(4), 10–16.

Brice, R. (2004). *Identification of phonemes and graphemes in Spanish-English and English speaking kindergarten students.* Doctoral Dissertation. University of Central Florida. Orlando, FL: UMI Proquest.

Brisk, M. E., & Harrington, M. M. (2000). *Literacy and bilingualism: A handbook for ALL teachers.* Mahwah, NJ: Lawrence Erlbaum.

Burnette, J. (1998). *Reducing the disproportionate representation of minority students in special education* (ERIC/OSEP Digest #E566). Arlington, VA: ERIC Clearinghouse on Disabilities and Gifted Education.

Carillo, M. (1994). Development of phonological awareness and reading acquisition: A study in the Spanish language. *Reading and Writing, 6*(3), 279–298.

Carlisle, J. F., & Beeman, M. M. (2000). The effects of language of instruction on the reading and writing of first-grade Hispanic children. *Scientific studies of reading, 4*, 331–353.

Carlisle, J. F., Beeman, M., Davis, L. D., & Spharim, G. (1999). Relationship of metalinguistic capabilities and reading achievement for children who are becoming bilingual. *Applied Psycholinguistics, 20*, 459–478.

Chiappe, P., Siegel, L., & Gottardo, A. (2002). Reading-related skills of kindergarteners from diverse linguistic backgrounds. *Applied Psycholinguistics, 23*, 95–116.

Cisero, C. A., & Royer, J. M. (1995). The development and cross-language transfer of phonological awareness. *Contemporary Education Psychology, 20*, 275–303.

Cummins, J. (1984). *Bilingualism and special education: Issues in assessment and pedagogy.* San Diego, CA: College-Hill Press.

Denton, C., Anthony, J. L., Parker, R., & Hasbrouck, J. E. (2004). Effects of two tutoring programs on the English reading development of Spanish-English bilingual students. *The Elementary School Journal, 104*(4), 289–305.

Denton, C., Hashbrouck, J., Weaver, L., & Riccio, C. (2000). What do we know about phonological awareness in Spanish? *Reading Psychology, 21*, 335–352.

Dickinson, D. K., McCabe, A., Clark-Chiarelli, N., & Wolf, A. (2004). Cross-language transfer of phonological awareness in low-income Spanish and English bilingual preschool children. *Applied Psycholinguistics, 25*(3), 323–347.

Donovan, M. S., & Cross, C. T. (Eds.) (2002). Representation of minority students in special and gifted education. *Minority Students in Special and Gifted Education* (Full online text), 35–89. Retrieved on July 5, 2003, from http://www.nap.edu/openbook/0309074398/html/R1.html.

Durán, E., & Shefelbine, L. (2003). Reading and literacy instruction for Spanish-speaking students. In E. Durán, J. Shefelbine, L. Carnine, E. Maldonado-Colón, & B. Gunn (Eds.), *Systematic instruction in reading for Spanish-speaking students* (pp. 85–137). Springfield, IL: Charles C. Thomas.

Durgunoglu, A. Y. (2002). A cross-linguistic transfer in literacy development and implications for language learners. *Annals of Dyslexia, 52*, 189–204.

Durgunoglu, A. Y., & Öney, B. (2000). Literacy development in two languages: Cognitive and sociocultural dimensions of cross-language transfer. *A Research Symposium on High Standards for Students from Diverse Language Groups: Research, Practice, and Policy, 1*, 78–99.

England, G., Collins, S., & Algozzine, B. (2002). Effects of failure free reading on culturally and linguistically diverse students with learning disabilities. *Multiple Voices, 5*(1), 28–37.

Escamilla, K. (2000). Bilingual means two: Assessment issues, early literacy and Spanish-speaking children. *A Research Symposium on High Standards for Students from Diverse Language Groups: Research, Practice, and Policy, 1*, 100–128.

Figueroa, R. A., & Ruiz, N. T. (1997, January). The optimal learning environment. Paper presented at the Council for Exceptional Children Symposium on Culturally and Linguistically Diverse Exceptional Learners. New Orleans, LA.

Fletcher, J. M., Simos, P. G., Shaywitz, B. A., Shaywitz, S. E., Pugh, K. R., & Papanicolaou, A. C. (2000). Neuroimaging, language and reading: The interface of brain and environment. *A Research Symposium on High Standards for Students from Diverse Language Groups: Research, Practice, and Policy, 1*, 41–58.

González, J., & Garcia, C. (1995). Effects of word linguistic properties on phonological awareness in Spanish children. *Journal of Educational Psychology, 87*(2), 193–201.

Gottardo, A., Chiappe, P., Yan, B., Siegel, L., & Gu, Y. (2006). Relationships between first and second language phonological processing skills and reading in Chinese-English speakers living in English-speaking contexts. *Educational Psychology, 26*(3), 367–393.

Grandmaison, E., Cormier, P., Comeau, L., & Lacroix, D. (1996). *Longitudinal relationships among phonological awareness, verbal working memory, lexical access, and reading achievement in English-speaking children placed in French immersion.* (ERIC Document Reproduction Service No. ED403774). Washington, DC: U.S. Department of Education.

Graves, D. (1985). All children can write. *Learning Disabilities Focus, 1,* 36–43.

Hakuta, K. (1986). *Mirror of language: The debate on bilingualism.* New York: Basic Books.

Hulme, C., Hatcher, P., Nation, K., Brown, A., Adams, J., & Stuart, G. (2002). Phoneme awareness is a better predictor of early reading skill than onset-rime awareness. *Journal of Experimental Child Psychology, 82,* 2–28.

Illes, J., Francis, W., Desmond, G. H., Gabrieli, J. E., Glover, G. H., Poldrack, R., Lee, C. J., & Wagner, A. D. (1999). Convergent cortical representation of semantic processing in bilinguals. Brain and Language, *70*(3), 347–363.

International Reading Association. (2003). *The role of reading instruction in addressing the overrepresentation of minority children in special education in the United States: A position statement of the International Reading Association.* Newark, DE: Author.

Lindsey, K. A., Manis, F. R., & Bailey, C. E. (2003). Prediction of first-grade reading in Spanish-speaking English language learners. *Journal of Educational Psychology, 95*(3), 482–494.

Lipka, O., Siegel, L. S., & Vukovic, R. (2005). The literacy skills of English language learners in Canada. *Learning Disabilities Research and Practice, 29*(1), 39–49.

Lyon, G. R. (1998, April). *Overview of reading and literacy initiatives.* Statement presented to the Committee on Labor and Human Resources, Washington, DC. Retrieved August 13, 2003, from http://www.readbygrade3.com/lyon.htm.

Manrique, A., & Gramigna, S. (1984). Phonological segmentation and syllabication in preschool and 1st grade children. *Lectura y Vida, 5,* 4–13.

McEwan, E. K. (2002). *Teach them all to read: Catching the kids who fall through the cracks.* Thousand Oaks, CA: Corwin Press.

Miller, J., F., Heilmann, J., Nockerts, A., Iglesias, A., Fabiano, L., & Francis, D. J. (2006). Oral language and reading in bilingual children. *Learning Disabilities Research and Practice, 21*(1), 30–43.

Moats, L. C. (1999). *Teaching reading* is *rocket science: What expert teachers of reading should know and be able to do.* Washington, DC: American Federation of Teachers.

National Reading Panel. (2000). *Report of the National Reading Panel teaching children to read. An evidence-based assessment of the scientific research literature on reading and its implications for reading instruction. Reports of the subgroups.* Rockville, MD: National Institute of Child Health and Human Development.

Navarra, J., Sebastián-Galles, N., & Soto-Franco, S. (2005). The perception of second language sounds in early bilinguals: New evidence from an implicit measure. *Journal of Experimental Psychology: Human Perception and Performance, 31,* 912–918.

Office of Bilingual Education and Minority Languages Affairs. (2000). Summary Report. In A. M. Love (Ed.), *Proceedings of a Research Symposium on High Standards in Reading for Students from Diverse Language Groups: Research, Practice & Policy.* Washington, DC: April 19–20, 2000.

Ortiz, A. (1992). Assessing appropriate and inappropriate referral systems for LEP special education students. *Proceedings of the National Research Symposium on Limited English Proficient Student Issues.* Washington, DC: September 4–6, 1991. *Focus on Evaluation and Measurement: Volumes 1 and 2* (pp. 315–342). (ERIC Document Reproduction Service No. ED349819).

Padolsky, D. (2002). How has the English language learner (ELL) student population changed in recent years? Retrieved November 10, 2003, from http://www.ncela.gwu.edu/askncela/08leps.htm.

Palmer, B., Chen, C., Chang, S., & Leclare, J. (2006). The impact of biculturalism on language and literacy development: Teaching Chinese English language learners. *Reading Horizons, 46*(4), 239–265.

Pugh, K. R., Sandak, R., Frost, S. J., Moore, D., & Menel, W. E. (2005). Examining reading developmental and reading disability in English language learners: Potential contributions from functional neuroimaging. *Learning Disabilities Research and Practice, 20*(1), 24–30.

Ramírez, J. D. (2000). Bilingualism and literacy: Problem or opportunity? A synthesis of reading research on bilingual students. *Proceedings of a Research Symposium on High Standards in Reading for Students from Diverse Language Groups: Research, Practice & Policy.* Washington, DC: April 19–20, 2000.

Riccio, C., Amado, A., Jiménez, S., Hasbrouck, J., Imhof, B., & Denton, C. (2001). Cross-linguistic transfer of phonological processing: Development of a measure of phonological processing in Spanish. *Bilingual Research Journal, 25*(4), 417–437.

Shaywitz, S. E. (1996). Dyslexia. *Scientific American, 276*(5), 98–104.

Signorini, A. (1997). Word reading in Spanish: A comparison between skilled and less skilled beginning readers. *Applied Psycholinguistics, 18*, 319–344.

Simos, P. G., Billingsley-Marshall, R. L., Sarkari, S., Pataraia, E., & Papanicolaou, A. C. (2005). Brain mechanisms supporting distinct languages. *Learning Disabilities Research and Practice, 20*(1), 31–38.

Snow, C. E., Burns, M. S., & Griffin, P. (Eds.) (1998). *Preventing reading difficulties in young children.* Washington, DC: National Academy Press.

Spafford, C. S., & Grosser, G. S. (1996). *Dyslexia research and resource guide.* Boston, MA: Allyn & Bacon.

Thomas, W. P., & Collier, V. P. (2002). *A national study of school effectiveness for language minority students' long term academic achievement.* Center for Research on Education, Diversity and Excellence and the Office of Educational Research Improvement. (ERIC Document Reproduction Service No. ED 475048).

U.S. Census Bureau. (2001). *The Hispanic population in the United States: Population characteristics.* Washington, DC: Author.

U.S. Census Bureau. (2003). *The Hispanic population in the United States: Population characteristics.* Washington, DC: Author.

U.S. Department of Education. (2002). *No Child Left Behind: A desktop reference.* Washington, DC: Author.

U.S. Department of Education. (2003a). Background Information Framework for the National Assessment of Educational Progress. Adopted August 1, 2003, by the National Assessment Governing Board. Washington, DC: Author.

U.S. Department of Education. (2003b). Institute of Education Sciences. National Center for Education Statistics: *The Nation's Report Card: Reading 2002, NCES 2003.* Washington, DC: Author.

Vandergrift, L. (2006). Second language listening ability or language proficiency? *The Modern Language Journal, 6*, 6–18.

Vaughn, S., Mathes, P. G., Linan-Thompson, S., & Francis, D. J. (2005). Teaching English language learners at risk for reading disabilities to read: Putting research into practice. *Learning Disabilities Research and Practice, 20*(1), 58–67.

Verhoeven, L. (2000). Components in early second language reading and spelling. *Scientific Studies of Reading 4*(4), 313–330.

Wagner, R. K., & Torgesen, J. K. (1987). The nature of phonological processing and its causal role in the acquisition of reading skills. *Psychological Bulletin, 101*, 192–212.

Wilkinson, C. Y., & Ortiz, A. A. (2003, April). *Best practices in eligibility assessment of English language learners.* Paper presented at the 2003 Council for Exceptional Children Annual Conference. Seattle, WA.

Winzer, M. A., & Mazurek, K. (1998). *Special education in multicultural contexts.* Upper Saddle River, NJ: Prentice-Hall.

Chapter 9

Writing Development

Patricia Crawford

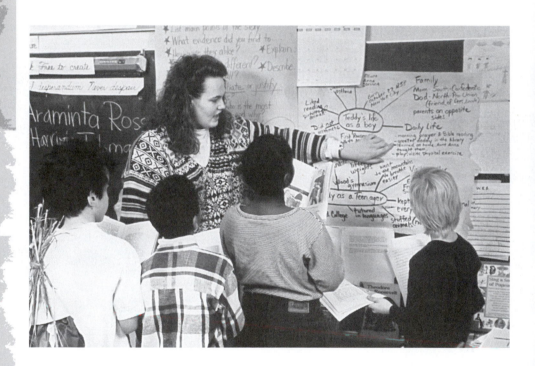

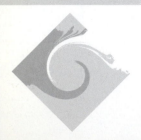

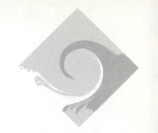

CHAPTER OUTLINE

INTRODUCTION

In accounts of American schooling, the curriculum has traditionally been said to focus on the three R's of reading, writing, and arithmetic. In spite of this reported focus, writing instruction has often been given little attention in the elementary grades. Clearly, historical evidence points to the importance of writing as a communication tool and the centrality of writing instruction as a key component of a well-rounded academic life (Bloodgood, 2002). However, instruction in this area has often taken a backseat to both reading and mathematics in American schools. Until recent years, authentic writing instruction has frequently been overlooked as a key curricular component.

When adults are asked to recall how they learned to write, many respond with stories of how they mastered the forms of manuscript print and cursive writing. Others talk about memorable assignments from their grade-school years. Still others will recall red-ink stories: tales of a teacher's negative feedback scrawled on their written work. Few, however, are able to detail either the pedagogical techniques or thought processes that helped them to become writers.

This disconnect is not surprising. Historically, teachers have been quick to give writing assignments, but they are less likely to actually teach the craft of writing, that is, the techniques through which students can approach the act of writing and that they can then utilize to make their own writing better (Fletcher & Portalupi, 1998). Likewise, when writing instruction has been offered, it has often been presented as a one-shot activity. Students were assigned a particular writing task, which was completed, graded, and then returned to the student or filed away by the teacher. Students have had few opportunities to revisit these writing pieces, nor have they been offered invitations to consider ways in which their writing could be strengthened. This approach to writing indicates a **product orientation,** in which the main focus is placed on the actual writing piece, typically generated in a single writing session. Little attention has been given to the process in which the writer developed that product. Consequently, few opportunities were provided to improve the piece of writing after the initial draft.

The lack of attention to authentic writing instruction and the importance of tapping into the processes that aid students' writing development was initially brought into focus through the groundbreaking work of Emig (1971) and Graves (1975; 1983) on the nature of children's composition processes. Emig's (1971) work with adolescents demonstrated that young writers found more success and satisfaction in writing when they had multiple opportunities to work on a piece and approach their writing through a series of recursive steps. Likewise, Graves's (1975, 1983) work in elementary schools indicated that young writers benefited from classrooms guided by a similar **process orientation.** In such classrooms, writers were invited to approach writing as an ongoing process instead of a one-shot task. They were given the necessary support to revisit pieces of writing and improve them through a series of flexible, recursive steps prior to the development of a final piece of work. Graves, who has frequently been referred to as the father of the writing process movement, dedicated many years to both outlining the process in which writers engage and clarifying ways in which this process can be used to support writers (Graves, 1983, 1994; Murray, 1995).

THE WRITING PROCESS

In general, the writing process refers to the series of steps in which writers engage when they compose text. During the early years of the writing process movement, researchers identified the following core steps in the process (Graves, 1975, 1983): (1) prewriting, (2) drafting, (3) revision, (4) editing, and (5) publication.

Prewriting

Prewriting refers to everything that takes place before the actual writing of a draft. It is the stage in which writers identify topics that are important to them and explore a whole range of possibilities for writing about these topics. Often referred to as **rehearsal,** this stage involves trying out ideas and thinking about ways that these ideas might be represented on the written page. Prewriting can take a variety of forms with young writers. For example, some students may benefit from brainstorming lists of topics and ideas. Others might find concept mapping, graphic organizers, or

FIGURE 9–1
Prewriting Strategies

- Having quiet "think time"
- Brainstorming lists
- Webbing
- Reading books about the writing topic
- Reading books written in the genre in which the author intends to write
- Drawing
- Building with blocks
- Free-writing
- Free play
- Taking notes
- Outlining
- Storyboarding
- Using graphic organizers
- Talking with a classmate
- Conferring with a more experienced writer from an upper grade
- Conferring with a teacher
- Interviewing a firsthand source
- Consulting with an expert outside the class
- Organizing papers and sources
- Listening to music
- Reviewing pieces of writing developed previously
- Using software to help organize thoughts

outlining to be good aids in the process. Other students may enjoy representing their initial ideas through verbal or artistic means. Though strategies can and should vary at this stage, the important point is that students need time to gather their thoughts, organize ideas, and plan for the next step when they actually begin to draft their writing piece. Figure 9–1 lists a variety of prewriting techniques.

Unfortunately, because of time constraints and a desire to move quickly to the actual writing of text, some writers and teachers of writing have viewed prewriting as being superfluous or unnecessary for the writing process. This is unfortunate because prewriting constitutes important thinking time and significantly affects the development, content, and organization of the final text. Murray (1985) suggests that 70% of the time devoted to writing should be devoted to prewriting.

Drafting

Drafting refers to the actual generation of text. It is the step where students put pencil to paper, or fingers to keyboard, and create a body of text. During the drafting stage, attention is placed on getting ideas down on paper so that the writer can eventually work with these thoughts and refine them into a final piece at a later time. At this point, students' attention should be on concepts and the generation of a complete piece of text. Concerns about grammar, mechanics, and spelling should be minimized at this stage. There will be time to address these issues at a later point in the process.

Revision

Revision is the stage in which the writer takes a closer look at both the concepts and form of the draft. The word *revision* comes from the root that gives us the word *vision*. Thus, revision literally means "to see again." This stage is an opportunity for writers to look at the initial draft (and in some cases, each successive draft) in a new way and consider how to improve it. At this point of the process, the focus is on content and big ideas, rather than on spelling and mechanics. Writers may look for gaps in the information presented; consult other resources; and depending on the situation, reshape or fine-tune the information presented. Likewise, writers might also look at elements of style and organization. For example, after reviewing an initial draft of a story, the writer might take the same central ideas and recast them into a poetic format. When the writer, usually in consultation with the teacher, has a sense of satisfaction with the overall content and organization of the piece, it is time to move on to editing, which is the next stage in the process.

Editing

Editing is the stage in the writing process in which the writer begins to focus on specific issues of mechanics. Unlike revision, which focuses on overarching elements of content and organization, writers edit for specific elements of grammar, spelling, punctuation, and a whole range of mechanics. If students are using a word-processing program, they might be urged to use spelling and grammar checks. Students should also utilize the classroom writing community, that is, ask peers to help them proofread, offer suggestions, and help edit their pieces. The goal at this stage is to move the piece toward final draft format, where it is ready to be shared with others.

Publication

Publication literally means to "make something public." Because writing is primarily a form of communication, most writers enjoy and appreciate having the opportunity to share their work and celebrate their writing with others. Publication can take many different forms. A simple method of publication can occur when pieces of writing are posted on a class bulletin board. Special writing pieces can be presented in more formal ways. Displaying short writing samples in frames or binding longer pieces into spiral-bound books helps make the publication a special and more authentic experience, while at the same time honoring both writers and their work. Young authors can also publish their work by reading it aloud. In this case, school professionals (i.e., speech-language pathologists, special-education teachers, or general-education teachers) often make use of the author's chair concept, in which a special chair or place of honor is designated for classroom authors who wish to share their work. The class gathers around the author's chair to listen, respond to, and celebrate their classmate's work.

Although each discrete step of the writing process should be understood in its own right, it is important to recognize that in practice, the steps are intertwined and recursive in nature. For example, some students who are at the point of drafting may find it helpful to return to prewriting strategies to develop or refine ideas that have been introduced in the text. Likewise, some students may find it necessary to stop and revise sections of text before they can complete a full version of an initial draft. Although publication is the last step of the process, most writers value and benefit from the opportunity to make their work public and share it in informal ways during the writing process. This allows them not only to gain confidence, but also to gather input from fellow writers in the classroom.

WRITER'S WORKSHOP

Process-oriented writing classrooms are typically organized around the format of a writer's workshop. Like most workshop environments, writer's workshops are busy places where people come to learn, develop skills, and create products in which they can take pride. Writer's workshop differs from the traditional image of composition classrooms in a number of ways. In this type of structure, the elements of time, ownership, and materials all play key roles (Atwell, 1998; Calkins, 1994).

Time

In workshop classrooms, school professionals try to provide large blocks of time for students to write on a regular, if not daily, basis. This use of time provides a challenge for general-education classroom teachers who are required to cover extensive amounts of material and meet the requirements of already overburdened curricula. However, experts emphasize that students should have multiple opportunities to engage in authentic writing during the school day. In addition, they need to have quality writing time, a minimum of four times per week, for writer's workshop to be effective (Graves, 1985).

To ensure that students have an opportunity to write each day, speech-language pathologists or special-education teachers may want to include journal writing as part of the curriculum (Fulwiler, 1987). Journals have proven to be an effective means for helping students not only to develop a routine of daily writing, but also to move into writing in a pleasant and nonthreatening manner. As anyone who has ever kept a diary can attest, a journal can serve varied purposes and be a great asset to the author at both the time of writing and in the future when the journal is reread. Journals can take many forms. In the most basic sense, a journal might be a regular chronicle of events, a written record of the important and not-so-important happenings of each day. These types of journals can serve as safe and important places for writers to put their deepest feelings, interests, questions, and passions onto paper.

While many journals are open-ended, others may have a sharper focus. For example, some journals may take the format of a **learning log,** that is, a record of a students' learning or research about a specific topic. Learning logs can be used in any subject area and may include words, illustrations, and diagrams to help document a student's learning. Young writers might also enjoy keeping a variety of other journals, such as travel logs, to capture vacation or field-trip memories, or literature logs to tease out important ideas and themes from favorite books. This type of expressive writing might be authentically connected to other areas of the curriculum through the development of **simulated diaries,** that is, pseudo-journal entries in which the writer takes on a different persona. Students might imagine that they are a character in a favorite book or television show and develop an entry that they think the character might write in response to a particular set of circumstances. To make a social studies connection, students can imagine that they are an historical figure or a person who lived during another era. They might then create journal entries that would be typical of that person, that is, his or her life during that time period.

Although journal writing is generally considered to be a personal and private activity, this type of writing experience can be modified to be more social in nature through the creation of **dialogue journals,** in which journals are passed from one writer to the next, allowing each participant to read and respond to selected entries through writing. Whatever format journals take, their incorporation into the curriculum ensures that time will be allotted for students to write each day of the school year.

Ownership

In traditional general-education classrooms, the bulk of the instruction tends to be teacher-initiated and -directed, with teachers standing in front of the class and delivering information to a large group of students. In writer's workshop, school professionals organize time in a variety of different ways and share their authority with students in the classroom, allowing students to make appropriate choices about the form and content of their writing pieces. This element of choice allows students to have a greater degree of ownership in their work. When students have this sense of personal investment in their writing, they tend to take their writing more seriously and be more apt to work toward developing a high-quality product in which they can take pride.

While speech-language pathologists and special-education teachers provide **direct instruction** (i.e., specific instruction usually involving step-by-step directions) of content, they typically do so on a limited basis and in the form of mini-lessons. **Mini-lessons,** also called craft lessons, are short (5- to 15-minute) lessons that focus on a specific topic that is relevant to students' learning. For example, mini-lessons might focus on a range of topics, including (1) specific prewriting strategies; (2) ideas for writing in a particular genre or form of writing; (3) specific methods for revision; (4) exploration of literary devices; (5) ideas for tackling editing by focusing on a particular skill, such as the use of quotation marks or capitalization of proper nouns; or (6) the use of paragraphing. The ideas for mini-lessons are endless and should flow from a balance between curricular mandates and unique writer needs. While some mini-lessons are presented in a large-group format, many school professionals find it to be equally or more effective to present these lessons to small subgroups of students who have common interests in writing or who are struggling to implement a particular skill in their writing (Calkins, 1994).

The concept of ownership plays a key role in the ways writers identify topics for writing. In this regard, there is a distinction between the practices in traditional classrooms and those in writer's workshop classrooms. In traditional general-education classrooms, topics for writing are usually provided by the teacher in a direct manner (e.g., "Today we are going to write about penguins" or "Please write a 100-word essay on the best thing that happened during summer vacation") or in the guise of creative formats designed to link writing with other parts of the curriculum (e.g., "Write a funny story that uses all 20 of this week's spelling words" or "Choose a story starter from the box. Copy it and complete the rest of the story"). Conversely, in workshop classrooms, students are encouraged to think like authentic authors who generate their own topics.

In writing process classrooms, students are encouraged to write about issues that matter so that they may have an authentic sense of ownership of their work (Atwell, 1998; Avery, 2002; Calkins, 1991, 1994; Graves, 1994). Particularly during the early years of the writing process movement, students were urged to write about personal experiences that were significant to them. This resulted in a considerable amount of writing presented in the form of personal narrative or memoir, with children writing about their daily experiences; personal relationships; and other aspects of their home, family, and school lives.

While this type of expressive writing is very important, other research has also shown the importance of supporting children's writing in a variety of genres that extend beyond personal writing (Dyson, 1997, 1999; Newkirk, 1989, 2001). Many students prefer to write about topics that are less realistic, dabbling in genres such as fiction and fantasy. Young writers often find a sense of freedom and empowerment when they are able to create written scenarios in which anything is possible. By writing in a variety of genres, students also become more attuned to audience awareness; that is, they develop the recognition that writing topics and styles may need to be adjusted to meet the needs and expectations of a particular readership.

Students' choices in genre often affect not only their topics, but also the forms of their writing. For example, students who find enjoyment in reading comic books and **graphic novels** may also enjoy writing in these formats. This type of writing will naturally have a different tone than traditional prose, and the balance between graphics and written text will be affected. Likewise, artistic presentation of the final published draft might be an important element for young writers. Speech-language pathologists and special-education teachers can help accommodate students' needs in these areas by sharing excellent models of writing with students through the incorporation of various forms of high-quality children's literature throughout the curriculum. Students also need to have a sufficient amount of work time and a supply of appropriate art supplies to create a publishable, final draft.

Materials

Materials play a key role in the writing classroom. Like all who practice a craft, writers can practice their craft with more ease and success when they have all of the necessary tools to do the job well. At first glance, it would seem that few materials are needed for the writing classroom. After all, what else is necessary besides paper and pencils? A closer look reveals that a full range of materials is necessary to stock a well-equipped classroom for writers. Among these materials are items that contribute to setting the tone and creating a literary environment, that is, actual tools of the trade for producing writing, and ample supplies for celebrating the writing of members of the writing community.

Writing flows most easily within a literary, **print-rich environment,** that is, a place stocked with inviting and engaging texts. In classrooms, these type of texts might consist of interesting and developmentally appropriate children's literature that can serve as writing models, reference materials to help writers track down information related to their pieces, and helpful information attractively presented and posted around the classroom. (See the Instructional Strategies box for more details on creating a positive writing environment.)

INSTRUCTIONAL STRATEGIES

Suggestions for Establishing a Positive Writing Environment

Speech-language pathologists, special-education teachers, and general-education classroom teachers can help not only to nurture children's writing abilities, but also help them to enjoy and value writing through the creation of a positive writing environment. To build this type of environment, it is important that the classroom be print-rich, which means that the classroom should contain a wide variety of texts that will be attractive to young readers and writers. Books from various genres, magazines, and newspapers all provide models of different writing genres for children to value and emulate. Dictionaries, thesauruses, phone books, and atlases are among the many texts that can serve as writing references for classrooms at a range of levels. Young children will benefit from the use of pictionaries, which help to span the gap as children move from interpreting visual images to written text.

Posters, printed directions, and bulletin board displays are all tools that communicate the message that the written word is valued. Labeling items with flashcards can be very helpful for writers in early childhood classrooms or environments in which children are just learning to speak English. Likewise, word walls can be a tremendous help for students who are mastering sight words, as well as those who need help in learning vocabulary, including words about specialized topics.

Displaying children's writing and illustrations is another important factor in establishing a positive learning and writing environment. When final drafts are published and shared (by way of posting or through inclusion in the classroom library), students develop a sense of audience, see themselves as authors, and understand that their written work has value. The experience of authorship can be made more authentic through the development of nicely bound student-authored books and by including these texts as part of the classroom library. In sum, this practice helps to reinforce the notion that even young writers have the potential to be authors and to contribute to the literary world.

Suggestions for Helping Students to Navigate the Writing Process

For writers both young and old, the writing process can be a daunting set of procedures. Initially, the series of steps required to produce a final draft can seem overwhelming. School professionals can take a number of steps to help students better understand, utilize, and embrace the writing process.

To do this, speech-language pathologists, special-education teachers, and general-education classroom teachers must first be completely familiar with the process themselves. They must engage in the act of writing so that they know the benefits and challenges posed by the task of formalized writing. If speech-language pathologists and teachers are writers, they will be better able to understand, support, and teach young writers who are faced with similar dilemmas in developing their drafts. Students will gain confidence in the teacher's understanding and approach when the teacher "dares to share" his or her own writing with the class. This can be done by modeling the writing process on an over-head projector and providing think-aloud commentary during the composition process, or simply by sharing completed pieces of writing during publication celebrations. School professionals need not be professional authors; they must simply be willing to engage in the writing process on a regular basis in an appropriate genre (e.g., newsletter articles, e-mails, short stories, poems, journal entries, etc.). Speech-language pathologists and teachers can help students embrace the writing process by making sure that the steps are clearly understood. The steps in the writing process should be posted in the classroom so that writers can use them as a guideline. Additional guidelines such as "five steps to editing" or a "how to get published" checklist can also provide very helpful, tangible support for writers.

Beyond the presence of print materials that set the tone for writing, students also need materials that will help them participate and find success in the writing act. The establishment of a class writing center can be very helpful in this regard (Diller, 2003). A writing center is a type of learning center, that is, a designated area in the classroom where students can engage in independent learning. In some classrooms, students simply go to the learning center during their free time when their assigned work has been completed. In other classrooms, students go to particular learning centers when the materials and planned experiences there will help them better approach their assigned work. Finally, the school professional in some classrooms designs a rotation system so that each student gets to visit and take advantage of the materials and experiences provided at the learning centers at varied intervals.

Writing centers should contain materials that help students enjoy writing and make their writing times more productive. For example, most students enjoy experimenting with a variety of writing materials (e.g., pencils, pens, markers, crayons, glitter pens, etc.). Scissors, scotch tape, and paper clips are invaluable items for young children who are learning about revision because these materials allow them to physically cut, paste, and insert items as part of the revision process. Other artistic materials, such as paints and items for collage, can be helpful for students who wish to illustrate their work. Hanging folders and file boxes make it possible for students to organize their work so they can return to it easily another time. Binding materials such as staplers, hole punchers, metal shower rings, yarn, string, and spiral rings can all be valuable items for binding a student-authored book. Finally, technological resources such as computers with developmentally appropriate word-processing and writing-support programs can make the actual mechanics of writing easier and, as a result, make children's work time less stressful and more productive. See Figure 9–2 for additional suggestions on creating a classroom writing center.

FIGURE 9–2
Key Considerations for Creating a Classroom Writing Center

- Space: The writing center does not have to be large, but it should be a designated place set apart from the hustle and bustle of the classroom. A small corner, nook, or table would be a good choice for the designated center.
- Materials: Fill the writing center with supplies to make the work of young writers easier and more inviting. Reference materials and a variety of papers, pens, pencils, crayons, markers, staplers, tape, Post-it Notes, glue, and other relevant items are all helpful materials for those who write.
- Environment: To be most effective, learning centers should be places that are attractive, inviting, and engaging. The environment can be enhanced by including attractive displays, comfortable seating areas, low lighting, and well-organized systems for storing and using materials.
- Connections: Although the focus of the center should be writing, it is helpful to make natural bridges with other areas of learning. For example, materials that link to other curricular areas involving writing, high-quality children's literature, and technology resources such as computers, Alphasmart units, and appropriate software are all welcome additions to the writing center.
- Organization: Organization is a crucial element in any type of learning center. If students are supposed to complete certain tasks at the writing center, make sure that clear directions are posted and easily accessible. Have clear guidelines for the efficient storage of materials and written works in progress.

WRITING AND SPELLING DEVELOPMENT

Children acquire control over written language forms in many of the same ways that they acquire control over verbal forms. From the time that they are born, young children are exposed to oral language. Parents and other caregivers attend to young infants, making eye contact, cooing, and repeatedly trying to engage them in conversations (e.g., "You're such a big boy, aren't you?" "Do you want that ball? Yes, you do! Here comes the ball!"). Children gradually make meaning from oral language and respond to it in a series of approximations, i.e., linguistic responses that, though not entirely correct, are children's best efforts at coming close, or approximating, the appropriate response.

Children's development of written language follows a similar progression. Children begin to experience and interact with written language from their earliest years. Exposure to bedtime stories, nursery rhymes, and other literature helps children understand that printed text has meaning that can be understood by others (Bissex, 1980; Dragan, 2001; Holdaway, 1979). Early experiences with drawing and then later writing helps children understand that they have the ability to communicate ideas to others by making marks on a page. As in the use of oral language, children who are beginning to write typically do so by using a series of approximations that, with experience and guidance, become closer and closer to accepted, conventional forms of writing. Children's early writing is referred to as **emergent writing** (Clay, 1991). This term is used to describe children's development and their emerging development as writers. Obviously, emergent writers do not have the experience or sophistication to write in the same way as experienced writers. During the emergent writing stage, children use written approximations to express their thoughts, gradually approximating conventional writing (Clay, 1991; Teale & Sulzby, 1989).

Although no two children (nor their progress) are alike, children's writing development tends to unfold through a series of predictable stages (Hall, 1987; Spandel, 2004; Gentry, 1982). When children begin to make marks on paper, their first efforts typically appear to be a series of scribbles that are initially random and then become more controlled over time. Eventually, children's writing begins to look less like scribbles and comes to take on the appearance of mock letters, that is, letterlike symbols that share many of the qualities of written language. Eventually children begin to use real letters. Their writing begins to grow in complexity and take on the form of conventional, rather than emergent, writing.

Spelling development also emerges in a series of approximations. These approximations are known as invented spelling because children construct or invent the spelling based on their knowledge of language in general, and sound-symbol relationships in particular. According to Gentry (1982), spelling development typically progresses through a series of flexible yet predictable stages. In the **precommunicative** stage, children use letters, but there is no sound-symbol correlation between the letters and the sounds they are meant to represent. In the **semiphonetic** stage, children show a beginning understanding of sound-symbol relationships. At this stage, children often represent whole words with a single letter, usually the initial consonant sound (e.g., "M" equals "Mike"). Later, children begin to incorporate final sounds, and medial sounds appear later still. In the **phonetic** stage, young writers demonstrate a general understanding of the alphabetic principle and can represent the sounds they hear in a logical fashion, in spite of the fact that they do not use conventional spelling. In the **transitional** stage, children demonstrate an increasing understanding of the conventions of written language. Their spelling, though not fully correct, is closer to conventional. Finally, in the **correct** stage, writers have a number of spelling words in their repertoire and know and apply many of the rules that govern conventional spelling. At this stage, the writer's attempts at spelling are usually correct.

CASE STUDY PERSPECTIVES

Both case studies in this chapter illustrate how best practices and strategies may be implemented by parents, classroom teachers, and other school professionals.

Case Study One Background: Simon

Simon, a monolingual speaker of English, is an active and enthusiastic learner in a local kindergarten class. At the end of the first month of school, Simon appears to have made a smooth and positive adjustment to school. He enjoys engaging in free play and takes particular pleasure in building elaborate block structures. During writing time, Simon works diligently, quickly putting pencil (or crayons) to paper. Each piece is dominated by elaborate pictures of monsters that are attacking large buildings. Although he works diligently, his "written" work typically only includes pictures and is rarely accompanied by any conventional text. When text is included, it is limited to his first name written in capital letters: S-I-M-O-N.

Simon's teacher, Ms. Hollander, is pleased that her student appears to enjoy writing time, but she is concerned with the writing he is developing. She consistently praises his efforts in an attempt to support his affinity for writing time and affirm his richly detailed illustrations. However, she worries that he is not willing to attempt conventional writing and wonders when he will make the transition from the illustration stage.

Ms. Hollander has taken a number of steps to support Simon's move into conventional writing. First, in an effort to make the text-illustration connection, she regularly uses big books during shared reading time. She points to each word of the text as she reads and frequently models the connection between text and illustration through the use of think-alouds (e.g., "I see a big dog in the picture. I wonder if the words will tell us what he's doing here" or "Let's read the words to find out why the man looks so grumpy"). Ms. Hollander has also encouraged the children in her classroom to work in collaborative groups and to share their work with other writers ("Don't forget to share the words and pictures from your stories with your neighbors"). She hopes that the modeling of the other students will motivate Simon to "join the writer's club" and add text to his illustrations. Although Simon appears to be happy, capable, and engaged in literacy learning, Ms. Hollander wonders if she should contact the guidance counselor to obtain a referral for special education for Simon so that he can receive additional support for his writing development.

Case Study One Comments: Simon

Simon's progress is not atypical of many kindergarteners. Young children enter school with varying levels of literacy experiences. Many children come to school having heard thousands of stories, while others come with a very limited repertoire of literary experiences. And while many children have had extensive experiences with writing, others come with almost none.

Ms. Hollander is taking many positive steps regarding Simon's learning. She should continue to make verbal and pedagogical connections between both reading and writing and the relationship between text and illustrations. Furthermore, she should help Simon develop as a writer by helping him set goals that are both attainable and developmentally appropriate. For example, one week she might encourage Simon to label one important feature in his illustration (e.g., monster). The next week, she might invite him to label three items within his illustration (e.g. monster, building, fire). The next week, she might encourage Simon to write down one thought about his picture (e.g., The monster breathed fire). Because of Simon's age and developmental level, Ms. Hollander should not expect or demand that Simon use conventional spellings. Such demands may result in Simon becoming reluctant to take risks and/or attempt new words or conventions in his writing. Ms. Hollander can assess Simon's progress by helping him maintain a portfolio of his writing pieces that include different artifacts that demonstrate his growth and control of a particular sound, word, or convention. In addition, examples of Simon's invented spelling collected over time will serve as powerful evidence of progress and the possible need for support in specific areas.

Ms. Hollander might implement several approaches within the curriculum. To help Simon develop the skills he needs to successfully transition from texts with solely visual components to ones with written words, journal writing may help Simon to view writing as a safe and predictable event. In journal writing, Simon can record his thoughts without fear of criticism.

Because Simon will be more likely to attempt to write new words, he will be gaining valuable experience in refining his knowledge of sound-symbol relationships and effective ways of communicating his thoughts.

In addition to providing Simon with opportunities to write, Ms. Hollander should also include times in the school day when she models writing for the students so that they can see her process. By using the language experience approach (LEA) (i.e., an approach that uses the child's experiences for content in writing), she can record events and opinions related to classroom happenings. Because the students' oral language is recorded directly in the language experience approach, the teacher will have the opportunity to model the idea that oral language can be written down and later read by either the writer or another audience.

Ms. Hollander might also build on Simon's natural interests in play and building. For example, she might create purposeful opportunities to include writing within the framework of free play. Paper and writing tools might be included within the housekeeping center so that the students can make shopping lists, record telephone numbers, or leave notes for others. In addition, Ms. Hollander might engage Simon in a verbal conversation about play and then invite him to later write about it (e.g., "You seemed so excited during playtime. Can you write about the things you did so that we don't forget them?"). Instant or digital photography could also be used to capture the structures that Simon builds. These images could be printed and incorporated into writing pieces ("Here's a great picture of the big castle you built with Dionne. Would you like to write a story about it?").

At this point, it does not seem that Simon needs additional interventions beyond those provided by the classroom teacher. His positive attitude toward school and his active engagement with activities related to reading, writing, and learning are all positive signs. Ms. Hollander should continue to encourage Simon, try interventions such as the ones described above, and engage in ongoing assessment activities that will help her monitor his progress in writing. If Simon does not respond to the interventions provided and fails to show growth in his ability to write over time, Ms. Hollander should then consider referring him for speech-language or special-education testing.

Foundations of Spelling

Spelling is certainly not the only or most important aspect of writing instruction. However, it is one aspect that receives a lot of attention. One reason for this is the high visibility of spelling (Kervin, 2002; Rosencranz, 1998). Though correct spelling usually goes unnoticed in the work of mature writers, incorrect spelling stands out as glaring errors. The media frequently calls attention to problems with spelling among school children and adults. For better or worse, parents and school professionals alike tend to equate the ability to spell with the ability to write effectively.

In the writing process, classroom teachers encourage children to write first and to worry about spelling and other editing issues later. They urge children to deal first with the matter of content, that is, to strive initially to get their ideas written in the form of a workable draft (Atwell, 1998; Calkins, 1994; Graves, 1984, 1994). The fact that children are encouraged not to worry about spelling in the initial stages of writing does not mean that the ability to spell correctly is not a matter of concern for teachers. It simply means that when children engage in the writing process, mechanics (including spelling) become a focus later when children edit their work.

There has been a tremendous amount of research related to the teaching of spelling and the ways in which students acquire related skills in this area (Chandler & the Mapleton Teacher-Research Group, 1999; Gentry, 1982, 1997; Groff, 1986; Hughes & Searle, 2000; Read, 1971; Treiman & Bourassa, 2000). Although there are many points of disagreement about the best way to approach spelling in the elementary classroom, there are a number of general principles on which educators can agree:

1. *Spelling is related to reading.* Students who spell well tend to be proficient readers. This makes sense because reading provides writers with ongoing authentic models of the ways in which sounds and letters are combined to represent meaning. However, being a good reader does not necessarily ensure that a student will be a good speller (Hughes & Searle, 2000).

2. *Spelling is related to writing composition.* Students who are proficient writers and who frequently engage in writing also tend to be proficient spellers. Those who enjoy writing typically have a desire to communicate with others and come to view proper spelling as an element that makes their communication more effective (Hughes & Searle, 2000; Kervin, 2002; Routman, 2005).

3. *Spelling is related to handwriting.* Students who are good spellers also tend to have good handwriting skills. It is not necessary for children to have beautiful handwriting; however, it is important for their handwriting to be legible enough that it can be read clearly. Children who do not have legible handwriting often are unable to read the spelling of words they have copied and then later recopy them incorrectly.

4. *Spelling is a meaning-making activity.* Even young children can identify patterns in written language and attempt to create patterns in their own writing (Clay, 1991; Holdaway, 1979; Treiman & Bourassa, 2000). Children attempt to find meaning in these patterns and to communicate meaningfully with others through their invented spellings.

5. *Learning to spell is a complex activity.* The ability to spell correctly is affected by a number of factors, including children's backgrounds with literacy, their knowledge of spelling strategies, their attitude, the ways in which spelling is approached in the classroom, and other factors (Rosencranz, 1998; Routman, 2005). Traditional weekly spelling lists of predetermined, decontextualized words are often of little help to students. These lists can be overwhelming for those who struggle with spelling. Therefore, teachers need to look beyond this traditional practice. Because of the complexity involved in spelling, there is no guaranteed approach to the teaching of spelling. Therefore, effective speech-language pathologists and teachers should use a variety of strategies to help their students become proficient spellers and to apply this spelling within the meaningful context of their writing.

Strategies to Support Spelling Development

To teach spelling effectively, speech-language pathologists and special-education teachers must help young learners understand the purpose of spelling. Children need to know that spelling is an important skill that enables them to communicate more effectively through their writing. When spelling is viewed in this context, it comes to be seen as a courtesy to the reader and an important part of the editing process. In short, children gradually come to understand that they must move from invented to conventional spelling so that their readers will be able to understand the full meaning and intentions of their writing.

Speech-language pathologists and special-education teachers who wish to support their students' spelling abilities should create a positive, print-rich learning environment, that is, a classroom that is full of helpful resources for spelling correctly. Print-rich classrooms have been described as environments that are brimming with meaningful examples of written language.

Word walls are one aspect of a print-rich environment that can aid children in their spelling and writing. A **word wall** is simply a classroom display that features relevant words for the members of the classroom writing community. These words are typically written on individual flashcards so that they can be grouped and organized in a variety of ways. The content of word walls varies according to the children's developmental levels and the school's curriculum. Some words that might be featured on classroom word walls may include (1) sight words, (2) names of students in the classroom, (3) words related to a particular topic of study in the content areas, (4) words with particular spelling patterns, (5) words that children discover in conversations or books, and (6) intriguing words.

When developing word walls, it is important to make sure that the children are aware of the purposes of this activity, that is, that the word wall contains words relevant to learning and that the word wall can be accessed as a valuable resource for spelling and writing. To help students understand these points, it is important to engage them in the actual creation of the word wall (Routman, 2005). Ask the students for words that should be included, call attention to each word when it is added, and purposefully arrange and rearrange the words so that they are most helpful for students. Words on the word wall might be arranged alphabetically or they might be grouped by theme. The important point is that students must view the word wall as a usable resource.

Students also benefit from other collections of words, such as word banks. A **word bank** is a collection of spelling words maintained by individual students within the classroom. Words are usually selected by the students themselves or in collaboration with the teacher. Word banks can be maintained in the form of individual cards placed in a small container or in the form of a notebook. In either case, the words should be organized alphabetically. With the box method, the word cards can be organized and rearranged at will. With the notebook method, each page should be labeled with a different letter of the alphabet. Students can then add new words to the notebook, recording each one by initial letter under the appropriate letter of the alphabet. In either case, speech-language pathologists and teachers should emphasize the importance of recording the word accurately and legibly (Rosencranz, 1998). As with word walls, the purpose of a word bank is to provide a ready spelling resource for students to assist them in their writing.

In addition to being immersed in a print-rich environment and having access to helpful resources, students benefit from seeing correct spelling modeled within the context of authentic writing. Speech-language pathologists and teachers can help accomplish this by modeling their own writing on an overhead projector or via computer projection.

When doing this, it is helpful for the teacher to provide a think-aloud, that is, thinking through and verbalizing decisions as they are being made ("I want to write a note about a surprise party, but I can't remember if the word *surprise* has an *s* or a *z* near the end. So I think I better check the word wall to make sure. Oops, I almost misspelled the word *principal* by putting a *-ple* at the end. I usually remember it by thinking that the principal is our pal") (Chandler & the Mapleton Teacher-Research Group, 1999). As speech-language pathologists and teachers think through their spelling dilemmas, students witness tangible demonstrations about how they might answer their own spelling questions.

In addition to teacher modeling, most students also need to engage in some type of word study to become proficient and confident spellers. Word sorts are one pedagogical tool that can be employed in this regard. Word sorts provide students with the opportunity to look closely at texts and to apply principles of word study where they are presented with a number of words written on individual cards and asked to sort them. In an open sort, students are asked to identify their own criteria for sorting words into subsets. They are urged to explore the words that share a common feature that they have discovered. In a closed sort, students are given predetermined criteria and asked to sort their word cards in a specified way. Word sorts may be based on either meaning or orthographic features. Possible sorts include grouping words by (1) initial sounds, (2) final sounds, (3) number of syllables, (4) types of prefixes or suffixes, (5) root words, (6) vowel sounds, or (7) any other identifiable pattern. Word sorts help students analyze written language and discover patterns that will aid them in both reading and spelling of words (Bear, Invernizzi, Templeton, & Johnston, 2004).

CASE STUDY PERSPECTIVES

Both case studies in this chapter illustrate how best practices and strategies may be implemented by parents, classroom teachers, and other school professionals.

Case Study Two Background: Christina

Christina is a monolingual speaker of English who has consistently struggled in the areas of reading and writing. Christina was retained in the second grade because of poor progress in these areas. In the third grade, Christina was tested and diagnosed with a learning disability. Now a ten-year-old, Christina has just started the fourth grade and continues to struggle with reading and writing.

When questioned, Christina reports that she does not enjoy writing time in school. She says that she "feels dumb" in spelling and is "always behind" the other students in writing class. By this, she means that she achieves low scores on weekly spelling tests and that it takes her much longer than her peers to complete writing assignments. To complete her written work, she usually needs additional time and sometimes misses recess or library time.

Neither Christina's parents not her teacher, Mr. Krummel, are pleased with the progress she is making in writing. They are concerned that her writing pieces often go unfinished, with her early drafts abandoned before they can be revised and transformed into a final draft.

Mr. Krummel is also frustrated with the mechanical problems in her writing. In spite of frequent reminders to proofread, Christina's papers are full of punctuation and spelling errors, and in many cases, they lack a sound organizational structure. When reminded to revise and edit, Christina appears to be frustrated and often simply recopies her draft, including the same mistakes she made in the previous copy.

Although Christina is in an inclusive general-education classroom, she does receive support services from the reading specialist. She does better with her written work when she works on a one-to-one basis with the specialist. During these sessions, however, she often misses valuable instruction and writing time in her own classroom, which puts her even farther behind in completing assignments. Christina's parents are displeased with her progress and fault the school system. At the last parent-teacher conference, Christina's mother remarked, "Teachers are supposed to actually teach kids what they need to know. No one's doing that for my daughter. What's wrong with this school?"

Case Study Two Comments: Christina

Christina has found school difficult and continues to struggle. Although she did not like writing before, chances are that she will like it even less in her current situation. She is overwhelmed by assignments that seem too difficult. Because she frequently spends recess and other enjoyable activities engaged in tediously recopying her work, she has begun to equate writing with punishment. Unless something changes, she will probably try to avoid having to write at all and receive less practice at using the skills that are so crucial to the writing process. Some other type of intervention needs to take place for her to succeed.

The first change that needs to take place is in instruction. Christina's learning disability means that she may learn differently than the majority of the students. Her diagnosed disability most likely means that she needs additional time to complete certain educational tasks to be successful. Clearly, writing is one of these tasks.

In light of this, Mr. Krummel should look closely at his assignments and consider how they might be modified to meet Christina's extended time needs. For example, if a spelling list of 20 words is too difficult, the list might be modified to include only five or ten words that Christina can actually learn and retain. She would benefit more from learning the majority of the words on a shorter list, than from learning just a fraction of the words on a longer list.

Likewise, if the assigned goal is to write an extended piece in a particular genre, the assignment might be modified by removing the length requirement. By writing a shorter piece, Christina can still have the valuable experience of engaging in the writing process and learning about the qualities of this particular genre. And the shorter assignment will probably mean that she will not feel overwhelmed and fall behind in her other work.

Christina's learning experiences and progress could also be positively affected through greater collaboration among the school professionals responsible for her education. Mr. Krummel and the reading specialist should work to coordinate their schedules better so that Christina no longer leaves the classroom during the important times of writing instruction and implementation. Co-teaching in the general-education classroom is one possibility (see Chapter 11 for further information about co-teaching). Finally, Christina's parents need to be kept informed of her progress and invited to support and reinforce the instruction that she is receiving at school through activities at home.

MODIFICATIONS FOR CHILDREN WITH DISABILITIES

Though writing is a challenge for most students, it is even more so for children who have some type of language-learning disability (Marchisan & Alber, 2001; Schirmer & Bailey, 2000; Scott & Vitale, 2003). Because of these challenges, some school professionals have speculated that the writing process is too difficult for students with language-learning disabilities. They argue that students with language-learning disabilities and other disabilities need more guidance than can be provided in open-ended steps. Yet others argue that children with special needs respond particularly well to the collaborative nature of writer's workshop; they also argue that the emphasis on the importance of personal ownership and the progressive yet recursive nature of each step in the writing process provides students with special needs the extra support they need to be successful (Graves, 1985; Marchisan & Alber, 2001).

In many cases, students with disabilities spend large quantities of time working on isolated skills. Engagement in writing experiences may enable them to learn the skill of writing within a meaning, purposeful, and sensitive context (Graves, 1985). However, for students with disabilities to benefit fully from these experiences, the speech-language pathologist (SLP), the special education teacher, and the general education classroom teacher may need to make some accommodations to meet their needs. Collaboration among school professionals is recommended because the student will benefit from the combined efforts. (Refer to Chapter 11 for additional information regarding collaboration.) Some possibilities for accommodations include the following:

1. *Provide guidance in choosing topics.* Choosing a topic with little guidance can seem like an overwhelming task. To help students in this area, demonstrate a number of specific prewriting strategies for topics that have personal significance for them. Ideas include brainstorming lists of favorite people, places, and things; rereading journal entries to find topics that recur; or developing lists of areas in which the student is knowledgeable or has expertise.

2. *Help students to plan effectively for writing.* After students identify a focus topic, they are ready to plan for their draft. Students with disabilities may need extra guidance at this point in the process. SLPs and teachers should help students brainstorm words that they associate with the topic, develop webs that reflect the breadth of information about which they might write, and/or develop a list of priorities among their subtopics. Beware of presenting too many prewriting strategies within a short period of time. Students with disabilities may need to practice using one strategy several times before they can feel confident with it and use it effectively.

3. *Set workable goals.* For some children with disabilities, the idea of engaging in a large writing project may seem so overwhelming that they do not know where to start. Teachers can help students in this area by helping them to plan, record, and work toward a series of attainable goals.

4. *Provide clear guidelines and criteria for assignments.* Students with language-learning disabilities will have greater success if the expectations for an assignment are clearly outlined for them. Speech-language pathologists and teachers

can help in this area by providing appropriate checklists and assessment rubrics in advance, and then helping students develop a plan to meet these objectives.

5. *View editing as a series of substeps.* Students with language-learning disabilities often struggle with the conventions of print. Therefore, editing can be an overwhelming process. These students will be more successful if editing is approached as a series of substeps. For example, one editing session might focus only on the proper use of quotation marks. A second session might focus only on the proper use of *their* versus *there* if these words are consistently used incorrectly in the draft. A third session could focus on spelling. This type of progression will make editing proceed smoothly and help the students to find success (Brice, 2004).

6. *Develop a plan for solving problems.* All students want to know what to do when they hit a roadblock. This is especially important for students with disabilities. Assistance can be provided to students in the form of strategies that will help them solve problems that they may encounter. For example, the following set of suggestions could be given to students when they are unable to spell a word:

1. Try to sound it out.
2. Check the word wall.
3. Check the word bank.
4. Try to write it and see if it looks right.
5. Ask a friend.
6. Ask the teacher.

For students with motor impairments, the very act of writing can be problematic. Students with mild forms of these disabilities may be aided by the use of simple adaptations such as special pencil grips. Other students may benefit from using word-processing programs instead of writing on paper. A number of assistive technology devices have been developed recently that can enable students with even severe motor disabilities to communicate with greater ease and effectiveness through computers.

CONCLUDING REMARKS

As previously noted, writing instruction in U.S. schools has historically been approached from a product-oriented approach, where the emphasis was placed simply on the quality of the writing piece produced by a student. The topics for these pieces were traditionally assigned by the school professional, with the writing generated in a single draft. More recently, a process-oriented approach has been taken in the teaching of writing, with emphasis placed on the ways in which students went about writing their work. Students were encouraged to choose their own topics and to engage in the writing step process for bringing a work to fruition (Graves, 1983; Calkins, 1991, 1994).

As the writing process was implemented in classrooms throughout the country, a number of concerns arose. Some educators were concerned that an overemphasis on process would take away from a commitment to teaching the mechanics of writing and negatively affect the quality of the writing product. Others argued that the process approach was inappropriate for students with disabilities and other children (e.g., English-language learners), who might need more explicit guidance and a stronger support system in the language arts classroom (Schirmer & Bailey, 2000). On the other hand, proponents of the process approach to writing expressed concern about the ways in which the process was implemented in the classroom, fearing that it was often implemented as a formulaic process that did not afford writers, learners, or teachers freedom of choice (Murray, 1995).

In reality, speech-language pathologists and teachers cannot subcribe to an orientation that is solely process or product. To be effective, school professionals must help students see themselves as genuine writers by (a) engaging in the writing process, (b) using strategies effectively to improve their craft, and (c) working toward the goal of developing high-quality writing in which they can take pride. By taking this approach, speech-language pathologists and all teachers will play a part in helping students develop the inclination, skills, and habits that will assist them to be effective and thoughtful lifetime writers.

REFLECTION QUESTIONS

1. What is the difference between a process orientation and a product orientation in the writing classroom?
2. What are the characteristics of emergent writers?
3. In Case Study One, Simon's teacher seems to want to take a hands-off approach. Why is this problematic?
4. In Case Study Two, Christina's parents appear to feel disenfranchised from the school system. If you were Christina's speech-language pathologist, special education teacher, or classroom teacher, what changes would you make to work more closely with them and to help them to gain confidence in their daughter's education?
5. Why can spelling be considered a meaning-making activity?
6. What can speech-language pathologists, special education teachers, and classroom teachers learn by looking at children's inventive spellings?
7. Why is the concept of ownership so important in a writer's workshop?

REFERENCES

Atwell, N. (1998). *In the middle: New understandings about writing, reading, and learning.* Portsmouth, NH: Heinemann.

Avery, C. (2002). *. . . And with a light touch: Learning about reading, writing and teaching with first graders.* Portsmouth, NH: Heinemann.

Bear, D., Invernizzi, M., Templeton, S., & Johnston, F. (2004). *Words their way: Word study for phonics, vocabulary, and spelling instruction.* Upper Saddle River, NJ: Merrill/Pearson.

Bissex, G. L. (1980). *GNYS AT WRK: A child learns to write and read.* Cambridge, MA: Harvard University Press.

Bloodgood, J. W. (2002). Quintilian: A classical educator speaks to the writing process. *Reading Research and Instruction, 42,* 30–43.

Brice, R. G. (2004). Connecting oral and written language through applied writing strategies. *Intervention in School and Clinic, 40*(1), 38–47.

Calkins, L. (1991). *Living between the lines.* Portsmouth, NH: Heinemann.

Calkins, L. M. (1994). *The art of teaching writing* (2nd ed.) Portsmouth, NH: Heinemann.

Chandler, K., & the Mapleton Teacher-Research Group. (1999). *Spelling inquiry: How one elementary school caught the mnemonic plague.* York, ME: Stenhouse.

Clay, M. M. (1991). *Becoming literate: the construction of inner control.* Portsmouth, NH: Heinemann.

Diller, D. (2003). *Literacy work stations: Making centers work.* Portland, ME: Stenhouse.

Dragan, P. B. (2001). *Literacy from day one.* Portsmouth, NH: Heinemann.

Dyson, A. (1997). *Writing superheroes: Contemporary childhood, popular culture, and classroom literacy.* New York: Teachers College Press.

Dyson, A. (1999). Coach Bombay's Kids learn to write: Children's appropriation of media material for school literacy. *Research in the Teaching of Literacy, 33,* 367–401.

Emig, J. (1971). The composing processes of twelfth graders. Urbana, IL: National Council of Teachers of English.

Fletcher, R., & Portalupi, J. (1998). *Craft lessons: Teaching writing K–8.* Portland, ME: Stenhouse.

Fulwiler, T. (Ed.). (1987). *The journal book.* Portsmouth, NH: Heinemann.

Gentry, R. (1982). An analysis of developmental spelling in *GNYS AT WRK. The Reading Teacher, 36,* 192–200.

Gentry, R. (1997). *My kid can't spell! Understanding and assisting your child's literacy development.* Portsmouth, NH: Heinemann.

Graves, D. H. (1975). The writing processes of seven-year-old children. *Research in the Teaching of English, 9,* 227–241.

Graves, D. H. (1983). *Writing: Teachers & children at work.* Portsmouth, NH: Heinemann.

Graves, D. (1984). *A researcher learns to write: Selected articles and monographs.* Westport, CT: Heinemann-Boynton/Cook.

Graves, D. H. (1985). All children can write. *Learning Disabilities Forum, 1,* 36–43.

Graves, D. H. (1994). *A fresh look at writing.* Portsmouth, NH: Heinemann.

Groff, P. (1986). The implications of developmental spelling research: A dissenting view. *The Elementary School Journal, 86,* 317–323.

Hall, N. (1987). *The emergence of literacy.* Portsmouth, NH: Heinemann.

Holdaway, D. (1979). *The foundations of literacy.* Sydney, Australia: Ashton Scholastic.

Hughes, M., & Searle, D. (2000). Spelling and "the second 'r.'" *Language Arts, 77,* 203–208.

Kervin, L. K. (2002). Proofreading as a strategy for spelling development. *Reading Online, 5*(10). Retrieved January 11, 2008, from http://www.readingonline.org/international/inter_index.asp?HREF=kervin/index.html.

Marchisan, M. L., & Alber, S. R. (2001). The write way: Tips for teaching the writing process to resistant writers. *Intervention in School and Clinic, 36,* 154–162.

Murray, D. (1985). *A writer teaches writing.* Boston, MA: Houghton Mifflin.

Murray, W. (1995, November–December). A talk with Donald Graves. *Instructor,* 42–43.

Newkirk, T. (1989). *More than stories: The range of children's writing.* Portsmouth, NH: Heinemann.

Newkirk, T. (2001). The Revolt against realism: The attraction of fiction for young writers. *The Elementary School Journal, 101,* 465–477.

Read, C. (1971). Pre-school children's knowledge of English phonology. *Harvard Educational Review, 41,* 1–34.

Rosencranz, G. (1998). *The spelling book: Teaching children how to spell, not what to spell.* Newark, DE: International Reading Association.

Routman, R. (2005). *Writing essentials: Raising expectations and results while simplifying teaching.* Portsmouth, NH: Heinemann.

Schirmer, B. R., & Bailey, J. (2000). Writing assessment rubric: An instructional approach with struggling writers. *Teaching Exceptional Children, 33,* 52–58.

Scott, B. J., & Vitale, M. R. (2003). Teaching the writing process to students with LD. *Intervention in School and Clinic, 38,* 220–224.

Spandel, V. (2004). *Creating young writers: Using the six traits to enrich writing process in primary classrooms.* Boston, MA: Pearson.

Teale, W. H., & Sulzby, E. (1989). Emergent literacy: New perspectives. In D. S. Strickland & L. M. Morrow (Eds.), *Emerging literacy: Young children learn to read and write* (pp. 1–15). Newark, DE: International Reading Association.

Treiman, R., & Bourassa, D. C. (2000). The development of spelling skill. *Topics in Language Disorders, 20,* 1–18.

Part 3

Home and School Language Programs

Chapter 10

Home and School Language Matches and Mismatches

Edward E. Heckler

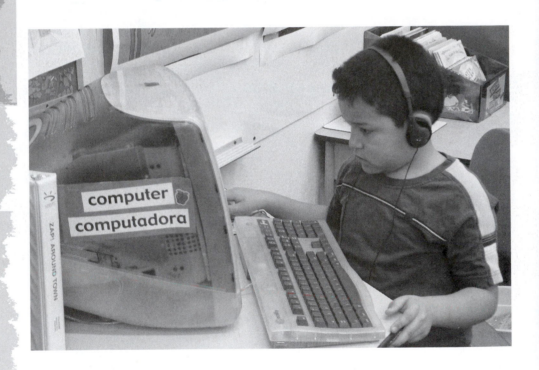

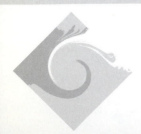

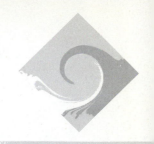

CHAPTER OUTLINE

CULTURAL INFLUENCES

Culture is a way of life for individuals who share a common heritage of beliefs, customs, and traditions. This shared heritage includes language, child-rearing practices, communication patterns, and literacy practices. The language in the following conversation clearly reflects the culture of the speakers, that is, of Spanish-English bilingual speakers from south Texas.

Along the United States–Mexico border, the following conversation occurred in a North-American supermarket:

Woman: ¿Dónde está el thin-sliced bread? [Where is the thin-sliced bread?]
  Clerk: Está en aisle three, sobre el second shelf, en el wrapper rojo.
    [It is in aisle three, on the second shelf, in the red wrapper.]
Woman: No lo encuentro. [I cannot find it.]
  Clerk: Tal vez estamos out of it. [Maybe we are out of it.]
    (Goldman, 1986, p.23)

Within a culture, individuals may share the same speech patterns and communicative systems, including languages and dialects. A **dialect** is a variety of a language that is mutually intelligible (understandable) to speakers of other varieties of the same language. A dialect is represented in this comment by an eighth-grade student from New York, "Dem dudes always be doin der thang," which other American-English speakers say as "Those guys are always doing their thing," (Smitherman, 1986, p.18). Most English speakers can understand this child's speech because it is a dialect of English and not a separate language such as Spanish, which would be unintelligible.

Every dialect reflects either the speech of a certain geographical area or of a social group. For instance, North Americans in various regions of the country label a carbonated soft drink differently: in New England it is a *tonic*; in the Midwest, *pop*; and in the South, *soda* or c*oke*. This same pattern occurs among speakers in different countries. In England the British eat *jacket potatoes* and buy *petrol* for their cars, while in the United States North Americans eat *baked potatoes* and buy *gasoline*.

Even in the same geographical region, however, members of different socioeconomic status speak differently. In the United States, the social dialect may reflect a speaker's level of education. The **prestigious dialect** is the formal language variety spoken in education, business, government, and the national media by the well-educated, influential members of a region. In contrast, a nonprestigious dialect or a vernacular dialect is a variety of the language.

Some dialects are based on the educational level of the speaker, while others may be based mainly on ethnicity. In terms of numbers of speakers, the two most important ethnic dialects in the United States are African American English and Spanish-influenced English (defined in a following paragraph). African American English (AAE) is the social variety of American English "spoken by African-Americans who are members of the working class" in large cities or the rural south (Green, 2002, pp. 5–6). Some of its basic traits are listed in Table 10–1. According to the 2000 U.S. Census, 12.3% of the U.S. population is African American, and they may speak African American English.

Another large ethnic group consists of Hispanics in the United States, whose ancestors came from Spanish-speaking countries, particularly from Mexico, Puerto Rico, and Cuba. According to the 2000 U.S. Census, the Hispanic population increased by 58% from 1990 to 2000. As of 2003, the Hispanic population comprised 12.5% of the total U.S. population (Marotta & Garcia, 2003, p. 16). Most Hispanics live in the western and southern United States, with nearly one-half residing in California and Texas. Among the Hispanic population, Mexicans comprise the largest group (58%); Puerto Ricans, the second largest (10%); and Cubans, the third largest (4%) (Marotta & Garcia, 2003, p. 17). These three groups display divergent living preferences, with most Mexicans in the West (55%), most Puerto Ricans in the Northeast (61%), and most Cubans in the South (74%) (Marotta & Garcia, 2003, p. 19).

Factors affecting Spanish in the United States are not simple; however, it should be noted that not all Hispanics are Spanish-English speakers. Spanish-influenced English is the social variety of American English "influenced by contact with Spanish, and spoken as a native dialect by both bilingual and monolingual speakers," especially in the Southwest (Fought, 2003, p. 1). Spanish-influenced English may be spoken by Latinos who are native English speakers and who may not know any Spanish. It does not refer to the speech of native Spanish speakers who are acquiring English as a second language but still may speak with mistakes as a result of some language interference. In contrast to the uniformity of African American English, the features of Spanish-influenced English vary considerably.

Besides African American English and Spanish-influenced English, other social English varieties exist; they are influenced by European languages such as French,

TABLE 10-1

Selected Contrasts Between Standard American English (SAE) and African American English (AAE)

(A) Phonology	SAE	AAE
Final consonant cluster reduction	hand, picked	han, pick
/b, d, g/ devoiced to /p, t, k/	cab, feed, pig	cap, feet, pick
/f/ or /t/ for /θ/ (*th* in *th*umb)	bath, with	baf, wit
/v/ or /d/ for /θ/ (*th* in *the*)	bathe, that	bave, dat
/l/ and /r/ liquids	help, four	hep, foh
/skr/ for /str/	street, straight	skreet, skraight

(B) Morphology	SAE	AAE
Noun plural -*s*	two puppies	two puppy
Noun possessive '*s*	mama's house	mama house
Third person singular present verb	She eats, runs.	She eat, run.
Past tense	John came.	John come.
Past and past participle verbs merge	saw, seen	seen, seen

(C) Semantics (lexicon)	SAE	AAE
	become engaged in some activity	get possessive pronoun–noun on
	(a) rest	(a) get my chill on
	(b) do an act like dancing with various partners	(b) get my mac on (usually males to females)
	(c) praise or worship	(c) get my praise on
	take advantage of, succeed by using wit but little effort	get over
	kiss	give someone some sugar
	slap my hand(s) in greeting	give me five
	press or apply light pressure to something	mash
	good, exciting	off the hook/chain

(D) Syntax	SAE	AAE
Omission of copula *be*	John is sick.	John sick.
Habitual *be*	Your phone bill is usually high.	Your phone bill be high.
bin for remote past	She has been running for a long time.	She bin running.
it and *dey* for existential "there"	There are usually knives in here.	It be knives in here.
	There is some coffee.	Dey some coffee.
Multiple negation	I don't ever have any problems.	I don't never have no problems.
Indirect questions with subject-verb inversion	Ask him if you can do it.	Ask him can you do it?

Source: Data from Green, 2002; Mufwene, 2001.

German, and Italian; by Asian languages such as Chinese, Japanese, and Tagalog; by Middle Eastern languages such as Arabic; and by Native American languages, including Cherokee and Navaho. Each dialect, whether regional or social, differs systematically from other varieties in the five subareas of language: phonology (sounds), morphology, semantics (lexicon), syntax (grammar), and pragmatics (use). To illustrate this, let us examine a few linguistic features of Spanish-influenced English, that is, how Spanish influences English or results in linguistic interference. Linguistic interference results because the speaker uses one set of language rules (e.g., Spanish) applied to their second language (i.e., English). This typically happens without the speaker's conscious knowledge.

Phonologically, the Spanish-influenced English dialect substitutes a /t/ for /θ/ (the voiceless interdental *th* in *th*umb) and a /d/ for /θ/ (the voiced interdental *th* in *th*e) in words like *tink* (think) and *dey* (they). The final consonant in a cluster is often deleted as in *star* (start). Some grammar rules differ because Spanish-influenced English may not morphologically use third person singular present *-s* verb forms, as in "He don't want" for the dialectally prestigious mainstream American English of "He doesn't want." Semantically, Spanish-influenced English defines some words differently, like *tell* for the standard *ask* in "She'll tell me how high" (see Table 10–2). Syntactically, Spanish-influenced English uses subject–verb inversion for indirect questions as in "And he told them who was it" for the standard "And he told them who it was," which retains the normal subject–verb word order.

Socioeconomic Status

Social attitudes concerning nonmainstream dialects often play a major role in communication and in education. One's speech identifies oneself; therefore, certain dialects have become associated with certain social groups. Some individuals from middle and upper socioeconomic levels regard lower socioeconomic speakers, in particular ethnic minorities, less favorably, and this attitude extends to their nonacceptance of social dialects.

Two basic views of vernacular dialects spoken by ethnically diverse minorities exist, that is, the deficit view and the difference view. The **deficit view** hypothesizes that the only acceptable dialect with "correct grammar" is considered to be the mainstream dialect or one being prestigious; other dialects (nonmainstream or nonprestigious) are considered to deprived, with unacceptable "bad grammar." On the other hand, linguists or language specialists advocate the difference view concerning vernacular dialects. The **difference view** hypothesizes that no dialect is deprived, with inadequate "bad grammar," because each dialect follows precise rules and can communicate messages clearly and logically. The latter view, the difference view hypothesis, is held by the American Speech-Language-Hearing Association (2003). Furthermore, the American Speech-Language-Hearing Association stated:

> It is the position of the American Speech-Language-Hearing Association (ASHA) that no dialectal variety of American English is a disorder or a pathological form of speech or language. Each dialect is adequate as a functional and effective variety of American English. Each serves a communicative function as well as a social-solidarity function. Each dialect

TABLE 10–2

Selected Contrasts Between Standard American English (SAE) and Spanish influenced English (SPIE)

(A) Phonology	SAE	SPIE
Alternation of ch /tʃ/ and sh /ʃ/	chair, show	share, chow
/t/ for /θ/ (*th* in *th*umb)	think, thing	tink, ting
/d/ for /ð/ (*th* in *the*)	they, there	dey, dere
Final consonant cluster reduction	start, least	star, leas
Word final /z/ devoiced to /s/	was /z/, guys /z/	was /s/, guys /s/
/b/ for /v/	never	neber
/ɪ/ (as in *sit*) to /i/ (as in *seat*)	king /ɪ/	king /i/
Different stress patterns		
(a) noun compound stress on second word	Thanksgíving míniskirt	Thanksgivíng miniskírt
(b) verb compound stress on first word	sit úp, shów up	śit up, shów up
Final declarative intonation rise	He's a good studentᵛ.	He's a good studentᵒ.

(B) Morphology	SAE	SPIE
Third person singular present verb	He doesn't want	He don't want
Past and past participle verbs	I had come, it spun	I had came, it spinned
Reflexive *-self* pronouns	himself, themselves	hisself, theirselves

(C) Semantics (lexicon)	SAE	SPIE
(a) Different English vocabulary use		

	SAE	SPIE
borrow for 'lend'	Lend me a pencil.	Borrow me a pencil.
talk to for 'date'	I date his sister.	I talk to his sister.
tell for 'ask'	She'll ask me how high.	She'll tell me how high.
barely for 'just recently'	They recently graduated from high school.	They barely graduated from high school.

(b) Use of Spanish borrowings in English

South Texas examples:

	SAE	SPIE
a type of soup		menudo
a party, a barbecue, or a political meeting		pachanga
a fifteen-year-old girl's coming-out rite		quinceñera

(D) Syntax	SAE	SPIE
Multiple negation	I don't have any pain.	I don't have no pain.
Indirect questions with subject-verb inversion	And he told them who it was.	And he told them who was it.
Comparative *more* for *more often*	They use Spanish more often.	They use more Spanish.

(continued)

TABLE 10–2 *(continued)*
Selected Contrasts Between Standard American English (SAE) and Spanish influenced English (SPIE)

Prepositions *in* versus *on*	in June, on a beer run	on June, in a beer run
Others	They got out of the car.	They got off the car.
	get away from their problems	get out from their problems

Source: Data from Fought, 2003; Penfield & Ornstein-Galicia, 1985.

maintains the communication network and the social construct of the community of speakers who use it. Furthermore, each is a symbolic representation of the geographic, historical, social, and cultural background of its speakers (p. 1).

A few vernacular-dialect rules differ from those of the prestigious dialect; consequently, a vernacular dialect has "structural integrity" (Adger & Wolfram, 2000, p. 393). It is the social prestige of the speakers, not the grammar of a dialect, that determines its favorable or unfavorable status in society.

Religion

Of the many crucial factors in one's culture, religion plays a prominent role in American communities. In the African American community, the church has historically been "the most powerful and long-standing institution" (Moss, 2001, p. 195), with the preacher serving as the foremost spokesperson and even political leader. Most African Americans are Protestant Christians. The church, "the cultural womb" and support system, has noticeably influenced African American "music, drama, literature, storytelling, and even humor" (Moss, 2003, p. 18). Some African Americans, however, belong to the Nation of Islam. These Muslims study the Koran and adhere to its principles, espoused by the prophet Mohammed, that include abstinence from eating pork and drinking alcohol.

Religion plays an all-encompassing role within Hispanic culture as well. Most Hispanics are Christian Catholics with an increasing number of Protestants. Hispanic religious practices often center in the home, with great respect for the Virgin Mary. Different groups identify with different manifestations of Our Lady of Sorrows: Mexican Americans with Our Lady of Guadalupe; Puerto Ricans, Our Lady of Providencia; and Cubans, La Caridad de Cobre (Ryan & Kanellos, 1995). To the faithful, religious pilgrimages remain an important Christian tradition. Also belonging to the Hispanic spiritual tradition are folk religions, sometimes an adjunct to Christian beliefs, which arose from everyday practices. Santeria, a form of worship with African and Caribbean roots, has historically been a vital force in Cuba and Puerto Rico. Other folk practices include spells by faith healers known as *curanderos* (i.e., healers) and curing ailments with herbal medicines. In shops labeled *yerberías* (i.e., herbal medicines) by Mexican Americans and *botánicas* (i.e., pharmacies) by Caribbean Hispanics, herbal medicines can be found (Ryan & Kanellos, 1995).

Family Values

During a child's acquisition of language, the family plays a major role. Within the contemporary African American community, two traits remain salient, that is, single parenthood and the extended family (Lassiter, 1998). Compared to the European American family, the African American family frequently consists of only one parent, typically the mother. Along with single parenthood comes a greater likelihood of poverty. The extended family may involve several generations of members, with grandparents sometimes providing primary care for the children. Lassiter (1998) stated, "The African American child is taught to function in two different societies, the black society and the white mainstream society, while maintaining his or her identity and self-esteem" (p. 37).

The family, *la familia*, plays a major role in an Hispanic child's life. Compared to the European American family, the Hispanic family more frequently consists of a larger extended family. The extended family may consist of parents and other kin such as grandparents, uncles, and/or aunts who may provide essential support for the children. Contrasted with the more egalitarian African American family, the Hispanic family is traditionally dominated by the father in the male role of a strong decision maker (Ryan & Kanellos, 1995). The role of the selfless, acquiescent mother concerns caring for children and being an obedient wife. The traditional Hispanic family, very devout to Catholic tradition, includes *padrinos* (godparents), *comadres* (godmothers), and *compadres* (godfathers), who undertake "a co-parenting role" to nurture "the spiritual and worldly needs of the child" (Madding, 2002, p.72).

"The role of children in the traditional Hispanic family can best be described by the proverb: 'Children are to be seen but not heard'" (Ryan & Kanellos, 1995, p. 106). In general, Hispanic children are "treasured," supported, and expected to participate in family activities and celebrations like weddings (*bodas*) and birthdays (*cumpleaños*). Other family members besides parents, chiefly siblings, can exert their influence in family affairs. Hispanic males, even young ones, often protect their sisters. This sibling relationship likewise affects language acquisition because siblings, and not just parents, impart speech to the younger children (Fought, 2003).

To impart cultural values and tradition to their children, European American families frequently use proverbs like "The early bird catches the worm" and "A penny saved is a penny earned." Hispanics similarly use sayings or *dichos* "(a) to censure, (b) to teach, (c) to establish rapport, and (d) to entertain" (Barajas, 2005, p. 71). Two examples of Spanish dichos (sayings) are:

> *El que tiene hambre, le atiza a la olla.*
> [He who is hungry stokes (the fire for) the pot.]
> *Más vale solo que mal acompañado.*
> [Better to be alone than in bad company.]
> (Barajas 2005, pp. 68, 89. See also Brice, 2002)

In a study of Hispanic families in California, Fought (2003) noted that Hispanic children live at home longer than European American children. If children are spending more time at home, both daily and over their lifetimes, their parents and siblings may contribute more to their linguistic environment than do parents and siblings in a community where the peer group receives more emphasis. The family structure may also be a crucial element in bilingual acquisition (p. 31).

PARENTAL ROLES IN COMMUNICATION AND CHILD REARING

Communication is a social process in which the encoder, a speaker with information, shares it with the decoder, a listener whose task is to comprehend the intended meaning. Mastering any language to communicate well takes a child many years. Parental attitudes about nurturing and communicating with young children affect the process of language acquisition greatly because "how parents talk with their preschool children is widely held to be an important factor in children's acquisition of cognitive and linguistic abilities" (Eisenberg, 2002, p. 206).

In many cultures, the parents play the seminal role in fostering the language development of children. In middle socioeconomic status (SES) North America, the mother dominates as caregiver, whose task is to help the child acquire language by a dyadic conversation between herself and the child. According to behavioral theory, two essential tasks for the caregiver predominate: first, to provide linguistic input by speaking frequently to the child; and, second, to provide a correct model of language. Generally, middle socioeconomic status caregivers amend child-speech slips, especially those of semantics because the learner's inappropriate words in a conversation may likely cause miscommunication or even no communication at all. For example, the caregiver may provide the term *helicopter* for the child's inappropriate labeling of *plane*. Slips in grammar (morphology and syntax) are also modeled correctly but much less consistently. For example, the caregiver may amend the child's production of "I sleeped" by modeling the form of "I slept."

Conversing with young infants, a middle socioeconomic status caregiver uses special speech that was formerly referred to as motherese. This child-directed speech refers to the distinctive modified speech that caregivers use when communicating with infants and also nonnative speakers of English in order to be understood more easily. This targeted child-directed speech reveals "the emotions of the speaker" and helps the child "make discriminations between sounds and words" (Golinkoff & Hirsh-Pasek, 2000, p. 32). In fact, the child may even prefer this speech, which normally occurs only during the first few years of life.

Child-directed speech consists of the following communication characteristics. Phonologically, caregivers exaggerate the intonation, use a higher pitch, speak noticeably slower with longer pauses, repeat sounds more often, and articulate both vowels and consonants more clearly. An example would be "goood mooooorrrrn-ing" to a child and "good morning" to an adult (Golinkoff and Hirsh-Pasek, 2000). Semantically, caregiver speech simplifies and restricts the vocabulary to basic topics to include the here and now in the child's immediate environment, repeats the same word often, and uses specialized "child talk" terms like *doggie, horsie,* and *moo moo* (cow). Syntactically, sentences are grammatically correct and comprehensible yet less structurally complex, often shorter, and more repetitious. Unlike adult communication, child-directed speech emphasizes very frequent questions and imperatives (commands), some of which may be rituals. Syntactic examples of child-directed speech include *Where's Daddy? Look at* (the) *doggie,* and *Let's play with the blocks* (Clark, 2003, p. 42). Nonverbal body movements like heightened caregiver facial expressions typically accompany this type of speech.

The following is an example of child-directed speech of a mother conversing with her 13-month-old son, Keith, while they are looking at a wordless baby picture book:

See the *doggie*, Keith? Oh, he's so cute! He looks like the dog that Mr. Owen has, doesn't he? And there's a *car*! The doggie is driving a *car*! What is the doggie wearing? A *hat*!. . . . The doggie is driving a *car* and wearing a *hat*! (Golinkoff & Hirsh-Pasek, 2000, p. 100).

These are English examples. Child-directed speech traits have been observed in widely divergent cultures and languages throughout the world (for instance, Spanish, Arabic, Marathi, Comanche, and Chinese) (Farb, 1975; Clark, 2003; Ferguson, 1977). Apparently child-directed speech shares some universal traits. For instance, "studies have found that parental sounds of comfort, prohibition, and praise are remarkably similar" (Golinkoff & Hirsh-Pasek, 2000, p. 32). Despite these universals of caregiver–infant communication, some cultures and languages (for instance, the Piedmont Trackton culture in the United States) may not use child-directed speech to the same extent.

In a seminal study of three separate Carolina Piedmont communities, Brice-Heath (1983) delineated adult–child communication differences based on culture, socioeconomic status, and ethnicity. The Mainstream Piedmont community, whose members comprised middle socioeconomic status (SES) European American and African American townspeople, displayed a greater evidence of child-directed speech in communicating with their young children. The mothers stressed question-and-answer routines so that their children "act[ed] as conversation partners and information-givers" (p. 249). The nearby Roadville community, whose members comprised the European American working socioeconomic status, also used child-directed speech during the first years of a child's life. Roadville residents believed that preschoolers needed conversational skills "to communicate their own needs and desires" and "to be communicative partners in a certain mold" (p.127).

In the third Piedmont community, Trackton, whose members comprised the African American working socioeconomic status group, child-directed speech was not as evident. Unlike the mother–child communicative dyad of the Mainstream community, Trackton regularly immersed the child in the speech of the entire community, not just that of family members. Their young children were not deemed to be "suitable partners for a regular conversation," yet "they are expected to *become* information-knowers by . . . taking in the numerous lessons going on in their noisy multi-channeled environments" (p. 86). In short, the three Piedmont communities shared a common language, that is, English; however, their children developed different communicative competencies as a result of culturally divergent child-rearing practices.

The norms of language acquisition for all other cultures and languages do not always include a middle socioeconomic status dyad of a caregiver and a child. For instance, among the rural Kaluli of Papua New Guinea, the communicative norm is a triad of (1) a caregiver, (2) an infant language learner, and (3) a third participant who is often an older sibling or relative. Typically the Kaluli caregiver directly models for the infant what information to tell the third participant (see Clark, 2003).

Socioeconomic status plays a role in parental communicative practices. Compared to lower socioeconomic status and lower-middle socioeconomic status mothers, upper-middle socioeconomic status mothers use more wh- questions (wh- words like *who*, *where*, and *when*) that require a reply of specific information. Lower socioeconomic status mothers, on the other hand, use more imperatives (commands) in child-directed speech than middle socioeconomic status mothers, according to research studies (Clark, 2003). The quantity of parental input directed to children varies by socioeconomic status: middle socioeconomic status parents produce 2,100 words per hour; working socioeconomic status parents, about 1,200; and lower SES parents, only 600 (Clark, 2003; Hart & Risley, 1995). In short, middle socioeconomic status parents communicate more verbally. According to research studies, the features of "effective maternal instruction" more frequently correlate with middle socioeconomic status than with lower socioeconomic status (Eisenberg, 2002, p. 208).

Besides socioeconomic status, other factors such as ethnicity and parents' formal education level also play pivotal roles in caregiver communication patterns. Steward and Steward (1973) investigated how mothers taught a game to preschoolers. They concluded that the caregiver's ethnicity was a contributing factor because both Mexican American and Chinese American parents "culturally demanded" their children show "obedience and respect of elders" to a greater degree than European American parents did (p. 335). However, Laosa (1980), who studied the teaching strategies of Mexican American and European American families, concluded that the mother's level of formal education, not ethnicity, counted most of all.

The type of instructional task is also relevant in parental communication with young children. An investigation of Mexican American maternal teaching strategies revealed a difference in child-directed speech based on the specific instructional task (Eisenberg, 2002). During block building, the mothers asked their children more questions and gave more positive feedback than they did for biscuit making. However, the mothers used more complex sentences for biscuit making than for block building.

Also playing a role in the communicative teaching practices is the caregiver's place of birth (immigrant versus native-born). In a study comparing immigrant Mexican American mothers, native-born Mexican American mothers, and European American mothers, Chavez and Buriel (1986) concluded that caregiver communicative roles were complex. Under high-effort-failure conditions, both native-born Mexican American and European American caregivers communicated using many reinforcements; however, immigrant Mexican American caregivers differed, with fewer reinforcements. Under low-effort-success conditions, however, immigrant Mexican American and European American caregivers communicated similarly, using many more reinforcements than native-born Mexican American caregivers.

Gender in communication also plays a role in language development because children are taught gender-specific linguistic-speech roles from their caregivers. Zentella (1997) studied working socioeconomic status Puerto Rican communicative practices in New York City and delineated how children were socialized into gender-appropriate behavior. Young girls were taught traditional obedience, duty, and restricted physical movement while boys were given more latitude and freedom with less restricted physical movement.

In addition to monolingual language learning, some caregivers choose bilingualism for their children's linguistic upbringing. Bilingualism refers to the ability to know and speak two languages fluently (Macnamara, 1967). Second-language acquisition consists of simultaneous bilingualism and successive (sequential) bilingualism.

Simultaneous bilingualism refers to a child's acquisition of two languages before age 3, while successive (sequential) bilingualism refers to a child's acquisition of a second language after age 3, after the acquisition (although incomplete) of the first language has begun (McLaughlin, 1978). (Refer to Chapter 4 for discussion of bilingual language development.)

According to the 2000 U.S. Census, 17.9% of all Americans over 5 years of age speak a non-English language at home, with 76.5% of these non-English speakers conversing "very well" or "well" in English, while 7.0% know no English (United States Census Bureau 2003). Among Hispanics from 1990 to 2000, "the percentage of the total population speaking Spanish at home has increased consistently at the national and state levels. Nationally, it increased from about 7.5% to 10.7%" (Marotta & Garcia, 2003, p. 21). This increase in Spanish home-language use mainly resulted from increasing numbers of Spanish-speaking immigrants. At least one-fourth of the Hispanics in California (25%), New Mexico (28.7%) and Texas (27%) speak Spanish in the home (Marotta & Garcia, 2003).

Language use among Hispanic Spanish-English-speaking caregivers depends on many factors, including (1) the caregiver's language proficiency, (2) educational philosophy, (3) the majority/minority status of each language in the community, (4) language use by other close family-members, (5) cultural identification, and (6) the caregiver's place of birth. First-generation caregivers raised in another country, who do not know English, will promote their native language. Second-generation English-dominant caregivers raised in the United States favor speaking with their children in English. Zentella documents the case of Maria, a New Yorker of Puerto Rican heritage, whose parents considered it essential that their children have the capacity to *defenderse* ("defend themselves") and speak English well enough "to get along" (1997, p. 244).

Parents who educate their children bilingually employ diverse strategies to accomplish their linguistic goals (Cunningham-Andersson & Andersson, 1999; Grosjean, 1982; Harding-Esch & Riley, 2003; Romaine, 1989). These strategies consist of:

1. The one person/one language method, in which each parent speaks a different language to their children, who respond in the same language spoken by the parent.

2. The one language–one location method, in which both parents speak the minority language of the community at home and the children learn English outside the home at school.

3. The non-native parent method, in which both parents speak the same native language, the dominant majority language in the community; however, at home, one parent always speaks to the children in a minority language that is not the parent's native language.

4. The mixed language method, in which parents use two languages and code-switch.

5. The specific age method, in which one language is used when the child is born; when the child reaches a certain age (often 3 to 5), the second language is then introduced (an example of successive sequential bilingualism).

6. The language-time method, in which one language is used at a certain time (such as morning) and the other language at a different time (such as afternoon).

How well do these different strategies succeed? Since each strategy has both strengths and weaknesses, the answer is not readily apparent. What matters most for successful acquisition of bilingualism "is that the child feels the *need* to use two languages in everyday life" (Grosjean, 1982, p. 175).

Goodz (1994), researching French-English bilingual families, concluded that the use of communicative strategies like those listed above are at best irregular. Goodz stated, "the actual language behavior of parents in bilingual families is not determined by a simple decision to present the languages in a prespecified way" influenced by "the parent's level of fluency in each language as well as by such situational factors as the need to attract the child's attention, for emphasis, and to discipline the child" (p. 70).

ROLES OF CHILDREN IN COMMUNICATION

Children, like parental caregivers, have specific cultural roles in communication. Behavioral theory states that the main tasks of young language learners are to imitate, repeat, and practice and to engage in discourse supplied by their caregivers. The following is a sample conversation between Lois and Patsy, the adults, and Peter, a two-year-old who is playing with a dump truck.

Lois:	You're gonna put more wheels in the dump truck?
Peter:	Dump truck. Wheels. Dump truck.
[Later]	
Patsy:	What happened to it (the truck)?
Peter:	(looking under chair for it) Lose it. Dump truck! Dump truck! Fall! Fall!
Lois:	Yes, the dump truck fell down.
Peter:	Dump truck fell down. Dump truck.

(Lightbown & Spada, 1999, p. 10)

Peter is imitating the caregiver's model, which he has just heard.

Language learning, however, involves more than behavioral imitation and practice. The child's imitation of caregiver speech is not always apparent or present. It should be remembered that the learner actively creates language.

It is vital for young children acquiring two languages to develop metacognitive competence to realize that different languages exist. A child's awareness of different languages can emerge early, as illustrated by this conversation between a 3-year-old German child and his father:

Father:	Der Techniker an der Universität hat mein Radio repariert. [The technician at the university fixed my wireless].
Thomas (3;8,3):	Hast du Deutsch gesprochen? [Did you speak German?]
Father:	Nein, Englisch. [No, English.]
Thomas:	Kann der Techniker kein Deutsch? [Doesn't the technician know any German?]

(Saunders 1982, p. 227)

Fantini (1985) reports a similar metacognitive language realization for his 5-year-old Spanish-English bilingual Mario.

Being empowered with being bilingual, children translate reasonably well even if they are not always literal. Harding-Esch and Riley (2003, p. 67) related how a girl translated her Italian father's irate comments to an English-speaking Canadian:

Father (to little girl, in Italian):	Tell him he's a nitwit.
Little girl (to third party, in English):	My father won't accept your offer.
Father (to little girl, in Italian):	Why didn't you you tell him what I told you?

SCHOOL EXPECTATIONS

When children enter school, they need to communicate in the special academic register of the classroom, which is not always spoken at home. A **register** denotes a special type of language variation used in a certain situation by the participants. Among the many school registers are academic classroom discourse, peer-to-peer discourse, and sports discourse.

Speech-language pathologists and special education teachers expect that students understand and use academic discourse at school. This educational discourse typically involves a hierarchical conversation between a speech-language pathologist or special education teacher and students. Cazden (1988) illustrated this when she stated:

> Teachers have the right to speak at any time and to any person; they can fill any silence or interrupt any speaker; they can speak to a student anywhere in the room and in any volume or tone of voice. And no one has any right to object (p. 54).

When using an academic register, speech-language pathologists and special education teachers issue directives (commands) to students and questions for which the answers are often known beforehand. Striking similarities exist between the middle socioeconomic status caregiver child-directed talk and school professional academic discourse to young children because both involve "higher pitch, more exaggerated intonation and careful enunciation, shorter sentences and more frequent repetitions, and many more questions" compared to normal adult discourse (Cazden, 1988, p. 160). A study of secondary classrooms in Scotland (cited in Cazden, 1988) narrowed classroom academic discourse to eight functions: (1) attracting attention, (2) controlling speech, (3) confirming understanding, (4) summarizing, (5) defining, (6) editing, (7) correcting, and (8) specifying the topic.

Academic discourse demonstrates remarkable homogeneity in North American classrooms. Regardless of the geographical area, the ethnicity or the native language of the speech-language pathologist or special education teacher, or the subject being taught, school professionals commonly display similar academic discourse traits in schools throughout the country with minor variation (Adger & Wolfram, 2000; Cazden, 1988; Brice-Heath, 1992).

Most classroom discourse is conducted solely or mainly in the mainstream or prestigious American English dialect. Regardless of their home dialect, native-speaking children of English are expected to learn and use prestigious speech in the classroom. Native-speaking children of other languages (for instance, Spanish-speaking Mexican immigrants) are expected to acquire English as rapidly as possible for academic discourse.

Classroom researchers such as Sinclair and Coulthard (1975) and Mehan (1979) have found certain common uses of language in general education classrooms. These have included use of directives (commands), informatives (giving information), and elicitations (questions). The results of a study by Brice, Mastin, and Perkins (1997) in an English-as-a-second-language classroom concur with the previous findings. Thus, it appears that general language use in the English-as-a-second-language (ESL) classroom does not differ greatly from what has been observed for general education.

The language functions of the Brice et al. (1997) study found that the ESL classroom followed a less structured adherence to the curriculum than the general education classroom. It also fostered more opportunities for students to practice their English. Hence, informative statements are encouraged in the ESL classroom, whereas they may not be in other environments.

Overall, the ESL classroom appeared to be teacher-directed, as evidenced by a high degree of questions, commands, feedback, and provision of information. In general, the high number of questions validated the notion of the classroom being teacher-directed. When the students answered a question, it reflected the typical IRE pattern in which the teacher *Initiates*, students *Respond,* and the teacher *Evaluates* the response (Cazden, 1988).

Some cultures within North American society, especially middle socioeconomic status cultures, prepare their children well for school. An example is the middle socioeconomic status culture of the African American and European American Piedmont Mainstream community, whose child-rearing communicative practices mirrored the verbal skills favored by the school community. For instance, the mainstream community used child-directed speech that provided labels and answers to questions. Talk such as "What's this?" and "Who's that?" clearly prepares youngsters for future academic discourse in school, which also emphasizes providing labels and answering questions.

Besides preparing children for academic discourse, the Piedmont caregivers continuously introduced children to books and stressed the importance of literacy. Even before they could read, Piedmont youngsters participated in dialogue about reading materials. They discovered that written sources have a nonliteral framework; thus, they "learn the distinctions between contextualized first-hand experiences and decontextualized representations of experience" (Brice-Heath, 1983, p. 256). Consequently, they became "producers and consumers of literacy in a consistent, highly redundant and repetitive pattern in using oral language" (Brice-Heath, 1983, p. 256).

They saw both caretakers and siblings read daily, and they realized the relevance of both reading and writing. All this home focus on literacy predisposed the children to success in school, with its similar concomitant focus on literacy. In summary, the spoken and literate home practices of preschool caregivers mirrored school language practices.

Matches and Mismatches Between Home and School

Students entering school bring their home language with them and, for some of them, home language and school language result in a good match. Generally these are middle and upper-middle socioeconomic status children who speak the prestigious language and dialect. In middle socioeconomic status homes, the child-directed speech by caregivers basically mirrors the school speech-language pathologist's or special education teacher's question-and-answer classroom discourse. Moreover, these children, who have been introduced to literacy by their caregivers, typically recognize the importance of literacy, even if they have not yet started to read. Their home upbringing makes them linguistically prepared to learn at school.

Mismatches

For other students, however, a mismatch sometimes exists between home communicative behavior and school linguistic expectations. "A crucial question is the extent to which school socialization and experience are discontinuous with respect to that of the home" (Romaine, 1984, p. 166). A discussion of the main mismatches between home and school follows; they include limited English abilities, context embedded language, decontextualized language, nonprestigious dialects, and varying cognitive learning styles.

A serious mismatch occurs between home and school for non-English-speaking children who have limited English abilities. With the exception of foreign-language classes, English is the language of instruction at school. For students who have no English abilities or whose English-language ability is very limited, the problem is indeed serious because they cannot comprehend the in-class communication about course content. For speech-language pathologists or special education teachers who do not speak the student's home language, it is an extremely monumental challenge to communicate information to these students. The next section will provide some practical suggestions for speech-language pathologists and special education teachers to help alleviate this language-comprehension problem. In addition, students may experience social isolation if no classmate or only a few classmates speak their home language. Peer-group acceptance or rejection can have a major effect on students' academic performance.

A mismatch between home discourse and school discourse concerns context. At home most of the conversation is in the "context of practical activity" (Romaine, 1984, p. 167); that is, discourse concerns the children's immediate environment or a specific example. For instance, young caregivers normally restrict their early speech to actions and objects in the children's immediate physical surroundings (using context embedded language). In school, academic classroom discourse is much more abstract. Decontextualized language is removed from the immediate context, whereas only the message itself provides meaning. It does not restrict speech to the physical classroom environment. Children may encounter problems in adjusting to this disparity between the home, where language is contextualized, and the school, where it is decontextualized.

Although speech-language pathologists and special education teachers expect students to speak academic English, many students from lower SES homes may not have these language abilities. It should be noted that children who speak a non-prestigious dialect of a language may have some exposure to the prestigious dialect because of its widespread use in such entertainment media such as television, radio, and films. Some research studies have suggested that children who speak a non-prestigious variety of English are assessed more negatively. For instance, Spanish-English speakers who do not speak English with typical articulation "consistently receive more negative judgments on both personality and linguistic rating scales" (Bailey & Galván, 1988, p. 32). (See also Ramírez, Acre-Torres, & Politzer, 1982.)

Another mismatch concerns cognitive learning style, which may be considered "an individual's natural, habitual, and preferred way of absorbing, processing, and retaining new information" (Lightbown & Spada, 1999, p. 58). In a study of Mexican American and Puerto Rican fourth- and fifth-grade Spanish-English bilinguals, Baecher (1982) discovered differences in learning style. The "collective cognitive style" of both groups revealed "a definite preference for activities involving listening rather than reading for information;" however, "significant differences were found between both groups in listening ability (English and Spanish)," with Mexican Americans having a higher listening comprehension (p. 376).

These mismatches between home and school may result in low academic performance by minority students and particularly by Hispanic students. According to Baecher (1982), mismatches may account for low Hispanic school performance: "(1) language and cultural experiences, (2) socioeconomic status, (3) school experiences, and (4) inadequate testing" as well as inadequate "attention given to the cultural diversity and learning styles of bilingual students" (p. 368).

How to Bridge the Language and Communication Gap

With more children entering the classroom not speaking English as their first language, speech-language pathologists and/or special education teachers are challenged to facilitate the process of English-second-language learning. Several crucial classroom principles may provide optimum language success: (1) value the student's home language, (2) value the student's culture, (3) involve parents, (4) emphasize the learner's active communication in English, (5) use cooperative learning, (6) integrate academic content with meaningful language learning, and (7) have high student expectations (Díaz-Rico, 2004; Díaz-Rico & Weed, 1995; Freeman & Freeman, 2001; 2002).

One key principle is for the speech-language pathologist or special education teacher to value the student's home language (Díaz-Rico & Weed, 1995; Freeman & Freeman, 2001). A speech-language pathologist or special education teacher needs to use the learner's home language or dialect as a valuable teaching resource, even if the school professional does not know the home language. An effective language program will *add* English to the language(s) that students bring to school while encouraging them to continue developing their first-language oral and written skills. On the other hand, programs that attempt to replace students' first language with English may undermine the personal and cultural confidence that is essential to students' academic progress (Cummins, 1994).

The speech-language pathologist or special education teacher needs to value a student's home culture because it plays a crucial role in language learning

(Freeman & Freeman, 2001; Díaz-Rico & Weed, 1995; Pérez & Torres-Guzmán, 2002). "The acquisition of English alone in no way guarantees that every linguistic minority student will succeed academically . . . . the cultural messages received by children from both the school and the larger society may influence their feelings about school as well" (McKeon, 1994, p. 23). The speech-language pathologist or special education teacher should integrate the student's culture into the curriculum in a meaningful way. For example, the school professional may wish to utilize cultural integration following Banks's (1988) model. Under this model of cultural integration, instructional lessons follow a hierarchy of three steps:

1. The **contributions approach** focuses on the surface issues and incorporates only discrete elements (such as heroes, foods, music, dance, and holidays) into the curriculum. The traditional curriculum remains unchanged in structure, goals, or characteristics.

2. The **additive approach** adds content, concepts, and themes from other cultural groups. School professionals may add a book unit or course in the university curriculum that focuses on a diverse group or specific topic.

3. The **transformational approach** offers to change the structure of the curriculum and offer students the opportunity to view concepts, events, or themes from a different cultural perspective. Culture is viewed not as how one group has contributed to the mainstream, but rather as how each group has emerged from the contributions of the other cultures. Different themes pervade the curriculum.

Consequently, both the speech-language pathologist and special education teacher should learn more about the student's home culture and cultural interaction styles. Students of different cultures may have experienced classroom instruction differently too. For example, Native American children traditionally learn by being silent in class and listening; Asian children, often in large classes, are accustomed to teacher authority but limited student participation.

Hayes, Bahruth, and Kessler (1998) demonstrated a successful literacy program in rural south Texas that valued both the students' home language and culture. The students, Spanish-English-bilingual migrants considered at risk due to previous academic failure, ranked below grade level in language and reading abilities by the fifth year. When the teacher implemented linguistically, culturally, and pedagogically sound classroom instruction that used both languages and a copious amount of mainly English reading and writing, these at-risk students succeeded. In just that one year, the students averaged three years of reading growth. Due to the teacher's use of two languages, the students' reading and writing abilities improved (Hayes, Bahruth, & Kessler, 1998). These students successfully graduated from high school, with some entering community colleges and universities.

A crucial principle is for the speech-language pathologist or special education teacher to involve parents and families in the child's education (de la Luz Reyes & Halcón, 2001; Díaz-Rico, 2004; González, Huerta-Macías, & Tinajero, 1998). Most immigrant parents of second-language learners are genuinely interested in their children's progress; however, cultural differences or inadequate home–school communication can hinder their active participation. To communicate better with parents whose home language they may not know, speech-language pathologists and/or special education teachers should use interpreters, if they are available. Speech-language pathologists and special education teachers need to understand and value the practical and cultural knowledge that all parents possess. Parental participation in children's language and literacy development fosters student learning, and home–school cooperation is important for student success. By respecting the children's home culture, speech-language pathologists and/or special education teachers can help fulfill this genuine plea as exemplified by a Hispanic mother:

> Que los hijos no se avergüencen de sus padres porque no saben leer y escribir y por trabajar en el campo, y que les den su valor como padres.
>
> [That our children not be ashamed of their parents because they don't know how to read and write, and because they work in the fields; and instead, continue to value and honor them as parents.] (quoted by Ada & Zubizarreta in de la Luz Reyes & Halcón, 2001, p. 242).

Society values good English communication; therefore, some parents who are concerned that the home language may hamper second-language learning try to raise their children monolingually in English despite their limited English knowledge. In these situations, unexpected and even unsuccessful results may occur, including the children's inability to communicate effectively with their monolingual native-language-speaking relatives (Tse, 2001). It is more beneficial for the children if parents with a very limited English-language ability speak the home language instead. For language- and literacy-learning success, children need to be reared in a language-rich environment, whether in the home language or in the school second language (Coelho, 1994; Cummins, 1992; Tse, 2001).

An additional principle for successful language learning is that the learner actively communicate in English. To acquire communicative competence, the learner needs more than grammar and syntactic knowledge (Swain, 1985). Crucial components of "effective communication" include "learning to carry on conversations, modifying language to fit various contexts, and choosing the best style of speech for each interaction" (Díaz-Rico & Weed, 1995, p. 85). During language-instruction time, the learner should actively speak, read, and write in the second language for "authentic communication," which means that "language is used to communicate about real ideas to real people" (McKeon, 1994, p. 27). Meaningful topics from the learner's culture, family, and interests should be chosen for authentic communication in the classroom. Simple language exercises consisting of fill-in-the-blank and circle-the-correct-answer items should be used very sparingly because they do not provide authentic communication.

Two important types of language skills exist, that is, BICS and CALP. According to Cummins (1992), BICS refers to Basic Interpersonal Communication Skills, or conversational discourse, while CALP refers to Cognitive Academic Language Proficiency, or academic school discourse. Normally it takes a learner two years to acquire BICS, but it takes considerably longer, four to seven years, to acquire CALP. For school success, a learner definitely needs CALP as well as BICS (Collier, 1987; Ramírez, 2000; Thomas & Collier, 2002). (See Chapter 4 on second-language acquisition.)

It is essential to incorporate cooperative peer-group learning into classroom activities because authentic communication tends to be social, and this is the learning style that many culturally and linguistically diverse children display (Gonzalez et al., 1998; Gudykunst, 1991; Gudykunst, Ting-Toomey, & Chua, 1988; Pérez & Torres-Guzmán, 2002; Richard-Amato, 2003; Ting-Toomey, 1994; Triandis, 1995). Communication involves unconscious scripts that are habitual. These scripts may be unknown to the individual unless they are continually examined (Gudykunst, 1991). These unconscious scripts may become barriers to communication in the classroom environment. School professionals are often unsuspecting of the ways the scripts are used and to what degree culture influences their use. Gudykunst (1991) emphasizes this point: "When we engage in habitual or scripted behavior we are not highly aware of what we are doing or saying" (p. 26). He also maintains that when communicating with others of differing cultures, school professionals base their interpretations on their own cultural referent systems, which involve speaking-listening and verbal-nonverbal behavior scripts. Thus, ineffective communication may result. As Gudykunst states (1991), "Our culture and ethnicity influence the attributions we make about others' behavior" (p. 30). Cooperative learning may take the form of several students working together as a group to help each other learn more efficiently. Students who lack English second-language proficiency may not be satisfactory language models for each other. Therefore, a student with limited English ability can be placed with a more proficient language peer (Pérez & Torres-Guzmán, 2002). Research suggests that both the language learner and the more fluent peer mutually improve their content knowledge (Richard-Amato, 2003).

The speech-language pathologist or special education teacher can use cross-age tutors, that is, older students to coach younger students. "Cross-age tutoring provides an opportunity for Latinos to engage in a social pattern of learning that is quite familiar and comfortable for them" because traditional Latino families often stress the importance of cooperation with older siblings (Huerta-Macías in González et al., 1998, p. 36). (Also see Richard-Amato & Snow, 2005.)

In addition to cooperative learning, speech-language pathologists and/or special education teachers should integrate academic content with meaningful language learning. It can take a second-language learner four years or more to acquire adequate proficiency in classroom academic language (CALP). While second-language learners are acquiring their English CALP, the speech-language pathologist or special education teacher cannot suspend instructing content because language learners need to be concurrently taught academic content. Doing so requires classroom adjustments. (See Richard-Amato & Snow, 2005.)

Speech-language pathologists and special education teachers should have high expectations so that learners achieve their true academic potential (Darder, Torres, & Gutiérrez, 1997). Learners need "cognitively challenging work" even though their second language ability may be limited (González et al., 1998, p. 262). Too often school professionals restrict limited English-language-proficient students to basic activities and content, and use repetitive drills incorporating relatively low-level exercises like those in worksheets. Learners exposed only to such basic instruction will not be prepared to meet the cognitive challenges of advanced academic work in school.

INSTRUCTIONAL STRATEGIES

1. Use home-culture content in class. Students should interview parents about customs, traditions, and holidays of the country of origin and then report about them in their class.
2. Involve parents. Encourage parents to read traditional children's stories at home (if they can). Parents can teach children a skill (making tortillas) and children can report in class about what they learned.
3. Use written communication to develop the second language. Students can write to pen pals in another class and then meet.
4. Form peer-tutor groups. Pair an older or more fluent learner with a younger or less fluent learner to read stories or write journal entries.
5. Integrate course content and language. Stress key vocabulary in mini-lessons about the course subject.

Limitations

Although these crucial principles can foster the learner's second language, limitations still exist. Time is a major constraint when learners are not given adequate time for special second-language instruction to reach the academic proficiency level. Students may receive only one or two years of English-as-a-second-language instruction and then be expected to succeed in the all-English general education classroom. Classroom teachers may lack school time or training to give these learners any extra language assistance.

Speech-language pathologists and/or special education teachers who know the learners' first language can better understand the learners' linguistic challenges. Another related limitation is having a classroom of students who speak different languages so that even bilingual speech-language pathologists and/or special education teachers cannot address all the different language needs. In such cases, it may be especially difficult for school professionals to communicate with parents, resulting in decreased parental involvement.

CASE STUDY PERSPECTIVES

Case Study One Background: Roberto

Roberto, a native Spanish speaker from Mexico, arrived in the United States during the school year. His family comes from a lower socioeconomic status. Prior to his enrollment in high school in the United States, Roberto had only a second-grade education in Mexico. In addition, he has not been in school for the last six years. Now 16 years old, Roberto is learning English as a ninth grader. At high school he is enrolled for two hours daily in English as a second language (ESL) with individualized help from an instructional aide. He receives special English-language classes for one hour; for the rest of the day, he receives small-group instruction in core content classes such as science and math. Roberto is not assisted by a speech-language pathologist or special-education teacher. He has participated in several Saturday tutoring sessions for conversation, spelling, and reading.

Roberto's overall progress in learning English, however, has been labeled as "very slow" by his teachers, who have rated him to be considerably below average. Not surprisingly, Roberto has encountered problems in acquiring English phonology. In particular, he has problems distinctly articulating sh (/ʃ/ as in *shoe*), th (/θ/ as in *thin* and /ð/ as in *then*), z (/z/ as in *zoo*), and w (/w/ as in which). Besides phonological difficulties, he has problems with correct verb forms (such as present tense third-person singular -*s* as in *she eats*) and subject-verb agreement (especially for *be* and *have* verbs). His knowledge of English vocabulary is extremely limited, so his English-language reading proficiency is quite low, too. In short, Roberto can neither understand nor communicate in English very well.

Case Study One Comments: Roberto

Roberto's slow progress in English-language learning mainly stems from his very limited education in Mexico and some possible learning disabilities. Lacking an adequate background in Spanish, he could barely read or write in his first language, possibly due to some phonological awareness difficulties, limited letter knowledge, limited exposure to print materials, and limited oral and written vocabulary. Consequently, Roberto has not acquired decoding skills for reading. In addition, he lacks fundamental study habits that are requisite for educational success. Because he lacked academic skills in Spanish, he could not transfer Spanish-language academic knowledge to English.

Roberto is not performing academically at the ninth-grade level in either Spanish or English. Roberto should be referred for a response to intervention plan and possibly later for speech-language or special-education assessments. Acquiring English and succeeding in school will be challenging for him. Therefore, school professionals should focus on improving his English-speaking skills to enable him to become a proficient reader before he finishes school.

Case Study Two Background: Mayra

Mayra (not her real name), a native Spanish speaker from Mexico, arrived in the United States within the last year. Her family comes from a middle SES. She is 14 years old and learning English as a ninth-grade student. Her high school curriculum consists of two hours of English-as-a-second-language class with personalized support from an instructional aide, and small-group instruction in core content courses such as science and math for the rest of the day. Mayra receives no special-education services.

Outside the classroom, Mayra practices speaking in English as often as she can. She speaks to her friends in English, watches television shows broadcast in English, and reads books written in English. In contrast to Roberto's many language and learning difficulties (see Case Study One), Mayra has experienced no real difficulties in acquiring English phonology, morphology, semantics, and syntax. According to her teachers, her overall progress in learning English has been "extremely fast."

Case Study Two Comments: Mayra

Mayra's well-developed English likely originates from her educational background in Mexico. Before her arrival in the United States, she had been immersed in school culture and literacy, undertook good study habits, and acquired an eighth-grade education in her native country with no gaps in her education. Mayra can understand, read, and write fluently in Spanish.

Consequently, she could positively transfer this academic knowledge from her first language (Spanish) to her second language (English). After one year, her reading score test in English for students with limited English proficiency was ranked at the 90th percentile. In addition, Mayra continued her second-language learning outside school with wide-ranging English communicative activities involving friends, television, and books. Successful language learning, as indicated earlier, occurs when the learner actively communicates in English (see Diaz-Rico & Weed, 1995; McKeon, 1994). Mayra has demonstrated that she is indeed a very successful second-language learner.

CONCLUDING REMARKS

Of the many factors that may influence a child's acquisition of a language, the most important involve culture, family values, parental communicative roles, and the specific language situation (monolingualism versus bilingualism, standard versus nonstandard dialect). All of these factors play a pivotal role in determining whether a child's language and communicative behavior matches the school's expectations or whether a serious linguistic mismatch between home and school exists.

When a non-English-speaking child enters school, the teacher is challenged to implement pedagogically and linguistically sound strategies to foster optimum second-language development. Some of the most promising strategies, despite limitations, are home-language and home-culture appreciation, parental involvement, active learner communication, cooperative learning, academic content and language integration, and high student expectation.

Reviewing the evidence concerning immigrant English-language learning, one researcher reaches this optimistic conclusion: "Despite public perception to the contrary, children of immigrants are by and large learning English rapidly and succeeding in schools" (Tse, 2001, p. 29). The real challenge is to attain the same optimistic conclusion about the linguistic abilities of all culturally and linguistically diverse students.

REFLECTION QUESTIONS

1. A student's writings reveal many misspellings and other problems. How can a speech-language pathologist or special education teacher decide if this just indicates a beginner's home dialect or language use, or if this problem requires a speech-language pathologist or other specialist?
2. A student's parents know little or no English. What advice can a speech-language pathologist or special education teacher offer them about home first- and second-language use in order to help the student's communication skills?
3. A student's parents, both non-English speakers, have only a very limited education. What advice can a speech-language pathologist or special education teacher offer them to help improve their child's literacy skills at home?

4. How can a speech-language pathologist or special education teacher balance the need for a nonnative speaker to practice actual English communication that will include many errors with the need to learn grammatically correct English?

5. How can a speech-language pathologist or special education teacher integrate aspects of a student's home culture into meaningful classroom language activities?

6. Refer to Case Study One. Roberto, a native Spanish speaker with just two years of education, is now experiencing major problems adjusting to normal high school life and, in particular, learning English as a second language. For students like Roberto, what practical and beneficial strategies would you suggest to improve their English second-language learning?

7. Refer to Case Study Two. Mayra, a native Spanish speaker from Mexico, is very successfully acquiring English as a second language. Which teaching strategies are especially effective in helping students like her transfer first-language CALP academic knowledge to the second language?

REFERENCES

Adger, C., & Wolfram, W. (2000). Demythologizing the home-school language dichotomy: Sociolinguistic reality and instructional practice. In J. K. Peyton, P. Griffin, W. Wolfram, & R. Fasold (Eds.), *Language in action: New studies of language in society* (pp. 391–407). Cresskill, NJ: Hampton Press.

American Speech-Language-Hearing Association. (2003). Technical report. American English dialects. *ASHA Supplement, 23*, 1–3.

Baecher, R. (1982). The instruction of Hispanic American students: Exploring their educational cognitive styles. In F. Fishman & G. Keller (Eds.), *Bilingual education for Hispanic students in the United States* (pp. 368–383). New York: Teachers College Press.

Bailey, K., & Galván, J. (1988). Accentedness in the classroom. In D. Bixler-Márquez & J. Ornstein-Galicia (Eds.), *Chicano speech in the bilingual classroom* (pp. 29–40). New York: Peter Lang.

Banks, J. (1988). Approaches to multicultural curriculum reform. *Multicultural Leader, 1*(2), 1–2.

Barajas, E. R. (2005). Sociocognitive aspects of proverb use in a Mexican transnational social network. In M. Farr (Ed.), *Latino language and literacy in ethnolinguistic Chicago* (pp. 67–95). Mahwah, NJ: Lawrence Erlbaum.

Brice, A. E. (Ed.) (2002). *The Hispanic child: Speech, language, culture and education.* Boston, MA: Allyn & Bacon.

Brice, A., Mastin, M., & Perkins, C. (1997). English, Spanish, and code switching use in the ESL classroom: An ethnographic study. *Journal of Children's Communication Development, 19*(2), 11–20.

Brice-Heath, S. (1983). *Ways with words.* Cambridge, UK: Cambridge University Press.

Brice-Heath, S. (1992). Literacy skills or literate skills? Considerations for ESL/EFL learners. In D. Nunan (Ed.), *Collaborative language learning and teaching* (pp. 40–55). Cambridge, UK: Cambridge University Press.

Cazden, C. (1988). *Classroom discourse.* Portsmouth, NH: Heinemann.

Chavez, J., & Buriel, R. (1986). Reinforcing children's effort: A comparison of immigrant, native-born Mexican American and Euro-American mothers. *Hispanic Journal of Behavioral Sciences, 8*(2), 127–142.

Clark, E. V. (2003). *First language acquisition.* Cambridge, UK: Cambridge University Press.

Coelho, E. (1994). Social integration of immigrant and refugee children. In F. Genesee (Ed.), *Educating second language children* (pp. 301–327). Cambridge, UK: University of Cambridge Press.

Collier, V. (1987). Age and rate of acquisition of second language for academic purposes. *TESOL Quarterly, 21*(4), 617–641.

Cummins, J. (1992). Language proficiency, bilingualism and academic achievement. In P. Richard-Amato & M. Snow (Eds.) *The multicultural classroom.* (pp. 16–26). White Plains, NY: Longman.

Cummins, J. (1994). Knowledge, power, and identity in teaching English as a second language. In F. Genesee

(Ed.), *Educating second language children* (pp. 33–58). Cambridge, UK: Cambridge University Press.

Cunningham-Andersson, U., & Andersson, S. (1999). Growing up with two languages. London: Routledge.

Darder, A., Torres, R., & Gutiérrez, H. (Eds.) (1997). *Latinos and education: A critical reader.* New York: Routledge.

de la Luz Reyes, M., & Halcón, J. (2001). *The best for our children: Critical perspectives on literacy for Latino students.* New York: Teachers College Press.

Díaz-Rico, L. (2004). *Teaching English learners: Strategies and methods.* Boston, MA: Allyn & Bacon.

Díaz-Rico, L., & Weed, K. (1995). *The crosscultural, language, and academic development handbook.* Needham Heights, MA: Allyn & Bacon.

Eisenberg, A. (2002). Maternal teaching talk within families of Mexican descent: Influences of task and socioeconomic status. *Hispanic Journal of Behavioral Sciences, 24*(2), 206–224.

Fantini, A. (1985). *Language acquisition of a bilingual child: A sociolinguistic perspective.* San Diego, CA: College-Hill Press.

Farb, P. (1975). *Word play.* New York: Bantam Books.

Ferguson, C. (1977). Baby talk as a simplified register. In C. Snow & C. Ferguson (Eds.), *Talking to children: Language input and acquisition* (pp. 209–235). Cambridge, UK: Cambridge University Press.

Fought, C. (2003). *Chicano English in context.* Houndmills, UK: Palgrave Macmillan.

Freeman, D., & Freeman, Y. (2001*). Between worlds: Access to second language acquisition* (2nd ed.). Portsmouth, NH: Heinemann.

Freeman, Y., & Freeman, D., (2002). *Closing the achievement gap: How to reach limited-formal-schooling and long-term English learners.* Portsmouth, NH: Heinemann.

Goldman, L. (1986). Tex-Mex. *English Today, 5*, 23–26.

Golinkoff, R. M., & Hirsh-Pasek, K. (2000). *How babies talk.* New York: Plume.

González, M., Huerta-Macías, A., & Tinajero, J. (1998). *Educating Latino students: A guide to successful practice.* Lancaster, PA: Technomic Publishing.

Goodz, N. (1994). Interactions between parents and children in bilingual families. In F. Genesee (Ed.), *Educating second language children* (pp. 61–81). Cambridge, UK: Cambridge University Press.

Green, L. J. (2002). *African American English.* Cambridge, UK: Cambridge University Press.

Grosjean, F. (1982). *Life with two languages.* Cambridge, MA: Harvard University Press.

Gudykunst, W. (1991). *Bridging differences. Effective intergroup communication.* Newbury Park, CA: Sage Publications.

Gudykunst, W., Ting-Toomey, S., & Chua, E. (1988). Intergroup relationships. In W. Gudykunst & S. Ting-Toomey (Eds.), *Culture and interpersonal communication* (pp. 201–217). Newbury Park, CA: Sage.

Harding-Esch, E., & Riley, P. (2003). *The bilingual family: A handbook for parents* (2nd ed.). Cambridge, UK: Cambridge University Press.

Hart, B., & Risley, T. R. (1995). *Meaningful differences in the everyday experience of young American children.* Toronto, Canada: Brookes.

Hayes, C., Bahruth, R., & Kessler, C. (1998). *Literacy con cariño* (new ed.). Portsmouth, NH: Heinemann.

Laosa, L. M. (1980). Maternal teaching strategies in Chicano and Anglo-American families: The influence of culture and education on maternal behavior. *Child Development, 51*(3), 759–765.

Lassiter, S. M. (1998). *Cultures of color in America.* Westport, CT: Greenwood Press.

Lightbown, P., & Spada, N. (1999). *How languages are learned* (rev. ed). Oxford, UK: Oxford University Press.

Macnamara, J. (1967). The bilingual's linguistic performance: A psychological overview. *Journal of Social Issues, 23*, 59–77.

Madding, C. C. (2002). Socialization practices of Latinos. In A. E. Brice (Ed.), *The Hispanic child: Speech, language, culture and education* (pp. 68–84). Boston, MA: Allyn & Bacon.

Marotta, S., & Garcia, J. (2003). Latinos in the United States in 2000. *Hispanic Journal of Behavioral Sciences, 25*(1), 13–34.

McKeon, D. (1994). Language, culture, and schooling. In F. Genesee (Ed.), *Educating second language children* (pp. 15–32). Cambridge, UK: University of Cambridge Press.

McLaughlin, B. (1978). *Second-language acquisition in childhood.* Hillsdale, NJ: Lawrence Erlbaum.

Mehan, H. (1979). *Learning lessons: Social organization in the classroom.* Cambridge, MA: Harvard University Press.

Moss, B. J. (2001). From the pews to the classrooms. In J. L. Harris, A. G. Kamhi, & K. E. Pollock (Eds.), *Literacy in African American communities* (pp. 195–211). Mahwah, NJ: Lawrence Erlbaum.

Moss, B. J. (2003). *A community text arises.* Cresskill, NJ: Hampton Press.

Mufwene, S. S. (2001). African-American English. In J. Algeo (Ed.), *The Cambridge history of the English language:* Vol. 6. *English in North America* (pp. 291–324). Cambridge, UK: Cambridge University Press.

Penfield, J., & Ornstein-Galicia, J. L. (1985). *Chicano English: An ethnic contact dialect.* Philadelphia, PA: John Benjamins.

Pérez, B., & Torres-Guzmán, M. (2002). *Learning in two worlds: An integrated Spanish/English biliteracy approach* (3rd ed.) Boston, MA: Allyn & Bacon.

Ramírez, D. (2000, April). *Bilingualism and literacy: Problem or opportunity? A synthesis of reading research on bilingual students.* Research Symposium on High Standards in Reading for Students from Diverse Language Groups: Practice and Policy, Office of Bilingual Education and Minority Languages Affairs, Washington, DC.

Ramírez, A., Acre-Torres, E., & Politzer, R. (1982). Language attitudes and the achievement of bilingual pupils in English language arts. In J. Fishman & G. Keller (Eds.), *Bilingual education for Hispanic students in the United States.* (pp. 269–288). New York: Teachers College Press.

Richard-Amato, P. (2003). *Making it happen: From interactive to participatory language teaching* (3rd ed.). White Plains, NY: Pearson Education.

Richard-Amato, P., & Snow, M. (2005). *Academic success for English language learners.* White Plains, NY: Pearson Education.

Romaine, S. (1984). *The language of children and adolescents.* Oxford, UK: Basil Blackwell.

Romaine, S. (1989). *Bilingualism.* Oxford, UK: Basil Blackwell.

Ryan, B., & Kanellos, N. (Eds.). (1995). *Hispanic American almanac.* New York: U·X·L International Thomson.

Saunders, G. (1982). *Bilingual children: Guidance for the family.* Clevedon, UK: Multilingual Matters.

Smitherman, G. (1986). *Talkin and testifyin.* Detroit, MI: Wayne State University Press.

Steward, M., & Steward, D. (1973). The observation of Anglo-, Mexican-, and Chinese-American mothers teaching their young sons. *Child Development, 44*(1) 329–337.

Swain, M. (1985). Communicative competence: Some roles of comprehensible input and comprehensible output in its development. In S. Gass & C. Madden (Eds.), *Input in second language acquisition* (pp. 235–256). Rowley, MA: Newbury House.

Thomas, W. P., & Collier, V. P. 2002. *A national study of school effectiveness for language minority students' long-term academic achievement.* (ERIC Document Reproduction Service No. ED 475048).

Ting-Toomey, S. (1994). Managing intercultural conflicts effectively. In L. A. Samovar & R. E. Porter (Eds.), *Intercultural communication. A reader* (7th ed.) (pp. 360–372). Belmont, CA: Wadsworth.

Triandis, H. (1995). *Individualism and collectivism.* Boulder, CO: West View Press.

Tse, L. (2001). *"Why don't they learn English?": Separating fact from fallacy in the US language debate.* New York: Teachers College Press.

United States Census Bureau (2003, February 25). United States Census 2000: Summary tables on language use and English ability: 2000 (PHC-T-20). http://www.census.gov/population/www/cen2000/phc-t20.html.

Zentella, A. (1997). *Growing up bilingual.* Oxford, UK: Blackwell.

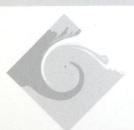

Chapter 11

School Language Programs for Language Learning Disabled and Exceptional Needs Children

Roanne G. Brice and Alejandro Brice

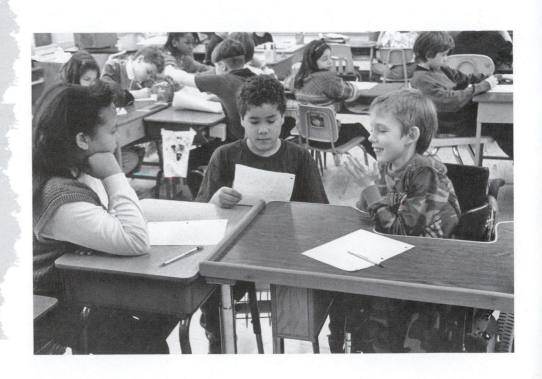

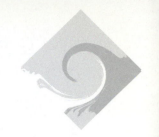

CHAPTER OUTLINE

INTRODUCTION

Speech-language pathology and special education instruction for students with disabilities have changed significantly over the last decade. Access to the general-education classroom via the inclusion movement has been at the forefront of this change. "**Inclusion** [emphasis added] has been used to describe the education of students with disabilities in general education settings" (Mastropieri & Scruggs, 2004, p. 7). The older term of mainstreaming may still be used by some education professionals. **Mainstreaming** refers "to the placement of students with disabilities—often part-time—into general class settings" (Mastropieri & Scruggs, 2004, p. 7). Hence, mainstreaming and inclusion can be considered similar. However, inclusion specifically provides accommodations and instructional strategies to students to facilitate their learning of the general curriculum (Vaughn, Bos, & Schumm, 2007). Inclusion can be further defined as either full inclusion or part-time inclusion. **Full inclusion** refers to instruction for students with disabilities in the general education classroom for the entire day (Vaughn, Bos, & Schumm, 2007). **Part-time inclusion** refers to instruction for students who are in the general education classroom for a portion of the school day and includes services provided outside the classroom in a speech and language therapy room or in a separate special education resource room.

The Council for Exceptional Children (1993, 2007) states that each child, to the maximum extent appropriate, should be educated in the school and classroom he or she would otherwise attend. It involves bringing support services to the child (rather than moving the child to the services). Inclusion means that instruction is provided in the general education classroom where additional supports are made available so that students learn and succeed in the classroom. Inclusion can be further defined as being either consultative or collaborative. Friend (2006) defined **collaboration** as "the way in which professionals interact with each other and with parents and family members as they work together to educate students with disabilities . . . it is the means of achieving goals" (p. 30). One of the philosophies of the inclusion movement has been the "zero rejection" belief. This belief centers around the premise that no student is too disabled nor is any disability too severe for the student to be included in the general education classroom. In agreement with the zero rejection philosophy is the Individuals with Disabilities Education Act (IDEA) definition of the least restrictive environment (LRE). Students with disabilities should be taught in the LRE possible. The **least restrictive environment** is the setting that best meets the educational needs of the student with disabilities and that is most similar to that of students who are not disabled (Vaughn, Bos, & Schumm, 2007). Inherent with the least restrictive environment is the notion of continuum of services. **Continuum of services** means that students with disabilities receive a full range of services, from self-contained classrooms to resource rooms, to general education classrooms. In addition, all educational programs for children with exceptionalities must be educationally relevant.

As early as 1992, the National Association of State Boards of Education stated that **mainstreaming** (where students were only partially included in general education environment for portions of the day) and labeling have been unsuccessful attempts for students served in special education (Kauffman, 1989). It is widely accepted that all students are more alike than they are different (Kauffman, 1989). The distinctions of special education versus general education have not always been beneficial for students and teachers. Stainback and Stainback (1984, 1987, & 1996) stated that labeling can be harmful to students with disabilities and also detrimental to their education. This reinforces the issue of the importance of establishing the least restrictive environment for students with special needs.

In recent years the focus of education has been to enhance the education of *all* students (Braaten & Mennes, 1992; Braaten, Kauffman, Braaten, Polsgrove, & Nelson, 1988; Friend, 2006; Kauffman, 1989; McGregor & Vogelsberg, 1998; Reynolds, Wang, & Walberg, 1987; Stainback & Stainback, 1996; Stainback, Stainback, Stefanich, & Alper, 1996; Wehmeyer, Lattin, Lapp-Rincker, & Agran, 2003; Vaughn, Bos, & Schumm, 2007). Consequently, most school districts have implemented inclusive and/or collaborative practices in their schools. As a result, the model of using self-contained classrooms and practices outside the classroom (e.g., resource and therapy classrooms) has diminished somewhat, with inclusive instruction in the classroom taking its place (Vaughn, Bos, & Schumm, 2007).

Inclusive instruction for students in the general education classroom is viewed as the least restrictive environment (LRE). Inclusion also seeks to reduce the notion of separate and distinct curriculums for students with disabilities. Over the last 20 years, the inclusion debate has shifted from *whether* inclusion should be the dominant teaching model to *how* inclusion and access to the general education classroom and curriculum can best be implemented. Inclusion and collaboration within the general education classroom can be defined as including four significant features: they (1) are integrated environments where all students learn together, (2) do not unnecessarily label or identify students as exceptional learners, (3) make the best use of educational benefits, and (4) reduce the need for a separate curriculum and assist students' access to the general education curriculum.

The separation of the general education curriculum from special education has led to certain inequalities in the education of students with disabilities. Consequently, some students have not had exposure to the general education curriculum. One solution to this predicament has been for school professionals to provide speech-language or special education supportive instruction in the general education classroom. This necessitates collaborative efforts between the speech-language pathologist (SLP) or special education teacher and the general education teacher. This reasoning is based on four key points: (1) the general education classroom is the most natural environment where language occurs, (2) generalization or carry-over is most likely to happen if instruction occurs in the general classroom, (3) other children in the classroom can benefit from SLP or special education instructional strategies presented, and (4) instructional success will be assessed by the students' academic success.

EDUCATION REFORM

The most recent legislative education reform (January 2002) was endorsed when President Bush signed into law the **No Child Left Behind (NCLB)** Act of 2001. The U.S. Department of Education (2002) stated:

> [S]ince the *Nation At Risk* report was issued nearly 20 years ago, there has been vigorous national debate over how to improve our nation's schools and our children's achievement. Out of these years of debate, a general consensus has emerged that schools and districts work best when they have greater control and flexibility, when scientifically proven teaching methods are employed, and when schools are held accountable for results. These are the guiding ideas behind the NCLB Act (p. x).

The reauthorization of NCLB specifies four major components: (1) a stronger accountability system for students' educational performance; (2) a greater flexibility for states, school districts, and schools to use federal funds; (3) increased choices for parents of children who are disadvantaged; and (4) an increased emphasis on teaching methodologies that are scientifically based and have been shown to be instructionally sound. According to the U.S. Department of Education (2002), educational accountability will be established when the "data will be disaggregated for students by poverty levels, race, ethnicities, disabilities, and limited English proficiencies to ensure that no child—regardless of his or her background—is left behind" (p. x). All students, regardless of their special needs placement, should receive their instruction in the general-education classroom whenever possible. This inclusive model requires collaboration and/or consultation with classroom teachers.

Types of Programs

Common models for inclusion of speech, language, and other instruction are to have SLPs and special-education teachers **collaborate** (i.e., assist and co-teach with the general-education teacher in the classroom) and/or **consult** (i.e., provide the teacher specific teaching strategies for children with disabilities). Typically, speech and language services have been provided in resource rooms, outside the classroom, or consultatively.

For some special-education students, **resource rooms** may be the least restrictive environment. The students may leave their general-education classrooms for periods of time for specific instruction, as designated on their individualized education plans (IEPs).

The **itinerant model** is used for students with particular disabilities that may require less therapeutic contact time. The itinerant SLP typically takes the student from her or his classroom to address specific speech (e.g., articulation, fluency, voice), language (e.g., oral language, written language skills), or hearing-related skills (e.g., auditory processing).

INCLUSION MODELS

The **collaboration** instructional model is defined here as a form of working together and/or co-teaching with other school professionals (Idol, Nevin, & Paolucci-Whitcomb, 2000). Collaboration may involve the speech-language pathologist in the resource room, the special education teacher in the general education classroom, or the speech-language pathologist in the general education classroom.

One person does not take the role of expert under the collaborative model. The focus is to facilitate instruction for special needs students. One type of collaboration is to provide instruction for these students in the general education classroom. This model is inclusive, where all school professionals share their expertise in their respective fields. A collaborator should be a facilitator and also function as a team member. Collaboration is a cooperative endeavor that focuses on problem solving (e.g., how to teach the student with disabilities in the general education classroom). Implementing teaching strategies is problem solving (Idol, Nevin, & Paolucci-Whitcomb, 2000). Collaboration is more of a direct service delivery model wherein school professionals are all in direct instructional contact with students. Collaboration needs to be defined separately from consultation.

The **consultation** model is defined here as education professionals (e.g., general- and special-education teachers, SLPs, school psychologists, counselors) sharing their knowledge and expertise in a common teaching/working relationship. The team recognizes that various viewpoints and types of knowledge are required to provide the most comprehensive support needed for each student. Consultation is a voluntary activity because the recipients (i.e., other team members) are not required to implement the suggestions. It is also important to note that team or consultative members should not present their expertise so that it would be perceived by others as authoritative. Consultation is an indirect service delivery model because the consultant does not directly teach the students with disabilities and/or disorders. Some obstacles to implementing the suggestions may include time, space or resource allocations, training of key personnel, and support for the key persons involved (i.e., the speech-language pathologist, special education teacher, general education teacher, students, family members, and other school personnel). However, the collaborative models are more commonly used to support students with disabilities. A discussion of several collaborative models follows.

Various Collaborative Models

One service-delivery model is not superior to another when providing speech-language or special education services (American Speech-Language-Hearing Association, 1999; Borsch & Oaks, 1993). Collaborative models may consist of (1) classroom-based team teaching or co-teaching, (2) classroom-based complementary teaching, (3) supportive teaching, (4) outside the classroom resource management, and (5) self-contained programs.

In **classroom-based team teaching** or **co-teaching,** the general education classroom teacher and the speech-language pathologist or the special educator alternately teach the content. In addition, they work together for lesson planning, progress monitoring, and decision making regarding instructional strategies and/or accommodations to be implemented in future lessons. **Classroom-based complementary teaching** occurs when the classroom teacher has the primary responsibility for teaching the general curriculum, and the SLP or special educator focuses on implementing specific instructional strategies or accommodations to adapt the lesson to the academic level of the student. In **supportive teaching,** the SLP or special educator incorporates supplemental information and/or instructional materials related to the class content either in the classroom or in a therapy room (i.e., outside the classroom). In **outside the classroom resource management,** the SLP collaborates with the classroom teacher. The SLP may observe the classroom; however, instructional support for the student is typically offered outside the general-education classroom. **Self-contained programs** are the most restrictive environment in a school setting. The SLP or special educator is the classroom teacher and is responsible for both academic content instruction and speech-language therapy. In some instances, students are mainstreamed for one or more classes as their academic skills improve. Students in a self-contained classroom setting should be included in the general education classroom and allowed access to the general curriculum to the highest extent possible.

Co-teaching is the equal sharing of classroom lessons and responsibilities between the SLP/special educator and the classroom teacher. Co-teaching seems to offer the most benefits to students by offering instructional strategies for all students in a classroom; it also enhances continuity of instruction because students do not lose instructional time by leaving the classroom. The co-teaching model is particularly beneficial for at-risk students who may be struggling or those who are not yet identified as needing special education services. In addition, co-teaching reduces any social stigma that students may experience by leaving the classroom. Instructional support from the speech-language pathologist and/or special educator and the general classroom teacher is enhanced through co-teaching activities (Bahamonde & Friend, 1999; Friend, 2006).

Co-teaching involves more time and planning than individual classroom lessons. Dieker and Barnett (1996) indicated that an important part of co-teaching is to devote weekly planning time to evaluation of the process, that is, how to (1) present the lesson, (2) adapt the instruction, and (3) evaluate student learning. Issues regarding discipline, instructional strategy adaptations, and assignment of grades need to be co-planned and discussed between the speech-language pathologist or special education teacher and the classroom teacher. These components can be grouped according to (1) sharing, (2) accommodations, and (3) enhancing (Deboer & Fister, 1998; Pearl, 2005).

Sharing involves a division of teaching responsibilities. The general education teacher may lead the classroom lesson, while the speech-language pathologist may assist with instructional support. The special education teacher circulates and assists with the classroom lesson. The speech-language pathologist or special education teacher also teaches lessons at classroom stations or teaches parallel lessons to small groups of students. Other options for instruction (e.g., alternate teaching, alternation sequence) are discussed later in this chapter.

Accommodations are implemented for students who require variations in instruction or test taking.

> Accommodations are provisions made in how a student accesses and demonstrates learning. Accommodations are changes to how students are expected to learn (instruction) and how they demonstrate what has been learned (assessment). The use of an accommodation does not change the standards, the instructional level, or the content and provides the student with equal access and equal opportunity to demonstrate his or her skills and knowledge (Florida Department of Education, 2000, p. 72).

Accommodations may include use of (1) highlighted texts, (2) manipulatives, (3) note-taking assistance, (4) extended time on assignments, (5) repeating instructions, (6) tests given orally, (7) assistive technology, (8) study aids (e.g., number chart, dictionary, map), (9) small-group instruction, and/or (10) preferential seating (Vaughn, Bos, & Schumm, 2007). The accommodation may involve changing the classroom environment to better meet the individual learning needs of students with exceptionalities. The environment can be adapted by seating the student in a non-noisy area with less disruption and reduced traffic. Time demands for completing assignments may either be removed or extended. Alternate assessments, such as an oral report instead of a written report, may be used to gauge student progress.

Enhancing involves providing additional strategies not typically used during classroom instruction. For example, visual aids (posters) or graphic organizers (flow charts) may be employed. Instructional learning strategies (e.g., audio recording of notes) may also be utilized. Use of peer buddy or peer-mediated instruction is another option.

The above-mentioned service delivery models may be used exclusively or in any combination. According to the Annual Reports to Congress on the Implementation of IDEA, a range of options, tailored to meet the individual needs of all students, continues to be the most effective approach (U.S. Department of Education, 1996, 2007). It is also important to remember that the general education classroom is usually the least restrictive environment (LRE) for students with disabilities. Therefore, speech-language or special education instruction should be provided in the general education classroom when it is the least restrictive environment.

According to the American Speech-Language-Hearing Association (1999), one service delivery model should not be used exclusively. It is recommended that instruction in spoken and written language be provided by speech-language pathologists, special educators, and classroom teachers in a variety of settings. It is essential to assess the specific needs of each student to determine the most appropriate least restrictive environment for providing the services needed in spoken and written language. Specific curriculum-based instruction can be developed by a team approach to meet the student's individual educational needs in accessing the general curriculum. Specific examples of collaborative teaching follow.

One example of collaborative teaching consists of **alternate teaching** (Montgomery, 1993). The SLP and/or special education teacher changes roles in aiding the general classroom teacher. The SLP may also aid the general education or special education teacher by outlining lecture notes on the chalkboard or whiteboard, underlining main points, spelling and defining new vocabulary, highlighting and sequencing main ideas, and generally offering learning strategies that can benefit all students in the classroom. Individualized education plan (IEP) objectives can be written so that instruction occurs in the general education classroom rather than the resource classroom. Skills such as oral and written language, attainment of main ideas, sequencing, and categorization can be targeted. Other examples may include reading fluently and/or oral and written comprehension activities.

Another collaborative example consists of a "three-week outside the classroom, one week in class" **alternation sequence,** as mentioned by Montgomery (1993). Using this strategy, the SLP or special education teacher provides therapy or instruction using an outside the classroom model or resource classroom model for three weeks. For the fourth week, the SLP or special education teacher observes the classroom and answers questions, assists in cooperative learning groups, conducts language-enriching activities, or promotes emergent literacy (e.g., she or he may support reading through phonemic awareness, phonics, vocabulary, or reading fluency activities). Literacy activities may include the following steps, in which the SLP and/or special education teacher assists the classroom teacher: (1) the SLP and/or special education teacher meets with the general education classroom teacher and investigates which core reading books are being used by the teacher, (2) all school professionals share their weekly lesson objectives, and (3) the SLP or special education teacher aids the classroom teacher on agreed-upon days when she or he teaches the lesson. Lessons may include story telling with semantic organizers. Examples of semantic organizers include story maps, web diagrams, or other aids that assist students in organizing or restructuring thoughts during speaking, listening, reading, or writing activities. Students are encouraged to apply their listening, oral comprehension, auditory memory, and visualization skills (Owens, 2004). Refer to Table 11–1 for an overview of different instructional models.

Becoming a collaborative professional means that certain procedural steps must be followed so that the classroom teacher's cooperation is obtained. In particular, the SLP or special education teacher should obtain students' class schedules from the general classroom teacher. It is important for the SLP or special education teacher to observe those classrooms to ascertain the language demands placed on the students (i.e., for listening, speaking, reading, and writing). This observation assists the SLP and teachers in recognizing the learning and communication demands expected of students. All school professionals must have good communication skills for collaboration to be

TABLE 11–1
Types of Instructional Models Employed by Speech-Language Pathologists and Special Education Teachers

Environment	Model	Speech-Language Pathologist's or Special Education Teacher's Role
General education classroom	Collaboration	Working with the teacher in the classroom.
General education classroom	Collaboration with supportive teaching	Assisting the general education classroom teacher.
General education classroom	Co-teaching	Sharing the responsibility of planning and teaching lessons.
Separate classroom	Resource room	Instruction in another classroom for a portion of the day.
Separate classroom	Self-contained classroom	Academic instruction and specialized instruction (e.g., speech-language or special education) is provided by the speech-language pathologist or special educator.
Therapy room	Outside the classroom or itinerant model	Instructional support is provided outside the classroom.
Outside the classroom	Consultation	Information is provided to the general education classroom teacher. No instruction is provided in the general education classroom, separate classroom, or therapy room.

Source: Brice, A., & Brice, R. (2007). School language and classroom programs for children with language impairments: Collaborating with parents and school personnel. In C. Roseberry-McKibbin (Ed.), *Language disorders in children: A multicultural and case perspective* (pp. 439–464). Boston, MA: Allyn & Bacon.

successful. Important communication skills include appropriate listening, effective questioning, respect and acceptance of others, and an ability to stay on task (Vaughn, Bos, & Schumm, 2007). Appropriate question use requires knowing when to ask open-ended questions (i.e., questions that prompt discussion) versus closed-ended questions (i.e., questions that typically require factual answers). In addition, respect and acceptance of the other school professional's opinion is essential to good communication. In conclusion, the team must preserve the joint focus of classroom collaboration.

Some obstacles for collaboration include the necessity of school professionals reformulating what their specific roles entail in regard to their role in collaboration. The team should realize that struggles in role expectations and role release can occur as a result of change. Therefore, active steps to initiate, choose, and maintain a collaborative program must be taken by the collaborative team. For school professionals who are accustomed to working separately and independently, a transition time may be necessary in learning to work collaboratively as a team member.

Successful collaboration involves the following attributes: (1) team members share common objectives, (2) all team members contribute equally, (3) leadership is distributed equally, and (4) team decisions are shared and implemented as a team. Because role release is an issue in successful collaboration, the following six steps are presented to facilitate collaboration (Montgomery, 1993):

1. **Role extension.** All team members examine how new information is presented and how the information can relate to the students' needs. They also examine how to make the classroom curriculum meet the students' needs.

2. **Role enrichment.** Each professional adds to his or her existing knowledge base from other disciplines. Examples include sharing and examining curriculum materials, attending meetings, conferencing with other teachers, and conducting classroom observations.

3. **Role expansion.** The SLP or special-education teacher develops new knowledge and information from the other's discipline in an effort to better teach the students.

4. **Role exchange.** The team members switch roles. For example, the SLP may assume the task of teaching the class lesson.

5. **Role release.** The school professional allows another team member to take his or her role. This translates into trusting this person.

6. **Role support.** Each school professional supports the collaborative team. Support occurs when each professional realizes that each team member brings wanted skills and knowledge to the team effort.

In conclusion, successful collaboration occurs when school professionals show conviction and commitment to the effort. Administrative support from the school principal is necessary for collaboration to be successful. Along with shared team responsibility, it is important for parents to be included in the educational decisions of their children. Respect between all and parents is an important aspect of successful collaboration (Martin, Donovan, & Senne, 2003). When successful collaboration occurs, then students gain from the experience. Communication with parents can also be incorporated into parent-teacher conferences, through the student's planners or through regular phone conversations.

CASE STUDY PERSPECTIVES

Three case studies are presented next to illustrate how best practices and strategies may be implemented with parents, classroom teachers, and other school professionals.

Case Study One Background: Joseph

Joseph has been enrolled in speech and language therapy for one year. Joseph is a monolingual middle school student with difficulties in both speech and language. His main difficulties include oral motor skills, articulation, language, and pragmatics. He is 13 years old and attends middle school as a seventh-grade student. During the past year, he has made gains, yet he still shows some difficulties in the targeted speech and language areas for which he is receiving therapy. Joseph has been able to increase external oral motor accuracy (tongue agility outside his mouth) to a higher level of accuracy. Internal oral-motor exercises were difficult to elicit because Joseph does not like to perform these exercises. Joseph has also been able to increase his articulation of /ɹ/ ("r") at the sentence level, /ʒ, θ/ ("th") at the phrase level, and /tʃ/ ("ch") at the sentence level. Production of "th" in the final position of words poses difficulty because Joseph substitutes an /f/ for /ʒ, θ/ ("th").

Joseph has been able to increase his attention to tasks and answer wh- questions (e.g., who, what, where, when, why) to stories with moderate accuracy. Multiple cues from the speech-language pathologist are sometimes necessary to obtain a response from Joseph. Joseph was able to increase turn-taking in therapy activities without any clinician prompts (i.e., not needing any solicitation from the clinician) with some accuracy. However, he continues to experience difficulties with classroom discourse and communicating in social situations. Joseph was able to increase his ability to sequence story events to almost 100% levels. In story accounting (telling a new story to the listener), Joseph can supply the setting, initiating event (conflict of the story), internal response of the character(s), and story consequence. Because Joseph was able to supply four story elements, this story is at the level of a primitive narrative (Stein & Glenn, 1975). Joseph does not provide any internal character plans (how the character was going to solve the story dilemma) or an ending to the story. Joseph's story development is appropriate but below grade level and needs further expanding.

Joseph has improved his use of language in interactions with others (i.e., pragmatics), yet he continues to have difficulties with initiating comments and using an appropriate loudness of voice; that is, he speaks too quietly. He also uses very little eye contact. He occasionally reverts to his previous behaviors of kicking his feet and not looking at the clinician, with his chin tucked into his chest. In conclusion, Joseph is a capable student showing progress for learning. Joseph's lack of motivation for learning and cooperation are concerns that should be addressed.

Case Study One Comments: Joseph

Joseph should continue to receive speech and language therapy services. If he is provided with appropriate accommodations and support, Joseph is capable of being successful in the general-education classroom. Because the classroom is the least restrictive environment, most instruction should occur there. His motivation for learning and cooperation are a concern. Joseph is a candidate for inclusive and collaborative speech and language instruction. Some instruction may need to take place outside the classroom because Joseph may need to be taught specific skills in isolation (e.g., oral language skills) that can later be reinforced in the classroom and generalized to other academic subjects in the classroom (e.g., written language skills) (Brice, 2004a). It was also noted that, due to his lack of motivation, Joseph may not do well being pulled from the classroom for speech and language therapy. The speech-language pathologist should attempt to involve the entire class in lessons that address more general speech and language skills so that Joseph is not singled out, which could cause him to receive excessive and/or unwanted attention.

Case Study Two Background: Esteban

Esteban is a bilingual Spanish-English-speaking student currently in second grade. Esteban is not a special needs student. He does not present with any language learning disability, attention deficit, or any type of disorder. It should be noted that any language- or learning-related difficulties that Esteban encounters are mainly attributable to learning English as his second language. Spanish is predominantly spoken at home. He receives ESL instruction outside the classroom for reading and mathematics. He receives his other instruction in the general classroom. He is assigned a Spanish-English-speaking paraprofessional to assist with mathematics instruction. He is also paired with another student (i.e., an English-proficient, Spanish-speaking student). He is seated at the front of the classroom near the teacher to minimize distractions. Esteban has been in an English-speaking environment for approximately two years.

The general education classroom consists of 25 students. Esteban and three other students in this classroom are bilingual Spanish-English speakers. Esteban is seated in a cluster of desks near the front of the classroom. Desks are arranged in a semicircle so that all students face each other. Most lessons are presented in one-hour blocks (e.g., science for one hour, mathematics for one hour). Due to delayed processing of English, Esteban's greatest obstacle in learning is understanding and following directions, and finishing classroom assignments. Classroom listening demands placed upon him are great. Esteban needs to understand lengthy, multistep instructions in English to successfully complete the classroom assignments. The following serves as an example of typical classroom instructions:

Teacher: "We're going to start our math lesson. Take out your books and turn to page 11. Remember that your book looks like this (the teacher holds up the book). It is the one with the castles on it. Do math problems 5 through 15 and also 25 to 40. I will walk around and check your work. Put your finished papers in the basket."

Directions and commands such as this are typical within the classroom, proceeding at a fast pace of instruction. Consequently, students need to possess enhanced auditory processing and listening skills to be academically successful (Brice, 2002; Brice, Mastin, & Perkins, 1997). Despite his learning English as a second language and the fast pace of instruction during most lessons, Esteban has been able to maintain his learning. In addition, he has been able to learn English, perform on grade level in this particular classroom, and achieve high grades.

Case Study Two Comments: Esteban

If Esteban is in a general education classroom where co-teaching occurs with other school professionals (e.g., SLP or special education teacher), then he can benefit from instructional strategies used and/or taught in lessons. The general education teacher should continue to use ESL strategies throughout her or his instructional practices.

Case Study Three Background: Juan

Juan is a bilingual student who was referred for comprehensive speech-language and special education evaluations. Juan's parents were concerned when he did not begin speaking until 5 years of age. Before 5, it was reported that he could say only *mother* (i.e., "mama") and *father* (i.e., "papa") in Spanish.

Juan is a Spanish-speaking ESL student currently in his fourth year at the local elementary school. Therefore, this is his fourth year of schooling and also speaking English. Juan's first year of school was in the second grade in the United States. He did not attend school in Mexico prior to this time. He was 10 years 8 months old at the time of the evaluation and was enrolled in fifth grade. It was reported by his parents (by means of a home language survey) that he spoke better Spanish than English. Spanish was the most frequently used language in the home, although he heard and spoke mainly English in school.

It was reported by his ESL and general education classroom teachers that Juan experiences great difficulty with reading and writing. His teachers have provided appropriate available resources (i.e., a Spanish-English-speaking paraprofessional that comes and assists the ESL and general classrooms for 20 minutes every afternoon).

Juan does not read or write in Spanish and has great difficulty expressing himself verbally (orally) in both Spanish and English. It was reported by the ESL and general education classroom teachers that his spoken vocabulary in both languages was limited. He was segmenting consonant and vowel sounds in reading and writing, yet he could not write a complete sentence independently. Juan is at risk for reading difficulties and possible academic difficulties (Brice, 2004b).

Juan was receiving services from the ESL teacher three times a week for approximately one hour per day. In addition, a paraprofessional worked with him 20 minutes every afternoon as ESL support. During math classes, Juan received additional support from the classroom teacher. For example, the teacher assisted Juan with spelling on the word math problems so that he could complete assignments. In addition, a volunteer came to his home four times a week after school to provide tutoring. Juan's classroom behaviors, as reported by his general-education fifth-grade classroom teacher, were deemed to be age- and socially appropriate (behaviors typically exhibited by fifth graders).

From classroom observations, it was noted that Juan spoke in the present tense form, omitting verb conjugations (e.g., "I watch that show last night"). A student should be able to converse with accuracy after two to three years of English exposure at school (Cummins, 1984; Thomas & Collier, 2002); however, Juan still experiences these difficulties after four years of English exposure. From the comprehensive speech, language, and special education evaluations conducted in both English and Spanish, the following conclusions were noted:

1. Juan presented with a language learning disability (LLD) that was not solely attributable to his learning and speaking English as a second language. This was drawn from the assessment results in English and Spanish, and from the ESL teacher's comments that Juan was not functioning at the same level as other English language learning (ELL) students, particularly when compared to his own siblings. Juan's level of performance, even after four years of instruction, was still well below grade level, even when his late start of school was considered (Collier, 1987; Cummins, 1984; Thomas & Collier, 2002).
2. Juan's disability is present in both languages. His communication skills in both Spanish and English were below expected levels. In addition, it should be noted that he did not begin speaking until after 5 years of age.
3. Results from the speech-language and cognitive evaluation conducted in Spanish and English indicated the following: (1) cognitive test results: auditory memory—significantly below average, short-term visual memory—significantly below average, visual processing of speech—below average, social reasoning skills to solve nonverbal problems—significantly below average, perceptual organization—significantly below average; and (2) vocabulary: difficulty expressing himself in Spanish, even with an interpreter's assistance. Overall, no mental impairment was found; however, he experienced difficulty in Spanish and English vocabulary.

Case Study Three Comments: Juan

Juan is a bilingual student with a language learning disability that is not primarily related to his learning and speaking English as a second language. Juan is not functioning at the same level as other ELL students. In addition, Juan does not read or write Spanish and has great difficulty expressing himself verbally (orally) in either Spanish or English. It was reported by his ESL and general education classroom teachers that Juan has experienced great difficulty with reading and writing. His teachers have provided adequate and necessary strategies to assist him in his learning, yet he has shown very limited progress. Based on the evaluation results, Juan qualifies for the specific learning disabilities program and speech and language services. It is most likely that the least restrictive environment is the general education classroom. The general education classroom teacher, the English-as-a-second-language teacher, the special education teacher, and the speech-language pathologist are all professionals who should collaborate and plan Juan's intervention plan.

INSTRUCTIONAL SUGGESTIONS

Suggestions for Inclusive Practices Working with School Administrators

Inclusion is not just placement in the classroom; it is a planned philosophy of instruction that is fostered throughout the entire school. Administrators can ensure that inclusion will work in their respective schools through the proper professional development training of SLPs and teachers. Many SLPs and teachers believe they have not been involved in the drafting of their school inclusion model. For inclusion to be successful (i.e., in meeting the education needs of all students), schools need to involve teachers in successful attainment of the collaborative model. Administrators should ensure that all educators have been provided the tools to be successful, and teachers must be strongly encouraged to implement the model of inclusion so that all students have access to the general curriculum.

Placement of any student in a "fully included" environment should occur only after the educational team (including the general education classroom teacher, special education teacher, speech-language pathologist, paraprofessional assigned to work with the student, and the parent or parents) have had the opportunity to discuss and design an inclusion plan that addresses the student's needs. The inclusion plan should specifically (1) designate the level of inclusion on a scale from physical inclusion to full academic participation with peers; (2) identify the amount of support from all educational staff, including paraprofessionals, that will be needed to maximize opportunities for the student to be successful in the inclusive setting; (3) provide specific training for the paraprofessional assigned to the students to facilitate quality instruction as well as continuity of instruction across academic settings; (4) identify who specifically provides what instruction and during what period of the school day; and (5) provide a plan for transitioning the student into a new environment. This may mean that the student begins by leaving the self-contained setting for one class period per day and then increasing the number of days per week until the student is in the general education classroom for that scheduled time all week.

Successful inclusion occurs only when the collaborative team meets formally and informally to discuss student progress. The student's inclusion plan must be monitored continually throughout the grading period so that any changes and corrections can be made as needed.

Inclusion requires that administrators allow for planning time so SLPs, teachers, and paraprofessionals can meet, plan, and modify lessons when necessary. Planning should not occur in isolation, but through a team approach. Successful collaboration takes commitment in the form of planning, time, and effort.

Suggestions for Collaboration with Families

Traditionally, the medical model has been used in speech and language therapy or instructional settings with all students from all cultural backgrounds. In the medical model, the speech-language pathologist assumes full responsibility for the entire process. For example, the speech-language pathologist determines the goals, selects the procedures, informs the students of those procedures, implements them, determines what changes need to be made, assesses progress toward goals, and counsels other school-related professionals regarding a student's communications (Creaghead, 1994). This model often fails to be family-friendly due to limited opportunities for interactions and family participation.

A more holistic and collaborative model, however, encourages family participation in educational and therapeutic decisions. Families from both individualistic and collectivistic (i.e., group-oriented) cultures benefit from a more holistic and collaborative approach to communication. This approach is characterized by shared problem solving. All participants, including family members and professionals, are involved in determining if a problem exists, its nature, intervention goals, and roles for implementing the solutions (Creaghead, 1994). Characteristics of successful collaboration include:

1. Team members sharing common goals
2. All team members contributing equally
3. Leadership distributed equally among the team members
4. Sharing of responsibility for implementing team decisions

Luterman (2001) stated that the notion underlying all family therapy is that the family is a system in which all components are connected and that any time a change occurs with one family member, then everybody in the family becomes involved. Involving educational professionals and all family members in the school and instructional process is part of the holistic and collaborative teaching systems model that can result in the following (adapted from Luterman, 2001):

1. A greater understanding of disabilities and people in general for the student and family
2. Increased compassion for the student
3. The family gaining an increased appreciation of their own health and well being

4. Increased sensitivity to the needs of a child with disabilities

5. The family coming closer together in a positive shared experience

The development of trust in working with families is the first step toward involving them in the child's educational decisions. Trust is a principal element in building the relationship with students and parents. For example, in a cross-cultural encounter, development of trust may be more difficult to establish because the two parties are from differing backgrounds. A presumed history of bias and ethnocentrism may be difficult to overcome. Developing trust is common among many group-oriented or collectivistic cultures. Hence, in learning about trust, the education professional can maximize teaching and family involvement. Luterman (2001) lists three elements in building trust: caring, consistency, and credibility. He also stated, "Caring is conveyed to the client [student or family member] in any number of ways, not the least of which is active and sensitive listening" (p. 37). Speech-language pathologists, special education teachers, and classroom teachers should become aware of the importance of listening and being able to take a "receiver attitude" such as that displayed by many group-oriented cultures.

Trust building can also be developed by nonjudgmental listening. From experience, it becomes evident that many families begin to display respect toward an SLP or teacher only after the school professional shows caring toward their child (Luterman, 2001). A caring attitude is a key component and should be a high priority in all educational and therapeutic settings.

Consistency and credibility are both important in developing trust. Consistency can be displayed by sharing the responsibility of learning objectives and/or benchmarks with students and by demonstrating the strategies used in the classroom to the family. By consistently working collaboratively with parents to achieve student academic success, a trusting relationship will develop over time. Credibility is initially garnered through use of a professional title or by academic degrees held. However, credibility can also be earned by demonstrating experience and expertise to family members and others in the community. Suggestions for building trust and maintaining credibility with families, particularly culturally and linguistically diverse families, include the following:

1. Provide written messages and materials—in the family's native language when possible.

2. Encourage families to share their view of educational experiences. This will reinforce that you are sincerely interested in their opinions.

3. Speak the family's native language whenever possible (even if it is only saying some greetings).

Open communication and optimal interactions are facilitated by the level of trust (Luterman, 2001). Family involvement requires respect and open communication. General suggestions for school professionals who want to maximize family involvement include (Brice, 2002):

1. Accept and appreciate families. Empower the family members in their roles in the child's educational plans and achievements.

2. Recognize and respect the rights and beliefs of parents and families.

3. Listen carefully and empathetically for the family's message and focus on positive hopes and aspirations for their child.

4. Assist families in feeling comfortable by sharing information and available resources. Prepare for all meetings so that your knowledge will be apparent at the appropriate time in the meeting.

5. Maintain trust by following through with stated agreements and plans.

What is notable about these interventions is that all SLPs and teachers can easily incorporate these family involvement practices.

Listening Skills Enhancement

In an early study by Griffin and Hannah (1960), it was reported that children spent up to one-half or more of their school day listening to teachers talk and teach. At home, children may be incessant talkers; however, at school they learn to become passive learners (Cazden, 1998; McDevitt & Oreskovich, 1993). A pattern can emerge in elementary school where children ask very few questions if they are not encouraged and facilitated. In some classroom settings, these instructional approaches have been noted by more current researchers as well (Brice, Mastin, & Perkins, 1997; Cazden, 1998, 2001; Dillon, 1982; Good, Slavings, Harrel, & Emerson, 1987).

It has been estimated that high school students may spend up to 90 percent of their school day listening to teachers talk. In addition, school discourse places great demands on students to comprehend lengthy sessions of classroom language. This becomes more apparent in the classroom as the student's age or grade level increases. Therefore, it is imperative that the SLP or special education teacher teach effective listening and auditory processing skills to all students, including both monolingual and bilingual students with disabilities (Brice, 2004b). Nelson (1991) stated:

> In addition to language use, the content of language events occurring in classrooms differs widely depending on grade level. Whereas in the earlier grades greater emphasis is placed on learning to read and write and perform basic mathematical computations, in the later grades much of teacher talk centers on topics of substance in the content areas of science, geography, social studies, and literature (p. 82).

Some educators believe that listening skills are a neglected area of the school curriculum (Donahue, 1997; Pearson & Fielding, 1982). Listening comprehension in schools is seldom the focus of classroom instruction and may not be actively addressed in therapy (Cazden, 2001; Wolvin & Coakley, 1988). However, listening is important because students are expected to listen and understand the academic content for a significant amount of time in the school day. In addition, listening comprehension abilities greatly influence a student's academic success (Cazden, 2001). Brice (2004b) stated that listening, phonemic awareness, and phonics skills were important skills for young bilingual children to use in accessing the general education curriculum. Speaking and listening are assumed to emerge and develop without any necessary instruction. However, some students with communication disorders or disabilities need specific instruction to improve their listening, communication, and comprehension skills.

Speech-language pathologists and teachers will find it useful to implement strategies to enhance perception and attention skills (Brice, 2004b). It has already been noted that school discourse and classroom instruction place great emphasis on listening skills. For example, student seating can be one way of maximizing listening abilities while minimizing auditory and/or visual distractions.

Classroom organization strategies for monolingual or bilingual students with language learning disabilities (LLDs) may also include use of advance organizers, lead statements, or preparatory sets. **Lead statements** are used to start lessons and orient the listener to what is to occur (Brice, Mastin, & Perkins, 1997). English-language-learning students and students with LLDs need more specific, step-by-step lead statements and explanations, rather than the use of single sentences, to be able to follow the teacher's directions. Directions may have to be repeated for some students. In determining the student's comprehension, ask for a brief summary of what was said. In addition, ask the student's opinion of the material. The SLP or teacher may use clarification requests to ensure student comprehension. For example, ask the student, "Can you tell me what you mean by. . .?" The following suggestions can make input more comprehensible to students: (1) slow the rate of verbal delivery of directions and content, (2) pause frequently to allow for more comprehension time, (3) use shorter sentences and phrases, (4) use fewer multisyllabic words, (5) avoid excessive use of slang or idiomatic speech (e.g., "She really put her foot in her mouth!"), and (6) emphasize key words through increased volume and slightly exaggerated rising intonations or variations in pitch.

CONCLUDING REMARKS

For inclusion, collaboration, and/or consultation to be implemented successfully in school, preparation needs to occur. School administrators must support inclusive or collaborative efforts for any significant student learning to take place. Collaboration will be successful only if it is implemented in an organized and coherent manner. If students are to benefit from enacted changes implemented under the Individuals with Disabilities Education Act (IDEA) or the No Child Left Behind (NCLB) Act, then students with exceptionalities must receive the most appropriate education in the least restrictive environment. It is important for general education teachers to have a positive attitude in serving the academic, social, and emotional needs of students with exceptionalities. It is expected that educators will become involved in how services are delivered, and that SLPs and teachers will receive adequate preparation. If both are accomplished, then education for students with disabilities can be sucessfully provided in the least restrictive environment. It is anticipated that all educators will provide inclusive classrooms where *all* children can learn.

INSTRUCTIONAL STRATEGIES

The following instructional strategies are for use in the general-education classroom during content instruction focusing on enhancing listening comprehension and interaction:

1. To enhance listening and auditory comprehension, make sure that instructions are presented during quiet times (Brice, Roseberry-McKibbin, & Kayser, 1997).

2. Students need to be encouraged to ask questions. Speech-language pathologists and teachers should avoid ambiguous questions and multiple questions because they limit classroom dialogue (Roseberry-McKibbin, 1995). In addition, multiple questions are hard to remember and to follow for students who need more processing time (i.e., students with CAPD or bilingual students). Vague questions may be hard to understand. Some culturally and linguistically diverse students may believe that it is rude to show that they did not understand and to ask for explanations (Roseberry-McKibbin, 1995).

3. Lessons should be shortened and scaffolded into progressive steps (Brice, Roseberry-McKibbin, & Kayser, 1997). In answering questions, keep in mind Bloom's hierarchy (1957) consisting of knowledge, comprehension, application, analysis, synthesis, and evaluation. Responses should be tailored to elicit these different levels, which promote various thinking levels. Montgomery (1993) adapted Bloom's taxonomy for use with special needs students:

   a. *Nonverbal responses (knowledge question).* "Show me the sailboat."
   b. *Yes/no questions (comprehension question).* "Did Thomas find the anchor?"
   c. *Embedded in the question (comprehension question).* A closed and forced choice is elicited. "Is this a life vest or a jacket?"
   d. *One word answer (knowledge question).* "What was under the tool box?"
   e. *Lists (application response).* "Name three ocean animals that people eat."
   f. *Elicit information (comprehension question).* "What happened to the sailboat during the storm?"
   g. *Analysis Question.* "Why is Thomas angry at the pirates?"
   h. *Synthesis Question.* "What does this story have that all stories have?"
   i. *Evaluation Question.* "Why is fresh water so important to survival at sea?"

4. Recount information related to students' experiences (Figueroa & Ruiz, 1997). Students remember content when information is related to their personal background and experiences (Gathercole & Baddeley, 1993).

REFLECTION QUESTIONS

1. Refer to Case Study One. Joseph is a monolingual middle school student with difficulties in both speech and language. His main difficulties include oral motor skills, articulation, language, and pragmatics. What strategies can be utilized in the classroom using co-teaching methods?

2. Refer to Case Study Two. Esteban is a bilingual student with some normal difficulties in learning English as a second language. He is receiving appropriate accommodation ESL strategies in the general education classroom. Esteban's greatest

hurdle in learning is understanding and following directions (e.g., teacher commands), which leads to difficulty in completing assignments. What strategies would you suggest to improve his listening, staying on-task, and completing assignments?

3. Refer to Case Study Three. Juan does not read or write in Spanish and has great difficulty expressing himself verbally (orally) in both Spanish and English. It was reported by the ESL and general education classroom teachers that his spoken vocabulary in both languages was limited. He will be receiving services in Spanish and English. The school district has no available bilingual special education teachers or bilingual speech-language pathologists. The school where you work has a part-time Spanish-English paraprofessional. As a monolingual special education teacher or speech-language pathologist, how can you provide part of his services in Spanish?

4. Classroom teacher Ms. Gardner is a seasoned teacher who does a good job of teaching fourth grade. One of her students, Tom, presents with some attention deficits and central auditory processing disorders. However, Ms. Gardner speaks very rapidly and in a low voice. How can you politely inform Ms. Gardner about the importance of slower speech and an adequate voice intensity to assist Tom's learning?

5. How can you earn the trust of your colleagues at school to gain entrance to their classroom when you are new and they are veterans in teaching?

6. Respond to the following comments regarding co-teaching: "I'm too busy to 'co-teach'"; "Oh, Ms. Jones tried that with Sally and Stewart in my classroom and it didn't work", "I already use all the learning accommodation strategies in my lessons."

7. What five qualities are important for a speech-language pathologist or special education teacher in working with parents or as a co-teacher in the general education classroom?

REFERENCES

American Speech-Language-Hearing Association. (1999). *Guidelines for the roles and responsibilities of the school-based speech-language pathologist.* Rockville, MD: Author.

Bahamonde, C., & Friend, M. (1999). Teaching English language learners: A proposal for effective service delivery through collaboration and co-teaching. *Journal of Educational Psychological Consultation, 10*(1), 1–24.

Bloom, B. (1957). *Taxonomy of educational objectives: The classification of educational goals by a committee of college and university examiners.* New York: McKay.

Braaten, B., & Mennes, D. (1992). A model of collaborative service for middle school students. *Preventing school failure, 36*(3), 10–15.

Braaten, S., Kauffman, J. M., Braaten, B., Polsgrove, L., & Nelson, C. M. (1988). The regular education initiative: Patent medicine for behavioral disorders. *Exceptional Children, 55*(1), 21–27.

Brice, A. (2002). *The Hispanic child. Speech, language, culture, and education.* Boston, MA: Allyn & Bacon.

Brice, A., Mastin, M., & Perkins, C. (1997). English, Spanish, and code switching use in the ESL classroom: An ethnographic study. *Journal of Children's Communication Development, 19*(2), 11–20.

Brice, A., Roseberry-McKibbin, C., & Kayser, H. (1997, November). *Special language needs of linguistically and culturally diverse students.* Paper presented for the American Speech-Language-Hearing Association Annual Convention, Boston, MA.

Brice, R. (2004a). Connecting oral and written language through applied writing strategies. *Intervention in School and Clinic, 40*(1), 38–47.

Brice, R. (2004b). *Identification of phonemes and graphemes in Spanish-English and English speaking kindergarten students.* Doctoral Dissertation. University of Central Florida. Orlando, FL: UMI Proquest.

Cazden, C. B. (1998). Two meanings of discourse. (ERIC Document Reproduction Service No. ED 420198).

Cazden, C. B. (2001). *Classroom discourse: The language of teaching and learning* (2nd ed.). Portsmouth, NH: Heinemann.

Collier, V. P. (1987). Age and rate of acquisition of second language for academic purposes. *TESOL Quarterly, 21*, 617–641.

Council for Exceptional Children. (1993). CEC policy on inclusive schools and community settings. *Supplement to Teaching Exceptional Children, 25*(4), 1.

Council for Exceptional Children. (2007). Inclusion. Retrieved on February 11, 2007, from http://www.cec.sped.org/Content/NavigationMenu/NewsIssues/TeachingLearningCenter/ProfessionalPracticeTopicsInfo/Inclusion/default.htm.

Creaghead, N. (1994). Collaborative intervention. In N. Creaghead & D. Ripich (Eds.), *School discourse problems* (2nd ed.), (pp. 373–386). San Diego, CA: Singular Publishing.

Cummins, J. (1984). *Bilingualism and special education: Issues in assessment and pedagogy.* San Diego, CA: College Hill Press.

Deboer, A., & Fister, S. (1998). *Working together. Tools for collaborative teaching.* Longmont, CO: Sopris West.

Dieker, L., & Barnett, C. (1996). Effective co-teaching. *Teaching Exceptional Children, 29*(1), 5–7.

Dillon, J. T. (1982). The multidisciplinary study of questions. *Journal of Educational Psychology, 74*, 147–165.

Donahue, M. L. (1997). Beliefs about listening in students with learning disabilities: Is the speaker always right? *Topics in Language Disorders, 17*(3), 41–61.

Figueroa, R. A., & Ruiz, N. T. (1997, January). *The optimal learning environment.* Paper presented at the Council for Exceptional Children Symposium on Culturally and Linguistically Diverse Exceptional Learners, New Orleans, LA.

Florida Department of Education. (2000). *Testing accommodations for students with disabilities.* Bureau of Instructional Support and Community Services Division of Public Schools and Community Education. Tallahassee, FL: Author.

Friend, M. (2006). S*pecial education: Contemporary perspectives for school professionals.* Boston, MA: Pearson Education.

Gathercole, S. E., & Baddeley, A. D. (1993). *Working memory and language.* Hillsdale, NJ: Erlbaum.

Good, T. L., Slavings, R. L., Harel, K. H., & Emerson, H. (1987). Student passivity: A study of question asking in K–12 classrooms. *Sociology of Education, 60*, 181–199.

Griffin, K., & Hannah, L. (1960). A study of the results of an extremely short instructional unit in listening. *Journal of Communication, 10*, 135–139.

Idol, L., Nevin, A., & Paolucci-Whitcomb, P. (2000). *Collaborative consultation* (3rd ed.). Austin, TX: Pro-Ed.

Kauffman, J. M. (1989). The regular education initiative as Reagan-Bush education policy: A trickle-down theory of education of the hard-to-teach. *Journal of Special Education, 23*(3), 256–275.

Luterman, D. M. (2001). *Counseling the communicatively disordered and their families* (4th ed.). Austin, TX: Pro-Ed.

Martin, S. M., Donovan, S. E., & Senne, M. (2003, November). *The heart of teacher preparation: Inclusion of families through curriculum module development.* Paper presented at the 2003 Teacher Education Division Conference, Biloxi, MS.

Mastropieri, M. A., & Scruggs, T. E. (2004). *The inclusive classroom. Strategies for effective instruction* (2nd ed). Upper Saddle River, NJ: Pearson.

McDevitt, T., & Oreskovich, M. (1993). Beliefs about listening: Perspectives of mothers and early-childhood teachers. *Child Study Journal, 23*, 153–172.

McGregor, G., & Vogelsberg, R. T. (1998). *Inclusive schooling practices: Pedagogical and research foundations.* Baltimore, MD: Brookes.

Montgomery, J. (1993). *Special education strategies: Shared goals. What's happening in curriculum and instruction?* Fountain Valley, CA: Fountain Valley School District.

Nelson, N. W. (1991). Teacher talk and child listening—Fostering a better match. In C. Simon (Ed.), *Communication skills and classroom success. Assessment and therapy methodologies for language and learning disabled students.* Eau Claire, WI: Thinking Publications.

Owens, R. E. (2004). *Language disorders. A functional approach to assessment and intervention* (4th ed.). Boston, MA: Allyn & Bacon.

Pearl, C. (2005, January). *Maximizing the potential of co-teaching as a service delivery model.* Paper presented at the Florida Division of Learning Disabilities Annual Conference, Orlando, FL.

Pearson, P. D., & Fielding, L. (1982). Research update: Listening comprehension. *Language Arts, 59*(6), 617–629.

Reynolds, M. C., Wang, M. C., & Walberg, H. J. (1987). The necessary restructuring of special and regular education. *Exceptional Children, 53,* 391–398.

Roseberry-McKibbin, C. (1995). *Multicultural students with special language needs: Practical strategies for assessment and intervention.* Oceanside, CA: Academic Communication Associates.

Stainback, S., & Stainback, W. (1987). Integration versus cooperation: A commentary on "Educating children with learning problems: A shared responsibility." *Exceptional Children, 54,* 66–68.

Stainback, W., & Stainback, S. (1984). A rationale for the merger of special and regular education. *Exceptional Children, 51*(2), 102–111.

Stainback, W., & Stainback, S. (1996). *Inclusion: A guide for educators.* Baltimore, MD: Brookes.

Stainback, W., Stainback, S., Stefanich, G., & Alper, S. (1996). Learning in inclusive classrooms: What about the curriculum? In S. Stainback & W. Stainback (Eds.), *Inclusion: A guide for educators* (pp. 209–219). Baltimore, MD: Brookes.

Stein, N. L., & Glenn, C. G. (1975). *An analysis of story comprehension in elementary school children: A test of a schema.* Educational Resources Information Center. (ERIC Document Reproduction Service No. ED 121474).

Thomas, W. P., & Collier, V. P. (2002). *A national study of school effectiveness for language minority students' long term academic achievement.* Center for Research on Education, Diversity and Excellence and the Office of Educational Research Improvement. (ERIC Document Reproduction Service No. ED 475048).

U.S. Department of Education. (1996). Eighteenth Annual Report to Congress on the Implementation of the Individuals with Disabilities Education Act. Washington DC: Author.

U.S. Department of Education. (2002). *No Child Left Behind: A Desktop Reference.* Washington, DC: Author.

U.S. Department of Education. (2007). Twenty-Fourth Annual Report to Congress on the Implementation of the Individuals with Disabilities Education Act. Washington DC: Author.

Vaughn, S., Bos, C. S., & Schumm, J. S. (2007). *Teaching exceptional students who are exceptional, diverse, and at-risk in the general education classroom* (4th ed.). Boston, MA: Allyn & Bacon.

Wehmeyer, M. L., Lattin, D., Lapp-Rincker, G., & Agran, M. (2003). Access to the general curriculum of middle-school students with mental retardation: An observational study. *Remedial and Special Education, 24,* 262–272.

Wolvin, A., & Coakley, C. C. (1988). *Listening* (3rd ed.). Dubuque, IA: W. C. Brown.

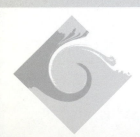

Chapter 12

School Language Programs for Bilingual Children

Elia Vazquez-Montilla

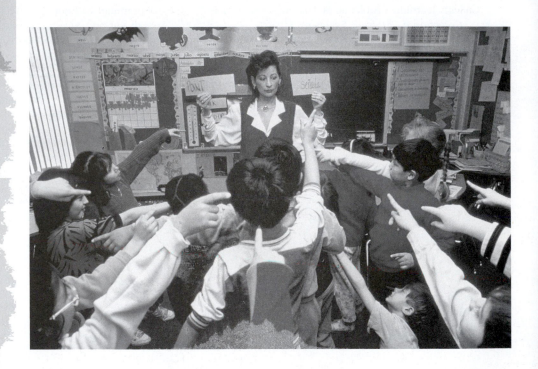

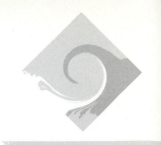

CHAPTER OUTLINE

INTRODUCTION

The success of school language programs for bilingual students continues to be observed by all individuals interested in the effectiveness of language programs in education. Recently there has been a noticeable shift away from programs that support bilingualism and consequently biliteracy (Coady & De Jong, 2004). Changes in the nation's political, social, and economic interests are currently redefining the national responses to language diversity and thus changing previous decades of bilingual program development and research (Ovando, 2003).

Research in the area of bilingual education shows that a variety of programs may effectively support the education of bilingual students (Echevarria & Graves, 2003; Genesee, 1999; National Clearinghouse for English Language Acquisition, 2006; Ovando, 2003; Ramirez, Yuen, & Ramey, 1991; Thomas & Collier, 1997). These results indicate support for programs that promote academic achievement while students are learning English. Programs for English-language learning (ELL) students can basically be divided into English-language development (ELD) programs versus bilingual programs. English-language development programs can include sheltered English and traditional English as a second language (ESL), English to speakers of other languages (ESOL), or transitional bilingual education (TBE) programs. Bilingual programs can include developmental bilingual, two-way immersion, or transitional bilingual education (TBE) programs. Note that the nature of TBE programs will depend on which language is used as the primary language of instruction (i.e., English or the native language).

All bilingual programs should include some English language development; that is, learning English should be one key component. For example, this may be accomplished by: (1) 80% of instruction in the first language (L1), while 20% of instruction is in English for grades K–1; (2) 60% of instruction is in L1, while 40% instruction is in English for the second grade; (3) 50% of instruction is in L1, while 50% of instruction is in English for the third grade; (4) 40% of instruction is in L1, while 60% instruction is in English for the fourth grade; and (5) 20% of instruction is in L1, while 80% instruction is in English for the fifth grade.

Consequently, language program choices are typically made by local school agencies. When making educational decisions, careful consideration must be given to district demographics, the specific language and learning needs of the students involved, and the range of services that can be supported by the available school resources (Rennie, 1993).

In terms of school demographics, there is a noted increase of language diversity throughout the schools in the nation (Vázquez-Montilla & Giambo, 2004). Thus, the challenge is in finding services for culturally and linguistically diverse (CLD) students that support learning, regardless of the home language and grade level. Research and demographic trends also describe CLD students as having a range of school-related distinctive characteristics that affect their learning needs, such as different academic preparation, varieties of language proficiency levels in both English and the home language, and an array of diverse school- and literacy-related experiences. In addition, social, economic, and cultural factors increase the number of variables that influence individual learning needs requiring careful consideration when providing educational services to CLD students (Genesee, 1999; Vázquez-Montilla & Giambo, 2004).

The challenge for schools today is to find ways to support quality educational programs that provide specific language services to increasing CLD student populations. Programs should integrate effective practices, support school contexts of academic achievement and excellence, and encompass the benefits of additive bilingualism.

EDUCATIONAL BILINGUAL PROGRAM OPTIONS AND INSTRUCTIONAL APPROACHES

A discussion of common programs (i.e., sheltered English programs, transitional bilingual programs, maintenance or developmental bilingual programs, and two-way instructional approaches) and essential instructional approaches will be presented. The following will be discussed for each program type: (1) a brief goal description and basic background information of the program, (2) important features and pedagogy of the program, and (3) resources and school support that are needed to implement the program.

English Language Development Programs: Sheltered English and Transitional Bilingual Programs

Changing patterns of immigration, international and global changes in government, and changes in national legislation have had an impact on the immigrant flow in the

United States (Ovando, 2003). National legislation such as the Refugee Act of 1980, the Immigration Reform and Control Act (IRC) of 1986, and the Immigration Act (IMMACT) of 1990 have also had a direct impact on the increase of CLD students in U.S. schools (Taylor & Whittaker, 2003).

Sheltered English and transitional education programs are specifically designed to address the immediate needs of recent immigrant students, especially those with limited or interrupted schooling in their home countries. Eligibility criteria for the programs include classification of students as limited English proficient (LEP) based on their standardized English test performances, less-than-age-appropriate education, lack of familiarity with the mainstream school system, documented personal trauma, and/or low self-confidence as a result of speaking English as a second language (Friedlander, 1991).

According to Genesee (1999), **sheltered English** is a widely used approach wherein academic subjects (e.g., mathematics) are taught in English. Instruction usually occurs in the general education classroom. Specific strategies are used for ELL students so that instruction is comprehensible. Attention is given to the English-language learner student's second-language needs. Strategies may include teacher scaffolding, frequent interaction, small-group activities, and use of meaningful activities (Brice & Perkins, 1997; Genesee, 1999).

Transitional bilingual education (TBE) programs are also referred to as early-exit education programs. Although the design and nature of the TBE program is to provide instruction in the native language, the reality is that many of these programs provide instruction in English. Therefore, TBE programs may provide instruction in English or in the native language. The focus of the TBE program is on exiting (i.e., transitioning) the student into the general-education classroom in a short period of time (e.g., one to two years) (Brice, 2002).

Consequently, these two program approaches support academic skills development along with a quick transition of students into the general education classroom (Center for School and District Improvement, 2004; Friedlander, 1991; Genesee, 1999). These short-term and compacted programs usually target recent-arrival students. However, if the school deems the students as needing specific English instruction, then the school can call on the federal definition and guidelines, which allow for participation of students who have been in the United States for up to three years.

Sheltered English and transitional programs focus on working with recent immigrants who most likely have limited exposure to mainstream schooling, limited literacy skills in their home language, and limited English proficiency. The key goals include the acquisition of functional English-language skills, along with basic core academic and literacy skills, and quick assimilation into the mainstream classroom.

Students with limited academic and language proficiency skills are not equipped to meet the academic demands of a typical general education classroom. This reality places them at risk for academic failure. Schools supporting these types of educational programs should develop strong literacy skills strategies to equip the ELL students with reading and writing skills necessary for the typical classroom. School professionals also need to be aware of the need to develop a sense of belonging and a culture of support for culturally and linguistically diverse students who have recently integrated into the school system. The assumption is that a strong connection among school, student, family cultural background, and community will lead to better opportunities for success.

School resources determine how the program will serve the CLD population (Short & Boyson, 2003). However, most of the sheltered English and TBE programs are designed to operate within an academic year. TBE programs are designed to facilitate the transition of CLD students to the general education classrooms within one to two years (or less). It is expected that, through TBE programs, students will continue acquiring grade-appropriate curricular and academic skills while learning English (Cummins, 1992; Cummins & Swain, 1986). Schools assume that students will not need additional support or assistance when they are transitioned to general education classrooms. Essential to any TBE program is having a core of trained English-as-a-second-language (ESL) or English speakers of other languages (ESOL) teachers as well as general education teachers to provide effective instruction after transition and to ensure academic success of mainstreamed ELL students. All school professionals need to have appropriate training in ESL/ESOL instructional strategies. In addition, school personnel need to be trained and familiar with the CLD students' needs and cultures.

The following is a list of important elements shared by most TBE programs:

1. Specialized instruction for a limited and transitional period of time.
2. Orientation to basic survival skills.
3. Specialized courses facilitating cultural integration and familiarization with U.S. cultural distinctions, including expected school routines and behaviors related to education.
4. Basic courses and strategy development for students with limited literacy skills or limited school experiences.
5. Sheltered instruction used as the prime instructional approach to initially promote basic core academic skills along with English language development and proficiency.
6. Transition to typical schools and classrooms is an essential goal.
7. Enhancement of self-esteem and access to support services such as tutoring and counseling.
8. Strong family involvement, where families are familiarized with school and community cultures and support services.

Developmental Bilingual Programs (DBPs)

Developmental bilingual programs (DBPs) are also known as maintenance bilingual programs or as late-exit bilingual education programs. Late-exit bilingual programs are designed to support students in the acquisition of English-language proficiency with use of the home language. Students receive instruction using their home language and English over a period of four to five years. Although the importance of bilingualism is well recognized, the politics of bilingual education still generates controversy among parents, schools, and politicians. The transformation of maintenance bilingual education into developmental bilingual education occurred when Title VII was introduced in 1984 (as part of the Elementary and Secondary Education Act) in an effort to eliminate negative political connotations. Long-term support is needed to ensure academic, cognitive, and linguistic development in CLD students, thus ensuring their academic success (Collier, 1989, 1992).

Developmental bilingual programs specify the need for long-term consistent teaching using both languages, that is, the home language and English (Cisneros & Leone, 1995). This program promotes high levels of achievement and proficiency in both languages. It also carefully considers cross-cultural communication and diverse cultural perspectives in both teaching and how curriculum materials are used. Many may consider DBP to be an enrichment program that supports additive bilingualism (Cummins, 1992), biliteracy, and biculturalism.

Research related to the length of time needed for CLD students to succeed in classrooms and on achievement tests (Collier, 1995; Thomas & Collier, 1997) supports the use of developmental bilingual programs. Students who are provided with continued challenging academic material, allowed to use their home language, and given consistent opportunities to learn academic content in English advance in achievement and academic performance.

Ideally, a developmental bilingual program begins at the lower elementary grade levels and continues to add a grade level every year. As a consequence, bilingualism and biculturalism emerge as strong components of this program. Important elements shared by DBPs include (Cisneros & Leone, 1995; Center for School and District Improvement, 2004; Dolson & Mayer, 1992; Genesee, 1999; Ramírez, Yuen, & Ramey, 1991):

1. The same status for both English and home languages as legitimate languages for teaching academic content.

2. Consistent use of cognitively challenging academic content, regardless of the language of instruction.

3. Same language used for extended periods of time to facilitate development of academic proficiency.

4. Content-based instruction supported with cooperative learning, sheltered instruction, and cognitive strategies.

5. Use of instructional materials showcasing and presenting multicultural and diverse perspectives.

6. Ongoing assessment to monitor academic progress and achievement of academic standards, and use of standardized tests to measure progress in comparison to the mainstream student population.

Developmental bilingual programs need long-term commitment from schools, families, and communities to succeed. There must be consistent academic instruction using both languages for many grade levels. Developmental bilingual programs also need a core of trained school professionals and teachers capable of effectively teaching all academic subject areas in both languages, along with the use of sheltered instruction strategies.

Two-Way Immersion (TWI) Programs

Two-way immersion programs are also known as two-way bilingual education or dual-language immersion. TWI programs differ from other bilingual programs because they serve both monolingual English speakers and speakers of the targeted minority language. Teaching employs both languages, and additive bilingualism and academic achievement is expected for all students (Morison, 1995). Consequently, students participating in TWI programs develop language proficiency in two languages, one being English. Cross-cultural understanding aptitudes also increase. Some schools recognize bilingualism as an asset and use TWI programs as a possible alternative educational program option.

Two-way immersion programs are long-term programs that aim toward bilingualism and high academic achievement for all students. Thus, the family and school's long-term commitments to this program are essential for its success. The focus on additive bilingualism is supported by integrated use of curricula where both languages are used with equal status as vehicles for teaching. The additive bilingualism emphasis implemented by these programs is supported by research on dual-language acquisition (Collier 1989, 1992, 1995; Cummins, 1992; Krashen, 1987).

Schools professionals expect students to be able to transfer literacy skills and academic learning skills to the learning of a second language once they have a strong foundation in their native language (Cummins, 1992). In addition, school expectations are for continuous and uninterrupted academic development resulting in the student's ability to speak, read, and write in two languages. By having two language groups and cultures represented, schools are providing a social milieu for students to understand other cultures and perspectives with regard to learning, problem solving, and social interactions. Two-way immersion programs are most commonly found in elementary schools, where a developmentally appropriate and nurturing environment encourages the bilingual environments needed to support the program (Cloud, Genesee, & Hamayan, 2000). Important elements shared by TWI programs include:

1. Equal number of students representing the targeted languages.
2. Languages considered equal in prestige.
3. Academic instruction provided in both languages for the same length of time.
4. Strong support for long-term and consistent cultural and bilingual academic environments.
5. Strategies supporting comprehensible input and development of background knowledge, including the use of thematic units and cooperative learning.
6. Two-way multiple opportunities for students to interact with peers who are native speakers of the targeted languages.
7. Students expected to read, speak, and write in both languages for social and academic purposes.
8. Ongoing assessment of grade-appropriate development, academic progress, and language proficiency development.

TWI programs need long-term commitment from schools, families, and the community. There must be a consistent academic instruction effort to use both languages for as many grade levels as possible to support bilingualism and biliteracy (Cloud, Genesee, & Hamayan, 2000). The integration and consolidation of two languages is basic to two-way immersion programs. Therefore, trained bilingual professionals capable of teaching academic subject areas in both languages are needed. In addition, a school's commitment to the program should be reflected in establishing communication with families using both languages, as well as obtaining equal involvement of families representative of the targeted languages.

FUNDAMENTAL INSTRUCTIONAL APPROACHES

For students learning English as a second language, the initial focus is on functional language acquisition rather than academic language. As the English language learner (ELL) gains in proficiency, however, the focus shifts from language learning to content learning, where students are expected to master grade-level-appropriate materials in English. This is apparent in the upper elementary, middle school, and high school grade levels, where content generates language needs. Consequently, when school professionals use English as the language of instruction, they must adapt their teaching to meet the different student language proficiency levels.

CRITICAL ISSUES

The nation's student profile indicates an increase in the CLD student population. School professionals are expected to diversify instruction to teach to different language proficiencies, different ranges of educational experiences and abilities, and different student learning needs. In addition, school professionals are responsible for providing educational opportunities that prepare students to meet curricular demands and increasing academic standards. Consideration of language issues, achievement gaps, special learning needs, and educational choices is critical in the school's ability to provide CLD students with equal opportunities.

INSTRUCTIONAL STRATEGIES

School personnel must become aware of social language to be able to assist all students with their education, particularly students who may be at risk for academic failure. These strategies have been modified to reflect a pragmatics nature:

1. Do not assume that similar behaviors have the same pragmatic intention. Assumptions may lead to miscommunications.
2. Suspend judgment. Avoid the tendency to stereotype behaviors and interpretations.
3. Recognize the vitality of diverse communication strategies. Language use will be different. The type of language use reflects cultural orientation.
4. Respect others by acknowledging their thoughts and desires.
5. Provide translation clues. Make your thoughts explicit.
6. Seek translation clues from others. Have others explain their actions.
7. Metacommunicate. Tell the other person how you interpreted the message or what she or he just said.
8. Expand your communication style repertoire. Say your message differently so that clearer communication may occur.

Closing the Achievement Gap in Older Students

Some students may immigrate to the United States in their adolescent years, making their educational transition to American schools difficult. These middle school and high school ELL students may find themselves in a quandary when they try to develop their English-language skills in conjunction with developing their academic language abilities. These students have to compete with their monolingual English-speaking peers (Freeman & Freeman, 2002; Walqui, 2000a) who are performing at a high academic level. The ELL students have a limited amount of time to develop strong language proficiency and meet the school's academic expectations (Chamot, 2000). In addition, school expectations generally assume that students will easily mainstream into general-education classrooms after completion of a basic functional language program. Schools should emphasize academic concepts, theme-based activities and curricula, students' background experiences, students' language and culture, and instruction to build on the students' English language proficiency (Walqui, 2000b).

Special Needs

Overrepresentation of CLD students receiving exceptional education services continues to be a recurring theme in education (Ortiz & Yates, 2002). Research suggests that school professionals continue to have difficulty differentiating between learning disabilities and learning difficulties related to second-language learning (Ortiz & Yates, 2002). Improving relevant assessment procedures to determine appropriate exceptional education placement is essential in providing suitable instruction for CLD students. Failure to use appropriate assessment procedures limits the use of intervention strategies (Ortiz, 2001).

Making Choices

Not all families who immigrate to the United States have sufficient knowledge regarding school policies and programs to make fully informed educational decisions. Families need guidance in making informed decisions related to what is appropriate for their child. If families lack understanding of the implications when making these decisions, then school professionals need to facilitate and guide the family members in this process. Table 12–1 summarizes various educational programs discussed in this chapter. The table and the following questions are intended to provide answers to some fundamental questions that may help families understand the scope of language programs available in school:

1. Is the program promoting bilingual literacy and proficiency while promoting academic development?
2. Is the program long term or short term?
3. What transition mechanisms are in place when the program is no longer available?
4. What kind of follow-up is available for students exiting the program?
5. What student population is primarily served?
6. What resources are available?
7. Are the school personnel bilingual and fluent in the child's native language?

TABLE 12–1

Educational Program Options for Culturally and Linguistically Diverse (CLD) Students

Language Used	Program	Students Served	Objectives	Transition Mechanisms	Resources Available	Personnel Training
L2 and L1	Transitional (early exit)	Students using the same L1.	English acquisition; L1 is developed to assist comprehension and to support the transition to the use of only English as a way of instruction; support and instruction for grade-level academics.	Use of English; efficient transition to the mainstream classroom within two years or less.	Transitional support and instruction provided for grade-level academics.	ESL/ESOL teachers and trained general-education teachers to ensure effective transition; trained in the use of sheltered instruction strategies; trained and familiar with CLD students needs and cultures.
L2 and L1	Developmental (late exit)	Students using the same L1.	Supports bilingualism, biliteracy, and biculturalism; use of L1 to support academic development; use of L2 increases as students gain in proficiency; supports cultural and diverse perspectives in the curriculum and class materials; provides consistent opportunities to learn academic content with either language; demonstration of academic language proficiency in L1 and L2.	Instruction is provided using both L1 and L2, with each given equal weight in the learning process; cognitively challenging experiences in both languages; content-based instruction.	Long-term support given to the program; content-based instruction is supported by cooperative learning and cognitive strategies; multicultural and diverse perspectives materials needed and used.	School professionals are expected to use both languages; trained bilingual teachers capable of teaching academic subject areas using both languages; also trained in the use of sheltered instruction.
L2 and L1	Two-way immersion	Monolingual English-speaking students along with students in the process of developing English proficiency; equal number of students of each language group preferred.	Targets additive bilingualism and academic achievement; uses both languages for instruction; aims for language proficiency in two languages, academic achievement, and cross-cultural understanding; increased abilities to read, write, and speak in both languages is expected.	Continuous uninterrupted academic development while in the process of language acquisition and development; integrated use of curricula for both languages.	Long-term commitment to the program is essential; mostly found in elementary schools; representation of two language groups and cultures; schools providing means for students to understand different perspectives of learning and social interactions; conducive to additive cultural and bilingual school environments.	Teachers are expected to use both targeted languages; trained in strategies that support comprehensible input; trained in sheltered English instructional strategies; equal involvement of families representing the targeted languages.

L1: home language; L2: English.

Given the limitations and challenges of schools, language programs for bilingual students are almost never implemented in a pure form. Modifications and changes usually are made as a result of difficulties in locating trained bilingual teachers or academic demands related to high-stakes assessments (Vázquez-Montilla & Giambo, 2004). Given the increasing numbers of CLD students, however, it is clear that these programs are essential.

CASE STUDY PERSPECTIVES

Case Study One Background: Carlos and Marcos

The Vázquez family (father; mother; twin boys, Carlos and Marcos; and the mother's parents) recently relocated from their native country of Colombia. The father did not finish college; however, he has taken extensive job-related training, including courses offered by his company in the United States. The mother graduated from college but has been a full-time homemaker ever since the twins were born. Both parents are Spanish speakers and have basic functional and conversational English skills. All their communication at home is in Spanish because the grandparents live in the home and speak only Spanish.

The mother visited the neighborhood school to register the children one month into the academic school year (i.e., September). The parents did not know that the school year began in August. The boys attended school in Colombia since kindergarten and are now in third grade. Their report card grades are satisfactory. However, teacher comments included "the boys need individual attention," "they are very energetic," "Carlos moves from one activity to the other without finishing the assigned task," "Marcos loses interest frequently," "Marcos likes to be the class clown," and "frequently the boys' behaviors disrupt the class."

Carlos and Marcos were placed in a third-grade general-education classroom where literacy and math skills are the target of the curriculum for most of the day. The classroom teacher thinks that Carlos and Marcos lack independent skills and display limited self-regulatory skills. However, the family is more concerned with raising bilingual children and keeping the home language intact. The parents also say that bilingualism will keep communication open with the grandparents at home and with their extended family in their home country.

After four months with Carlos and Marcos, the classroom teacher often finds herself having mixed feelings about the appropriate placement decisions considering school expectations, family expectations, and the well-being of the children. She believes that there is an underlying issue to their limited progress beyond their speaking English as a second language. In particular, Carlos seems to struggle not only with literacy skills but with numerical concepts. The teacher finds herself at a decision-making intersection. She wonders how to (1) advise and support the individual needs of these bilingual learners, (2) recommend appropriate services, (3) know which options will best support the boys' learning needs, and (4) advocate for culturally and linguistically diverse families.

Case Study One Comments: Carlos and Marcos

The following information provides a framework that will facilitate supporting the educational needs of the Vázquez brothers:

1. *Identify the problem.* Is there a learning discrepancy between what is expected and their achievement? What is known about Carlos and Marcos, the family, and the school program?
2. *Outline the problem.* What are Carlos and Marcos's individual issues and concerns? What are their individual needs? How can the problem be reframed to uncover essential educational issues?
3. *Explore options.* Identify possible experts to consult who may have had similar experiences. How can the school support the brothers' individual leaning needs? What are some short-term objectives for the students? What are some of the long-term goals?
4. *Develop an action plan.* Determine a sequence of priorities addressing specific activities and programs for effective implementation. Identify available resources.
5. *Reflect and evaluate progress.* Is the action plan working? Is the brothers' progress matching the established objectives? Are there new issues or challenges?

Case Study Two Background: Evelyn

Evelyn is a 14-year-old enrolled in the eighth grade (middle school) in southern Florida. She has been enrolled in the ESL program for three years. Her first language is Spanish and both parents continue to use Spanish in the home. Evelyn was born in Colombia and came to this country three years ago. Evelyn is receiving English-as-a-second-language (ESL) instruction for her content instruction. She is not receiving any other support services.

Evelyn was tested with the *Language Assessment Battery (LAB),* Spanish and English versions. Her performance indicates that all skills tested (i.e., listening, reading, writing) were higher in Spanish than in English. Her Spanish percentile score was 94, while her English percentile score was 38. An English *LAB* score of less than 40% indicates that an ESL student may have greater difficulty in transitioning from one language to another (Brice & Rivero, 1996). This is the case with Evelyn. In both Spanish and English, writing is her best ability, followed by listening and then reading.

According to district criteria in the state of Florida, Evelyn is ready to be exited out of the program, with a 33rd total percentile score on a standardized English assessment measure. However, she may still experience cognitive academic language proficiency (CALP) problems, as indicated by her lower English scores. Collier (1989) stated that an adolescent student may take up to seven years to acquire CALP proficiency in the second language when he or she has adequate proficiency in her or his first language. Thus, Evelyn may continue to experience language and academic problems. Listening skills seem to be a primary concern for Evelyn because most classroom instruction is very dependent on this skill (Secord, 1994).

Case Study Two Comments: Evelyn

The four basic strategies that will enable Evelyn to acquire better listening skills include rehearsal, elaboration, organization, and monitoring. Rehearsal strategies may include shadowing, where Evelyn repeats (in a whisper) what the teacher said or writes down key words from what the teacher has said. Elaboration tasks may include forming a mental image of two elements of what the teacher has said and generating a sentence that connects the two. In listening and remembering vocabulary, Evelyn may use the key-word method. This involves an acoustic link and an imagery link. For example, the word *disk* in *disk drive* is similar to the Spanish word of *disco* ("disk"). The acoustic link might be the word *disco*. The imagery link might consist of a disk or record driving a car. For an organization listening strategy, Evelyn might be taught to use clustering by having her organize items from a list into groups based on shared characteristics, for example, clustering items according to shape and size in a mathematics lesson.

Reading is another area of concern for Evelyn. A shared-book activity may be utilized with similar-level Hispanic students. The teacher should select a suitable story that possesses strong, temporal organization; is consistent with Evelyn's experiences; and is motivational. The teacher should have Evelyn (perhaps with a partner) highlight key words and phrases, develop physical props as backdrops for the story, and develop charts for the story relationship.

The teacher wants to develop a dialogue journal with Evelyn. The dialogue journal may be implemented as follows: (1) Evelyn and the teacher write each other on a regular basis on whatever Evelyn finds interesting; (2) all entries are confidential; (3) the teacher responds only to the content of the entry and not to grammar or spelling errors; (4) each entry should take five to ten minutes to write; and (5) the teacher comments, expands, or asks questions about the entry. Although the dialogue involves writing, it is being used here as a reading tool. Cognitive processing is also being addressed with more integration of information, more generalization, and a broader perspective.

In sum, Evelyn presents some normal difficulties in acquiring a second language, particularly with listening and reading skills. She does not present a language disorder.

CONCLUDING REMARKS

Although education of culturally and linguistically diverse students is a state and local responsibility, the federal government provides economic support and program guidelines to ensure that the educational needs of students with limited English proficiency are met (U.S. Government Accountability Office, 2001). Legitimate concerns include: (1) how long it takes to become English proficient, (2) identifying the best practices in meeting the CLD students' educational needs, and (3) how long students need to remain in any type of program before they are successful in school.

As the CLD student population increases, school districts are faced with the challenge of how to best meet student needs. Schools must find ways to support their CLD students' success in classrooms. School language programs for bilingual students serve to accentuate the dynamics of bilingualism, biliteracy, and biculturalism. The selected programs all share common characteristic that make them effective: (1) supportive school contexts, (2) high expectations for success, (3) academically challenging and engaging instruction, and (4) school staff development programs. A top language program is tailored to meet the linguistic, educational, and socioemotional needs of the CLD students. The program should provide instruction that allows students to succeed academically *and* socially.

REFLECTION QUESTIONS

1. What are the similarities and differences among the following programs: (a) sheltered English, (b) transitional bilingual education, (c) developmental bilingual education, and (d) two-way immersion programs?

2. What type of program would be most effective for an English language learning student in early elementary, upper elementary, middle school, or high school?

3. What are the advantages and disadvantages of each of the following programs: (a) sheltered English, (b) transitional bilingual education, (c) developmental bilingual education, and (d) two-way immersion programs?

4. The challenge for school professionals is in finding services for CLD students that support learning, regardless of the home language and grade level. What role does use of the native language play in learning for elementary school students versus middle school students?

5. Sheltered English is a program with instructional strategies to be implemented with English language learning students. What strategies might a general education classroom teacher employ?

6. Can sheltered English be used in developmental bilingual programs? If so, how?

7. Immersion programs in the United States have typically meant that English language learning students were placed full-time into general education English-speaking classrooms. How are two-way immersion programs different?

REFERENCES

Brice, A. (2002). *The Hispanic child: Speech, language, culture and education.* Boston, MA: Allyn & Bacon.

Brice, A., & Perkins, C. (1997). What is required for transition from the ESL classroom to the general education classroom? A case study of two classrooms. *Journal of Children's Communication Development, 19*(1), 13–22.

Brice, A., & Rivero, Y. (1996). Language transfer: First (L1) and second (L2) proficiency of bilingual adolescent students. *Per Linguam. The Journal for Language Teaching and Learning, 12*(2), 1–16.

Center for School and District Improvement (CSDI). (2004). *English language learner (ELL) programs at the secondary level in relation to student performance.* Portland, OR: Northwest Regional Educational Laboratory.

Chamot, A. U. (2000). *Literacy characteristics of Hispanic adolescent immigrants with limited prior education.* Proceedings of a Research Symposium on High Standards in Reading for Students from Diverse Language Groups: Research, Practice & Policy. (Washington, DC: April 19–20, 2000).

Cisneros, R., & Leone, B. (1995). The ESL component of bilingual education in practice: Critical descriptions of bilingual classrooms and programs. *Bilingual Research Journal, 19*(3–4), 353–367.

Cloud, N., Genesee, F. & Hamayan, E. (2000). *Dual language instruction: A handbook for enriched education.* Boston, MA: Heinle & Heinle.

Coady, M., & De Jong, E. (2004). Introduction to special topics issue SSTESOL Journal: Bilingualism and bilingual education. *Sunshine State TESOL Journal, 3*(2), 1–3.

Collier, V. P. (1989). How long? A synthesis of research on academic achievement in a second language. *TESOL Quarterly, 23,* 509–531.

Collier, V. P. (1992). A synthesis of studies examining long-term language minority student data on academic achievement. *Bilingual Research Journal, 16*(1–2), 187–212.

Collier, V. P. (1995). *Acquiring a second language for school.* (Directions in Language and Education Vol. 1, No. 4). U.S. Department of Education: National Clearinghouse for English Language Acquisition

(NCELA) and Language Instruction Educational Programs. Retrieved on January 24, 2006, from www.ncela.gwu.edu/pubs/directions/04.htm.

Cummins, J. (1992). Empowering through biliteracy. In J. V. Tinajero & A. F. Ada, (Eds.), *The power of two languages: Literacy and biliteracy for Spanish-speaking students* (pp. 9–25). New York: Macmillan/McGraw-Hill.

Cummins, J., & Swain, M. (1986). *Bilingualism in education: Aspects of theory, research and practice.* New York: Longman.

Dolson, D. P., & Mayer, J. (1992). Longitudinal study of three program models for language-minority students: A critical examination of reported findings. *Bilingual Research Journal, 16*(1–2), 105–157.

Echevarria, J., & Graves, A. (2003). *Sheltered content instruction: Teaching English language learners with diverse abilities* (2nd ed.). Boston, MA: Allyn & Bacon.

Freeman, Y. S., & Freeman, D. E. (2002). *Closing the achievement gap: How to reach limited-formal-schooling and long-term English learners.* Portsmouth, NH: Heinemann.

Friedlander, M. (1991). *The newcomer program: Helping immigrant students succeed in U.S. schools* (NCBE Program Information Guide Series No. 8). U.S. Department of Education: National Clearinghouse for English Language Acquisition (NCELA) and Language Instruction Educational Programs. Retrieved on January 16, 2005, from www.ncela.gwu.edu/pubs/pigs/pig8.htm.

Genesee, F. (1999). *Program alternatives for linguistically diverse students* (Educational Practice Report 1). University of California, Santa Cruz: Center for Research on Education, Diversity and Excellence (CREDE). Retrieved on January 23, 2006, from CREDE www.crede.org/products/print/eprs/epr1.shtml.

Krashen, S. (1987). *Principles and practice in second language acquisition.* New York: Prentice Hall.

Morison, S. H. (1995). A Spanish-English dual-language program in New York City. In O. García and C. Baker (Eds.), *Policy and practice in bilingual education* (pp. 85–92). Bristol, PA: Multilingual Matters.

National Clearinghouse for English Language Acquisition (NCELA). *Resources about language instructions programs.* U.S. Department of Education: National Clearinghouse for English Language Acquisition (NCELA) and Language Instruction Educational Programs. Retrieved on January 24, 2006, from www.ncela.gwu.edu/resabout/programss/index.html.

Ortiz, A. (2001). *English language learners with special needs: Effective instructional strategies* (Center for Applied Linguistics [CAL] Digest). Washington DC: Eric Clearinghouse on Languages and Linguistics. Retrieved on August 8, 2005, from www.cal.org/resources/digest/0108ortiz.html.

Ortiz, A. A., & Yates, J. R. (2003, April). *Serving English language learners: Trends and issues in general and special education.* Paper presented at the 2003 Council for Exceptional Children Annual Conference. Seattle, WA.

Ovando, C. J. (2003). Bilingual education in the United States: Historical development and current issues. *Bilingual Research Journal, 27*(1), 1–24.

Ramírez, J. D., Yuen, S. D., & Ramey, D. R. (1991). Longitudinal study of structured English immersion strategy: Early-exit and late-exit transitional bilingual education programs for language-minority children. *Bilingual Research Journal, 16*(1–2), 1–62.

Rennie, J. (1993). *ESL and bilingual program models* (Center for Applied Linguistics [CAL] Digest). Washington, DC: Eric Clearinghouse on Languages and Linguistics. Retrieved on August 8, 2005, from www.cal.org/resources/digest/rennie01.html.

Secord, W. (1994, March). *Developing a collaborative language intervention program.* Workshop presentation, Ft. Lauderdale, FL.

Short, D. J., & Boyson, B. A. (2003). *Establishing an effective newcomer program* (Center for Applied Linguistics [CAL] Digest). Washington, DC: Eric Clearinghouse on Languages and Linguistics. Retrieved on August 8, 2005, from www.cal.org/resources/digest/0312short.html.

Taylor, L. S., & Whittaker, C. R. (2003). *Bridging multiple worlds: Case studies of diverse educational communities.* Boston, MA: Allyn & Bacon.

Thomas, W. P., & Collier, V. P. (1997). *School effectiveness for language minority students* (NCBE Resource Collection Series No.9). Washington, DC: National Clearinghouse for English Language Acquisition (NCELA) and Language Instruction Educational Programs. Retrieved on January 24, 2006, from www.ncela.gwu.edu/pubs/resource/effectiveness/thomas-collier97.pdf.

U.S. Government Accountability Office. (2001). *GAO's 2001 Performance and Accountability and High-Risk Series.* Washington, DC: Author.

Vázquez-Montilla, E., & Giambo, D. (2004). Modifying foreign language programs in elementary schools:

Successes and challenges. *Sunshine State TESOL Journal, 3*(2), 29–38.

Walqui, A. (2000a). *Access and engagement: Program design and instructional approaches for immigrant students in secondary schools.* University of California, Santa Cruz: Center for Applied Linguistics and Delta Systems, Inc.

Walqui, A. (2000b). *Strategies for success: Engaging immigrant students in secondary schools.* (Center for Applied Linguistics [CAL] Digest). Washington, DC: Eric Clearinghouse on Languages and Linguistics. Retrieved on January 24, 2006, from www.cal.org/resources/digest/0003strategies.html.

Name Index

Subject Index